PLANT FOODS

for

NUTRITIONAL GOOD HEALTH

VEN HARI

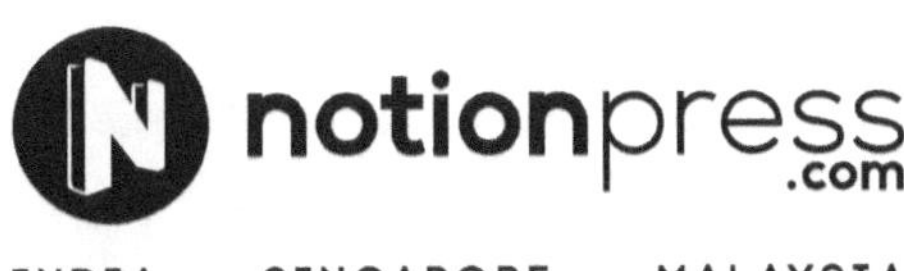

Notion Press

Old No. 38, New No. 6
McNichols Road, Chetpet
Chennai - 600 031

First Published by Notion Press 2019

ISBN 978-1-68466-906-6

Disclaimer

The information provided in this book have been derived from a number of sources including peer reviewed books and publications. The intention of this book is to provide information for educational, guidance and knowledge purposes and is not in any way intended to promote any products or to diagnose any disease and treatment options.

Dedication

I would like to dedicate this book to Mother Nature and the world of plants for providing food, shelter, clothes, medicine and the oxygen we breathe and to the great herbalists and teachers of plant biology.

Contents

Foreword

Plants serve as the source of nutrition for all and maintenance of good health. Health care providers as well as the public are increasingly becoming aware of the importance of proper nutrition. The term Nutraceuticals describes the importance of nutritional foods as drugs to keep us healthy. This book brings together information about the biology of plants that serve as sources of food, the nutritional value of foods and the various health related phytochemicals derived from edible plants. This book has the objective of reaching out to students in colleges as a text or reference book, to both readers with knowledge of plants and their uses and the public who have an interest in plants as they apply to the maintenance of good health. A substantial amount of information about botany and nutritional and health benefits derived from plant products have been included. Some of the information is technical but hopefully in simplified form.

Appreciation

I want to thank my wife Radha who encouraged me to write and edit this book and my son Raj who in his capacity as a physician shared his knowledge of medicine. I would also like to express my thanks to all my botanical and medical scientist friends for going over the various chapters and their comments.

Referances

This book is based on my own University lecture notes prepared over a period of over four decades with added information. All Web sites and books referred here were verified by cross Reference to original publications. In addition, I have cited important specific reviews, bulletins from Agricultural extension services and original publications have been and credited at the end of each chapter.

General Referances

Aykroid, W.R., Doughty, J., and A. Walker (1982): Legumes in human nutrition, FAO food and nutrition paper, 20, Food and Agriculture organization of the United Nations, Rome, Pp 152

Gopalakrishnan T.P. (2007): Vegetable Crops, New India Publishing, pp. 244–247, ISBN 9788189422417

Grubben, G.J.H. & Denton, O.A. (2004): Plant Resources of Tropical Africa 2, Vegetables, PROTA Foundation, Wageningen; Backhuys, Leiden; CTA, Wageningen

Heiser, Jr., C.B. (1979): The gourd book, Univ. Oklahoma Press, Norman, Oklahoma

Joshi, S.G. (2004): Medicinal Plants, Oxford & IBH Publishing Co. Pvt. Ltd., New Delhi, 2004, ISBN 81-204-1414-4, p.347.

Mader, S.S. (1998): Biology, sixth edition, WCB, McGraw-Hill, Boston, Pp 994.

Mauseth, James D. (2003): Botany: An Introduction to Plant Biology (third Edition), Jones and Bartlett Learning, 848 pages

National Research Council (2006): Lost crops of Africa: Volume II: Vegetables Washington, D.C.: National Academies Press, pp. 269–285, ISBN 0-309-66582-5

Nelson, D.L. and M.M. Cox (2000): Lehninger Principles of Biochemistry, Third Edition (3 Har/Com Ed.), W.H. Freeman, p. 1200, ISBN 1-57259-931-6

Nielsen, F.H. (1999): Ultra trace minerals. *In* Modern nutrition in health and disease/editors, Maurice E.S. et al., Baltimore, Williams & Wilkins, p. 283-303

Phytochemistry Reviews: Fundamentals and Perspectives of Natural Products Research, ISSN: 1568-7767 (Print) 1572-980X (Online)

Purves, W.K., Orians, G.H., & Heller, H.C. (1994): Life, the science of biology Sunderland, Mass: Sinauer Associates.

Raven, P.H., (2013): Biology of Plants – 8th edition, W.H. Freeman ISBN13: 978-1429219617

Salunkhe, D.K. and S.S. Deshpande (1991): Foods of Plant origin, Production, Technology and Human Nutrition, Van Nostrand Reinhold, New York, NY.

Salunkhe, D.K., and S.S. Kadam (1995): Handbook of Fruit Science and Technology: Production, Composition, Storage, and Processing, Marcel Dekker, Inc., New York, New York, Pp 632.

Salunkhe, D.K. and S.S. Kadam (1998): Handbook of Vegetable Science and Technology, Marcel Dekker, Inc., New York, Pp742

Singh, R.J., (2003): Plant cytogenetics, 2nd edition, CRC Press, Boaca Raton, pp385.

Smartt, J. and N.W. Simmonds, (1995): Evolution of crop plants, 2nd ed. Longman Scientific and Technical, New York

Taiz, L., Zeiger, E., Moller, I.M., and Murphy, A.M. (2015): Plant Physiology and Development, Sinauer Associates, Pp 761

Vaclav, V., Pimentel, M.H., Devine, M.M., (2013): Dimensions of Food: Edition 4, Springer Science & Business Media, 279 pages

Vaughan, J., and Geissler, C. (2009): The New Oxford Book of Food Plants, OUP Oxford, Aug 27, 2009 – Science – 288 pages.

Wiersema, John Harry; León, Blanca (1999): World Economic Plants: A Standard Reference, CRC Press, p. 661, ISBN 0-8493-2119-0.

World Health Organization (2004): Vitamin and Mineral Requirements in Human Nutrition, 2nd edition, World Health Organization, Health and Fitness, Pp 341

Web site references

http://www.tropicos.org/Project/IPCN

https://en.wikipedia.org.

https://www.mskcc.org/cancer-care/treatments/symptom-management/integrative-medicine/herbs/search

http://www.webmd.com/

http://www.plantgdb.org/

http://archive.gramene.org/resources/

http://www.ncbi.nlm.nih.gov/taxonomy

http://www.ncbi.nlm.nih.gov/genbank

http://www.fao.org/rice2004/en/aboutrice.htm

http://plants.usda.gov/alt_crops.html

http://www.k-state.edu/wgrc/Taxonomy/taxintro.html

http://plants.usda.gov/java/

http://www.prota.org/

http://anpsa.org.au/

http://irri.org/

http://www.cimmyt.org/en/

http://edis.ifas.ufl.edu./topics/agriculture/crops.html

http://plants.usda.gov/core/profile?symbol = MAUN4

http://www.nrcs.usda.gov/wps/portal/nrcs/detail/?ss = 16&nav-type = SUBNAVIGATION&cid = stelprdb1044954&navid = 120160320130000&pnavid = 120000000000000&position = Not%20Yet%20Determined.Html&ttype = detail&pname = PLANTS%20Interactive%20ID%20Keys:%20Introduction%20|%20NRCS

https://npgsweb.ars-grin.gov/gringlobal/search.aspx

https://www.croptrust.org/

http://www.bioversityinternational.org/

http://www.ars.usda.gov/main/main.htm

http://www.theplantlist.org/

http://www.floridata.com/plantlist/.

http://www.theplantlist.org/

http://www.kew.org/science-conservation

http://www.kew.org/science-conservation/plants-fungi/plants-roots-to-riches.

http://www.missouribotanicalgarden.org/plant-science/plant-science/about-plant-science.aspx

https://www.lsa.umich.edu/mbg/see/medgarden/ourgarden.asp?area = 15&plantID = 1

http://www.journals.elsevier.com/phytochemistry/

http://www.ncbi.nlm.nih.gov/pubmed

http://www.medline.com/research/library/

https://www.nlm.nih.gov/bsd/pmresources.html.

http://www.fao.org/ag/agp/AGPC/doc/Gbase/Default.htm

http://uses.plantnet-project.org/en/Main_Page

http://www.ntbg.org/

Nutrition tables: Modified from United States Department of Agriculture, Agricultural Research Service, United States Department of Agriculture, Agricultural Research Service, and USDA Food Composition Databases http://ndb.nal.usda.gov/ndb/foods

Photographs: the author snapped Photographs at indoor and outdoor farms, home garden, grocery stores and produce stores. I thank Vedic Farms LLC for permission to photograph some plants grown in their farm at Loxahatchee groves, South Florida.

Chapter 1

Introduction and History of Food Plants

The role of plants in maintaining good health through proper nutrition and use of plant products in treating disease have been a significant part of human history. Humans realized the use of various wild relatives of plants such as rice, wheat, barley, oats and other cereals as well as many legumes, oil plants and tubers as sources of food supplementing the flesh of animals for sustenance. As civilization advanced, many of these wild plants were domesticated and soon evolved into different species and varieties of food/nutritional plants. Certain plants evolved in specific regions of the earth and subsequently spread to other regions as animals and humans migrated.

The association of specific plants as a source for food, nutrition and general health for the general well-being of humans came from observation of the behavior of animals, by apparent trial and error, through folk lore, and through ancient books and reports. These ancient sources are, the hymns in the Hindu Vedas – Charaka Samhita between 760-200 BCE, Sushrutha Samhita 660 BCE, Ashtanga Samgraha ca 700 CE, Ashtanga Hridaya ca 800 CE from India. In addition, the sources include the Shennong documents from China dating back to about 2500 BC, the compendium of Materia medica compiled during the Ming dynasty as well as the Greek scientists-philosophers Hippocrates 460 BCE, Aristotle 384 BCE, Theophrastus, Galen 129–215 CE and Dioscorides, the Egyptian papyrus 1550B.C.and the canon of Medicine by Avicenna 980–1037 CE.

Plant based foods are derived from Cereals, Legumes, oil seeds, tubers, leaf, stem, root and fruit vegetables supplemented by nuts, culinary fruits, spices and condiments. Collectively, plant based foods provide carbohydrates, protein, fats, minerals, vitamins and many biochemicals that ensure proper growth and good health. Toxic principles found in certain plant foods may be removed by washing or cooking and processing. The importance of proper nutrition for good health was realized very early during the history of man. Thus, the Hindu holy texts known as the Vedas and Upanishads described food as the creator (Aham Annam, aham Annam). It states, "Those who know the real nature of food call it the medicament (aushadha) of all, because it affords a drink that can assuage the fire of hunger which would otherwise have to feed upon the very Dhatus or constituents of the body." The importance of proper food is further elaborated "Because food (Anna) is the eldest-born, the cause of all living beings therefore it is the medicament of all, as removing all diseases of samsara." The texts went on to describe how food is to be consumed, the honoring of cooking, the need to have good thoughts during eating etc. In the various Slokas (verses), these texts point out that we are derived from food and that we grow by eating food and eventually when we die our body made of food (Annamaya Kosha) returns back to the five elements –earth, water, air, fire, and space (Pancha bhutas). The great Ayurvedic texts written by Sushrutha and Charaka go on to describe the types of food that are important for good health and the need to show restraint in indulging in food which they refer to as mitha aahara or restraint in food. The diet and nutrition for pregnant women, nursing mothers and young children are described. It recommends milk, butter, fluid foods, fruits, vegetables and fibrous diets for expecting mothers along with soups made from jangala (wild animal) meat. In most cases, vegetarian diets are preferred and recommended in the Samhita. Sushruta Samhita also recommends a rotation and balance in foods consumed, in moderation. For this purposes, it classifies foods by various characteristics, such as taste. It lists six tastes – madhura (sweet), amla (acidic), lavana (saline), katuka (pungent), tikta (bitter) and kashaya (astringent). It then lists various sources of foods that deliver these tastes and recommends that all six tastes (flavors) be consumed in moderation and routinely, as a habit for good health. Similar descriptions on proper food and choice of food may be found in Chinese, Greek, Roman, Egyptian and Mesopotamian literature. Additional sources of information were derived from archeological studies and the careful scientific studies of Vavilov and others on the origin of cultivated plants.

Ancient man was essentially nomadic hunter-gatherers depending on animal food through hunting and gathering of nuts and wild fruits, leaves and roots as food sources. Being nomadic, they did not stay in any one place long enough to farm and cultivate specific plants for food. However, wherever they camped, they managed to supplement their animal based food with plant based food derived mostly from wild plants most of which we know today as ancient grains. The Angiosperms made up of dicotyledonous broad-leaved plants with two cotyledons and monocotyledonous plants with one cotyledon and parallel – veined narrow blade leaves are the main sources of plant food. However, a few gymnosperms such as the cycads and algae like chlorella and spirulina are also edible sources of food. The use of algal protein food is essentially a new development with restricted use. So, most of our food comes from Angiosperm sources. The grains of plants like Amaranth, Chia, Quinoa, Canihua, Hemp, Wild rice, Paddy rice (Oriza sp.), spelt (wheat), Teosinte (ancient corn), Buckwheat, were important sources of food initially. Some ancient grains that are now called pseudo-cereals are becoming popular as nutritional foods. As man graduated from being hunter-gatherers to a more settled life, they started to cultivate important food plants including modern day varieties of rice, wheat, corn, barley, oats, millets, oilseed plants, legumes, vegetables, nuts, fruits, spices and beverage plants.

The Origin and cultivation of plants for food seems to have been initiated in multiple regions on earth. Alphonse de Condolle in 1883 initiated the first studies on how cultivated plants originate. His ideas formed the nucleus for the more elaborate and detailed studies by the Russian Scientist N.I. Vavilov. Professor Vavilov concluded that the origin of cultivated plants coincided with the presence of the greatest diversity of the given species in that area. He then went on to identify six such centers of origin of various cultivated/domesticated plants initially and subsequently enlarged this to eleven such centers. Further ecological, phytogeography and DNA mapping by Restriction fragment length polymorphism (RFLP) studies enable us to conclude that centers of origin do not coincide with centers of diversity in all species although they do coincide in a few limited cases such as the origin of wheat.

Vavilov Centers: The list obviously includes primary centers of origin and domestication and secondary centers where plants probably were introduced deliberately or inadvertently and showed diversity in numbers of varieties. The examples below only concern food plants and does not include fibers or, intoxicants etc. The modern names of regions instead of the original names prevalent at the time of Vavilov are given here. The list shows overlaps between regions.

1. **China:** Vavilov listed 136 plants in this largest independent center, Inclusive of Fox tail millet, sorghum, soybeans, bamboo, onion, tea, rice, broomcorn millet, Japanese barnyard millet, Kaoliang, buckwheat, hull-less barley, adzuki bean, velvet bean, Chinese yam, radish, Chinese cabbage, , cucumber, pear, Chinese yam, , Chinese apple, peach, apricot, cherry, walnut, lychee, opium poppy, ginseng, camphor and hemp.

2. **India-Burma/Myanmar (Excluding North West India/ Pakistan):** One hundred and seventeen plants were listed as being endemic to this area. These included, rice, eggplant, sesame, mango, citrus, sugarcane, chickpea, pigeon pea, urad bean, mung bean, rice bean, cowpea, cucumber, radish, taro, yam, orange, tangerine, citron, tamarind, coconut palm, sesame, safflower, tree cotton, oriental cotton, jute, crotalaria, black pepper, gum arabic, sandalwood, indigo and cinnamon tree.

3. **South east Asia (Malaysian archipelago, Thailand, Cambodia, Laos, Vietnam, Indonesia):** Fifty-five plants including:

Rice, banana, coconut, cloves, cereals and legumes, Job's tears, velvet bean, pomelo, breadfruit, mangosteen, candlenut, coconut palm, clove, nutmeg, black pepper, manila hemp.

4. **Central Asia (Northwest India-(Punjab, Kashmir), Pakistan, Afghanistan, Tajikistan, Uzbekistan, and western Tian Shan, China)** 43 plants including: common wheat, pea, common millet, buckwheat, alfalfa Includes: club wheat, shot wheat, peas, lentil, horse bean, chickpea, mustard, flax, sesame, garlic, spinach, carrot, pistachio, pear, almond, grape, apple.

5. **Mediterranean (Egypt, Iraq, Syria, Israel, Jordan, Palestine, Italy, Greece, and regions bordering the Mediterranean sea):** 84 plants including: Durum and Emmer wheats, olives, rape, Polish wheat, spelt, Mediterranean oats, sand oats, grass pea, pea, lupine, flax, rape, black mustard, olive, garden beet, cabbage, turnip, lettuce, asparagus, celery, chicory, parsnip, rhubarb, caraway, anise, thyme, peppermint, sage, hops.

6. **Asia minor (Turkey, Iran, Armenia):** 83 plants including: Einkorn wheat, durum wheat, poulard wheat, common wheat, oriental wheat, Persian wheat, two-row barley, rye, Mediterranean oats, common oats, lentil, lupine, alfalfa, Persian clover, fenugreek, vetch, hairy vetch, fig, pomegranate, apple, pear, quince, cherry, hawthorn.

7. **Ethiopia/Abyssinia/Somaliland:** 38 species: Barley, sesame, castor bean, coffee, Abyssinian hard wheat, poulard wheat, emmer, Polish wheat, barley, grain sorghum, pearl millet, African millet, cowpea, flax, sesame, castor bean, garden cress, coffee, okra, myrrh, indigo.

8. **Meso America (Southern Mexico, Guatemala, Central America):** Forty nine plants including: Maize, bean, squash, sweet potato, red/chili pepper, papaya, guava, tobacco, lima bean, Tepary bean, jack bean, grain amaranth, Malabar gourd,

winter pumpkin, chayote, sweet potato, arrowroot, cashew, wild black cherry, cochineal, cherry tomato, cacao.

9. **South America (Peru, Equador, Bolivia):** 45 plants: Andean Potato, tomato, pine apple, cashew nut, starchy maize, lima bean, common bean, pumpkin, chili pepper,: cocoa, passion fruit, guava, cherimoya.

10. **Chiloe/Chile region of S. America:** 4 species inclusive of Common Potato,

11. **Brazilian/Paraguayan regions:** 13 plants: Peanuts (Ground nuts), cassava, cashewnut, pine apple, chili peppers, potato, manioc, peanut,

Other investigators modified the Vavilovian concepts using more modern methods such as carbon dating of buried seeds in archeological sites, restriction length polymorphism (RFLP), cite specific – genetic analysis, Random Amplified Polymorphic DNA (RAPDs), Amplified Fragment Length Polymorphism (AFLPs), Quantitative Trait Locus (QTL), Isozymes, Allozyme, and Zymograms suggested different proposals regarding the origin and domestication of cultivated plants. In summary, several long ranging diffuse areas could be identified for the origin of various plants that are cultivated now. These are:

1. **Fertile crescent (Iran, Iraq, Syria, Lebanon, Jordan, Israel, Southern Turkey/Anatolia):** wheat, barley, Flax, lentils, chickpeas, melons, olives, Figs, Dates, walnuts, Pigeon pea, cabbage, carrots, cucumbers, and melons; fruits and nuts and pistachios (about 11,000 years ago).

2. **Africa:** Pearl millet, Guinea millet, African rice, sorghum, cowpea, Bambara groundnut, yam, oil palm, watermelon, okra,

3. **The Eastern Asia ((includes China, Korea, Japan, Cambodia, Laos, Viet nam, Myanmar (Burma), Thailand):** Rice, soybean, Citrus, bamboo, oranges, Japanese millet

4. **South Asia: Indian Sub-continent including Sri Lanka, Malaya archipelago including Indonesia):** Paddy Rice *(Oriza sativa)*, various legumes such as cluster beans, horse gram, green gram, black gram, black pepper, cardomom (about 10,000–11,000 years ago).

5. **The Mesoamerican center (modern day Mexico, Brazil, Guatemala, Honduras, Venezuela):** corn (maize), the common bean (*Phaseolus vulgaris*), squash and pumpkins, chilli peppers, and tomatoes.

6. **Brazilian/Peru region:** Potato (Andes), Peanuts, Cashew nuts, Pineapple

7. **Tropical America, Tropical Africa and Polynesian, Australasian and in the Pacific Islands:** Root crops such as taro yams, bread fruit, Coconut palm in the pacific, sweet potatoes and cassavas in tropical South America and Yams in Africa, Macadamia in Australia have been domesticated.

Crop Selection, Hybrids, GM Crops and Organic Farming

Long before human intervention, plants were cross-pollinated by wind, insects, birds or other animals and those plants that were pollinated by compatible species resulted in the generation of hybrids with new characteristics. Very often, such cross-pollination occurred between two different wild species and the resultant hybrid produced edible grains or other edible parts of the plant. For example, natural crossing of a diploid species having genomes AA with another species with genomes BB results in a new tetraploid species with AABB genomes and if this tetraploid crossed with another species with genome DD , the result would be a hexaploid with genomes AABBDD. Natural selection then takes over and the diploid, tetraploid or hexaploid can be cultivated based on quality of the grain or other edible part produced. Such natural crossings have occurred naturally for all cultivated plants.

Subsequently, the intervention of man resulted in scientifically based crossing of different compatible species and selection of the ideal crop. Today, many species such as soybeans, corn and other plants have been genetically modified by inserting foreign genes from bacteria or other wild plants or by manipulating existing genes in the plant. These genetically modified plants (GMO) are modified to contain genes that confer resistance to insects, microbes or herbicides or have better shelf life, or delayed ripening of fruits or fruits with better qualities or with low or no toxic chemicals etc. These plants are now known as GM plants. In the USA, over 90 % of corn and soybeans are genetically modified strains using DNA recombinant technology.

GM plants do not necessarily mean that all GM plants contain foreign genes. In some cases, it involves simple silencing of specific pre-existing genes of the plant or introduction of an anti-sense m-RNA of a gene in the plant.

GM varieties of several plants have been developed and approved for cultivation and use. While some of these plants have been genetically modified (GM) by insertion of foreign genes from bacteria or viruses, others have simply been modified to alter or change the expression of pre-existing genes of the plant species of interest. In the case of herbicide tolerance, the plants were modified to express the 5-enolpyruvoyl-shikimate-3-phosphate synthetase (EPSPS) gene from bacteria that is resistant to glyphosate into these plants (eg. Corn, soybeans, cotton). Insect resistant plants were generated by introducing the thuringin genes from *Bacillus thuringensis* (Bt) that is toxic to insects but not to higher animals (Corn, Cotton, Soybeans). Generally, the recombinant GM plants expressed both herbicide tolerance as well as insect resistance. In the case of virus resistant plants, the plants were engineered to express the non-infectious coat protein gene of specific viruses that are the most common pathogens of these plants (eg. Papaya resistant to Papaya ring spot virus; tomato resistant to tobacco mosaic virus). In other cases, no foreign genes were introduced but the pre-existing genes of the plant were genetically modified by gene silencing, mutational methods, antisense m-RNA expression (e.g. Flavor saver tomato, non-browning arctic apples, and simplex low acrylamide potatoes). The GM plants that are currently listed by International Service for the acquisition of Agri-Biotech applications (ISAA) are:

1. Alfalfa: Herbicide tolerance

2. Apple (Golden delicious, Granny Smith): Prevention of browning

3. Beans: resistance to viruses

4. Canola: introduction of desirable oil components, herbicide tolerance

5. Cotton: Herbicide tolerance, insect resistance, (Bt-gene from Bacillus thuringensis)

6. Brinjal/Eggplant: Insect resistance

7. Chili pepper: Virus resistance

8. Corn/Maize: insect resistance, herbicide tolerance, increased lysine content, reduced phytate content.

9. Melons: delayed senescence

10. Papaya: Virus resistance

11. Potato: virus resistance, Insect resistance, fungal resistance, lowered acrylamide when cooked, modified starch

12. Plums: viral resistance

13. Soybeans: herbicide tolerance

14. Squash: virus resistance

15. Sugar beet: Herbicide tolerance

16. Sugar cane: Drought resistant

17. Tomato: Virus resistance, insect resistance

18. Wheat: Herbicide tolerance

The above crops and several others are being experimentally modified for delayed ripening of fruits, qualitative and quantitative changes in nutritional content, reduction of phytotoxicity and other traits. In the years ahead, more GM plants will be developed and approved for farming.

Until the advent of chemical fertilizers, weedicides and pesticides, agriculture depended mainly on inputs of organic animal and plant waste to fertilize plants and protect them from disease. In many countries, this is the main methodology for crop production. The introduction of chemicals into agriculture increased the yields of crops but at the same time posed dangers because of the toxicity of these chemicals. Therefore, there is an increased awareness of danger to health posed by crops that are produced after various chemical treatments. As a result, the consuming public has generated a huge market for crops produced without synthetic chemical usage and so organic farming or organic crops have become very popular. Thus, many vegetables, fruits, nuts and grains carry a special certificate (OMRI) if they are grown without usage of chemicals. The concern about pesticide residues in plant products grown under an umbrella of chemical usage is legitimate and hence, the switch to use of products from organically grown plants is understandable from the point of good health.

References

Candolle A. de (1883): Origine des plantes cultivées Paris: Ed. J. Laffitte, 1984

Centers of diversity and centers of origin: *In* genetic resources in plants – their exploration and conservation Ed. O.H. Frankel and E. Bennett, Oxford: Blackwell pp. 33–42

Flannery K.V. (1973): The origin of agriculture, Ann. Rev. of Anthropology 2: 271–310

Hancock, J.F. (2012): Plant Evolution and the Origin of Crop Species, 245 pp

http://avgwarrier.blogspot.com/2007/10/nourishment-is-brahman.html

http://www.vedarahasya.net/bhrigu.htm

http://www.isaaa.org/gmapprovaldatabase/cropslist/ (2015): Vavilovian Centers of Plant Diversity: Implications and Impacts, HortScience vol. 50(6)

Mangelsdorf P.C. (1974): Corn, Its Origin, Evolution, and Improvement Massachusetts: Harvard University Press, Cambridge 23

Poncept V., Robert T., Sarr A., Gepts P. (2004): Quantitative Trait Locus Analyses of the Domestication Syndrome and Domestication Process. Encyclopedia of Plant and Crop Science

Vavilov N.I. (1926): Studies on the origin of cultivated plants Trudy Byuro Prikl Bot. 16: 139–248. (Bull. Appl. Bot. Pl. Breeding, 16: 1–245)

Vavilov N.I. (1951): Phytogeographic basis of plant breeding, The origin, variation, immunity and breeding of cultivated plants Chronica Botanica 13: 1–366.

Chapter 2
Basic Plant Biology

Glossary of Scientific Words Used in Plant Science

Taxonomy: Classification

Algae: These are Unicellular, colonial, filamentous or leaf-like, photosynthetic organisms without xylem and phloem elements.

Angiosperms: Are plants that produce seeds that are covered by skin-like tissue. They are divided into Monocots and dicots (Eudicots)

Binomial Nomenclature: The system of naming biological organisms in Latin developed by Swedish scientist Carl Linnaeus in which the scientific name of an organism is a combination of two names, the first name being the generic name and the second the species name. The generic and species names are often followed by the name of the variety and or cultivar if applicable followed by a reference to the name of the person who named the organism.

Bryophyte: These are a group of non-vascular plants classified as mosses, hornworts and liverworts.

Clade: taxonomic hierarchy of a group of organisms classified together based on homologous features traced to a common ancestor.

Class: Category of taxa in a rank between division and order

Cline: continuous morphological variation in form within a species or sometimes between two species

Commercial name: Common and popular names of plants in English or local ethnic languages

Cultivar: denotes an assemblage of cultivated plants that are differentiated by one or more characters.

Cryptogams: This is an archaic term for organisms producing spores, without stamens, ovaries or seeds. They include algae, fungi, bryophytes and Pteridophytes (ferns).but not gymnosperms and angiosperms

Dicotyledonae/dicots: Now known as Eudicots, these are flowering plants with two cotyledons or seed leaves.

Division: The term used for the classification rank below kingdom in the taxonomic hierarchy.

Eudicots: The original Dicotyledonae renamed to reflect their morphology that consists of two cotyledons, netted leaf veins, presence of taproots, xylem and phloem arranged in distinct bundles in rings.

Family: A group of plants with many similar qualities and include many related genera and species.

Fungi: These are generally known as molds. These may be unicellular, multicellular, and filamentous or organized into macroscopic structures (Mushrooms, bracket fungi). These are not photosynthetic and may be saprophytes, facultative or obligate parasites.

Gametophyte: Refers to the haploid multicellular gamete-producing phase of the life cycle of algae and the lower and higher plants.

Genus: (plural, genera): Genus is the principal category of taxa intermediate in rank between family and species in the nomenclatural hierarchy.

Generic name: the name of a genus, for example Cucumis (Cucumber), Triticum (wheat) or Zea (corn)

Group: refers to an assembly of two or more cultivars within a species or hybrid. For example, bean group consists of *Phaseolus vulgaris* var cranberry, *P.vulgaris* var pinto etc.

Gymnosperms: Seed-bearing plants with naked ovules borne on the surface of sporophylls. Examples are conifers, Ginkgo, Gnetum and cycads.

Kingdom: This term refers to Category of organisms at the highest level in taxonomy for example, Kingdom: Plantae.

Monocotyledonae/Monocot: refers to angiosperms that have only one cotyledon in the seed. All grasses, all cereals, banana, bamboo, coconut are examples.

Nomenclature: in biology, it refers to the naming of all living organisms in Latin using the binomial system wherein, the organism has the name of the genus first followed by the name of the species and very often followed by the variety and cultivar as applicable. The first few letters of the person naming the organism is added at the end.

Order: In taxonomic hierarchy, this refers to a group below that of the Division (Division) and just above the family.

Pteridophytes: Includes all ferns but not gymnosperms or angiosperms.

Subgenus: is a further division of genus.

sp.: abbreviation of species often used when the genus but not the species is clear

spp.: plural of sp

Species: refers to populations of individuals that share common features and/or ancestry. Thus, a genus can include several species. Examples are *Triticum aestivum, Triticum vulgare* (wheats of two different species).

Subspecies: is a further grouping within a species. Its taxonomic rank occurs between species and variety.

Synonym: is an alternative name for the same taxon.

Taxonomy: is a term for classification of biological agents.

Type: This refers to a specimen in a herbarium that was the model for naming and describing an organism.

Var: (variety in common usage, abbreviated as var.): In the binomial system, a variety refers to a species with some distinct variation within the species.

Habitat

Aquatic: Plants whose natural habitat is water

Arid/semi-arid: Regions of dry weather with low rainfall under near desert conditions.

Community: refers to plants that characteristically occur together in nature.

Endemic: having a natural distribution restricted to a particular geographic region.

Epiphytes: are plants living on other plants but not parasitic on them. Many orchids are epiphytes.

Exotic: plants that are not native, introduced from another region or country.

Lithophyte: Plants that grow in rocky regions.

Population: all individuals, or of one or more species within a prescribed area.

Tropical and Sub-Tropical: Geographical areas with warmer temperatures usually near the equator and between the tropic of Cancer in the North and tropic of Capricorn towards the south.

Temperate: Geographical areas with lower/cooler temperatures.

Terrestrial plants: Land plants.

Growth types

Acropetal/Basipetal: Moving from roots to leaves (acropetal) or moving from leaves to roots or top to bottom (basipetal).

Annual/Biennial/perennial: Annual plants are those that complete their life cycle and dies within one year (Annual). Biennual plants complete life cycle in two years. Usually, they grow vegetatively during first year without flowering and flower and set seeds in second year. Examples are Carrots, Cabbage, and North-west European biennial cauliflower. Perennial plants live for an indefinite period of life growing vegetatively and setting flowers/fruits and seeds each year.

Apical meristem: the growing point at the apex of the plant.

Arboretum: a taxonomically arranged collection of trees.

Arborescent: Tree-like in growth or general appearance.

Decumbent: Branches growing horizontally on the ground, but turned up at the ends.

Evergreen: Plants that produce leaves all the year round.

Grassland: Vegetation dominated by grasses.

Groundcover: Dense vegetation that covers the ground.

Habit: the general external appearance of a plant, including size, shape, texture and orientation.

Habitat: is the place where a plant lives; the environmental conditions of its home.

Halophyte: a plant adapted to living in highly saline habitats like salt marshes, ocean beach shorelines.

Herb/Shrub/Tree/Vine/Succulents: Herbs are Vascular plants that do not develop a woody stem, for example, Corn, rice, chili pepper, tomato, eggplant, beans. Shrub is a woody perennial plant without a single main trunk, branching freely, and smaller than a tree. Trees are woody plants, usually with a single distinct trunk and generally several meters/feet tall. Vine is a plant that twines around a substrate like a pole, e.g. beans. Succulents are plants with thick leaves containing fluids such as Cactus.

Herbaceous: plants that are not woody, usually green, and soft in texture.

Herbarium: is a collection of preserved, usually dried, plant material. In addition, a building in which such collections are stored.

Indeterminate/determinate: Unlimited growth (indeterminate), limited growth (determinate).

Mangrove plants: are shrubs or small trees growing in salt or brackish water, usually characterized by pneumatophores that are breathing roots. The Everglades in Florida, USA, Sunderbans and Pichavaram in India are examples of Mangrove plants.

Marsh: a waterlogged area, swamp.

Meristems: are actively dividing regions in the plant that are responsible for overall growth of plant. Terminal meristems located at the apex of stem and roots of plants are responsible for growth in height. The axillary meristems located in axils of leaves give rise to branches and intercalary meristems give rise to growth in width. Leaf meristems located in the periphery of leaf blades are responsible for growth of leaves, and floral meristems give rise to flowers.

Perennial: plants whose life span extends over several years.

Persistent: remaining attached to the plant beyond the usual time of falling, for instance sepals not falling after flowering, flower parts remaining through maturity of fruit.

Procumbent: Spreading along the ground but not rooting at the nodes.

Prostate: plants lying flat on the ground.

Rainforest: a moist temperate or tropical forest dominated by broad-leaved trees that form a continuous canopy, includes epiphytes that live on other trees, shrubs and herbs.

Saprophyte/Epiphyte/Lithophyte/Parasite: Organisms deriving nourishment from decaying organic matter are Saprophytes; Plants living on the surface of another plant without being a parasite are Epiphytes. Plants that live in a rocky substrate are Lithophytes. Parasites are plants that derive all nourishment from another. Parasites may be facultative in which case they can either parasitize another plant or live like a saprophyte or they may be obligate in which case they are entirely dependent on the host for all their growth requirements.

Terrestrial: habitat, on land as opposed to water (aquatic) or on rocks (lithophyte), or other plants (epiphytic).

Weed: A weed is loosely defined as a plant growing where it is not wanted, (examples are Dandelions or Clover growing in lawns).

Xeromorph: a plant with structural features that prevent water loss by evaporation, usually associated with arid habitats.

Xerophyte: a plant that lives generally in a dry habitat having succulent stem and leaves.

Morphology of roots, stem, branches and leaves

Alternate: leaves or flowers borne singly at different levels along a stem.

Bark: The protective external layer of tissue on the stems and roots of trees and shrubs which are several layers thick and containing the food-conducting phloem elements.

Blade/Lamina: are the flattened part of a leaf, excluding the stalk.

Bole: refers to the trunk of a tree, usually below the lowest branch.

Bulb: Thick underground storage organ, consisting of a stem and leaf bases (the inner ones fleshy). Onion bulbs, tulip bulbs.

Climber: a plant growing more or less erect by leaning or twining on another structure for support, or by clinging with tendrils.

Compound leaves: Leaves composed of several leaflets.

Canopy: the branches and foliage of a tree generally at the very top of the plants.

Corm: Fleshy, swollen underground tuberous stem storing food reserves.

Dichotomous: is a term referring to forking into two equal branches. This kind of forked growth is seen in mosses and fern gametophytes.

Internode: is the portion of a stem between two nodes.

Laticiferous: are plants that are latex bearing, producing a milky juice.

Latex: is a milky fluid that exudes from plants such as rubber, figs, dandelions and milkweed.

Leaf: an outgrowth of a stem, usually flat and green, its main function is food manufacture by photosynthesis. Leaves may be simple with a single leaf blade or compound with multiple leaflets.

Leaflets: are the ultimate segments of a compound leaf.

Margin: Refers to the edge of a leaf blade.

Meristem: is an actively dividing tissue responsible for growth. Meristems are found in the margins of leaves, in the apex of the shoot, in the axils of the leaves, in the margins of stems and in the root.

Midrib/Mid-vein: is the central, and usually most prominent, vein of a leaf or leaf-like organ.

Morphology: refers to the form of an organism. In plants, it refers to the overall shapes of the whole plant as well as its parts.

Monopodial: is a mode of stem growth and branching in which the main axis is formed by a single dominant meristem.

Node: the part of a stem where leaves or branches arise.

Palmate: leaf with veins radiating out from a central point (usually at the top of a petiole), resembling spread out fingers pointing away from the palm. A compound palmate leaf has leaflets that radiate from a central point.

Petiole: is the stem-like stalk of a leaf.

Phyllode: a leaf with the blade much reduced or absent, and in which the petiole and or rachis perform the functions of the whole leaf.

Pinnate: divided leaves almost to midrib but segments still confluent.

Pneumatophore: is a vertical, aerial appendage to the roots of mangrove plants through which gases are exchanged. They are essentially breathing roots.

Primary vein: The single vein or array of veins that is conspicuously larger than any others in the leaf area are. In pinnate venation, the single primary vein is in the middle of the leaf. In palmate venation, several such veins radiate from a point at or near the base of the leaf.

Pulvinus: a swelling at either end of a petiole of a leaf or petiole of a leaflet,

Rachis: The axis of an inflorescence or a pinnate leaf; for example ferns; secondary rachis is the axis of a pinna in a bipinnate leaf distal to and including the lowermost pedicel attachment.

Rhizome: perennial underground stem usually growing horizontally.

Root hairs: are outgrowths of the outermost layer of cells just behind the root tips, functioning as water-absorbing organs.

Shoot: usually the aerial part of a plant; a stem including its dependent parts, leaves flowers etc.

Simple: undivided leaf.

Spine: is a stiff, sharp structure, formed by the modification of a plant organ that contains vascular tissue.

Sporophyte: This refers to the plant that produces spores in ferns or flowers and seeds in gymnosperms and angiosperms.

Stalk: the supporting structure of an organ, usually narrower in diameter than the organ.

Stem: refers to the plant axis that bears nodes, leaves, branches and flowers. Stems can be underground as in potato.

Stipule: a small appendage at the base of leaves.

Stolon: slender, prostrate or trailing stem, producing roots and sometimes-erect shoots at its nodes

Stoma: (plural stomata): a small microscopic hole in the surface of a leaf (or other aerial organ) allowing the exchange of gases between tissues and the atmosphere.

Taproot: is the main, descending root of a plant with a single dominant root axis.

Tendril: a slender organ used by climbing plants to cling to an object.

Terminal: any structure situated at the tip or apex.

Trichomes: Hair-like outgrowth from epidermis, e.g. a hair or bristle.

Tuber: an underground storage organ formed by the swelling of an underground stem which produces buds and stores food, forming a seasonal perennating organ, for example potato; yam. Very often swollen roots are also referred to as tubers.

Venation: is the arrangement of veins in a leaf. In dicots, the veins spread like the fingers in a human palm but in monocots, the veins are arranged parallel to each other as in all cereals, grasses, and banana.

Whorl: a ring of organs borne at the same level on an axis, for example leaves, bracts or floral parts.

Flowers

Androdioecious: are species where plants of same species bear only male flowers in some plants and bisexual in others.

Andromonoecious: are species, with bisexual flowers and male flowers on the same plant.

Androecium: are male parts of flower.

Apetalous: are flowers without petals.

Awn: are Long bristle-like appendage of some grass spikelets.

Bisexual: are flowers bearing both male and female reproductive organs.

Bract: modified leaf associated with flower or inflorescence.

Calyx: (plural calyces) the outer whorl of a flower, usually green; All sepals together are called calyx.

Catkin: refers to a spike, in which the mostly small flowers are unisexual and without a conspicuous perianth. The, catkins are usually shed as a unit.

Cyme: inflorescence in which the main axis and all lateral branches end in a flower (each lateral may be repeatedly branched).

Culm: is an aerial stem bearing the inflorescence.

Corymb: Inflorescence with branches arising at different points but reaching about the same height, giving the cluster of flowers a flat-topped appearance.

Dioecious: When male and female reproductive structures develop on different individuals, the plants are described as dioecious.

Glumes: bracts around a sedge, or similar plant; in grasses forming the lowermost organs of a spikelet.

Gynomonoecious: Species with bisexual flowers and female flowers formed on same plant.

Gynoecium: is a collective term for female parts of the flower containing the ovary with ovules and the style and stigma.

Gynodioecious: are species where some plants have bisexual flowers on same plants and others of same species have female flowers.

Inflorescence: several flowers closely grouped together to form an efficient structured unit, the grouping or arrangement of flowers on a plant.

Lemma: It is the lowermost of two chaff-like bracts enclosing the grass floret.

Monoecious: hermaphrodite, with all flowers bisexual; or with male and female reproductive structures in separate flowers but on the same plant; or of an inflorescence that has unisexual flowers of both sexes;

Nectary: is a specialized gland that secretes nectar, honey.

Papilionate: flowers that are butterfly-like with a corolla like that of a pea.

Pedicel: it is the stalk of a flower.

Peduncle: is the stalk of an inflorescence.

Perfect: Bisexual flowers with sepal, petals, stamens and pistil.

Perianth: is the collective terms for the calyx (sepals) and corolla (petals) of a flower. Abbreviation: P. For instance P 6 + six indicates the calyx and corolla each have six sepals + six petals.

Petals: are parts of a flower that give colors. Collectively a group of petals is called a corolla.

Polymorphic: refers to several different kinds of shape pand size, hence polymorphism. Monomorphic (a single type) and dimorphic (two types).

Protandrous: male sex organs maturing before the female ones, such as flower-shedding pollen before the stigma is receptive.

Protogynous: female sex organs maturing before the male ones, flower-shedding pollen after the stigma has ceased to be receptive, opposite of protandrous.

Raceme: is an indeterminate inflorescence in which the main axis produces a series of flowers on lateral stalks, the oldest at the base and the youngest at the top; cf. spike.

Sepals: are the outermost parts of a flower. These are usually light/dark green. Collectively sepals are called calyx.

Solitary: are single flowers that are not grouped into an inflorescence.

Spadix: is a spicate (spike-like) inflorescence with a stout, often succulent axis.

Spathe: is a large bract ensheathing an inflorescence.

Spike: an unbranched, indeterminate inflorescence in which the flowers are without stalks;

Spikelet: is a unit of the inflorescence especially in grasses, sedges and some other monocotyledons, consisting of one to many flowers and associated bracts (glumes).

Standard: is the large posterior petal of legume flowers.

Sympetalous: description of flowers with fused petals.

Unisexual: flowers of one sex, bearing only male or only female reproductive organs.

Umbel: a racemose inflorescence in which all the individual flower stalks arise in a cluster at the top of the peduncle and are of about equal length.

Fruits

Achene: Dry single seeded fruit.

Aggregate fruit: A cluster of fruits formed from the free carpels of one flower, blackberry, Mulberry, Boysenberry, and elderberry.

Berry: an indehiscent fruit, with the seeds immersed in the pulp, for instance tomato.

Capsule: is a dry fruit formed from two of more carpels that are united and dehiscing when ripe.

Cleistogamous: flowers that self-pollinate and never open fully, or self-pollinate before opening.

Cone: a fruit, usually woody, ovoid to globular, including scales, bracts or bracteoles arranged around a central axis, as in gymnosperms, especially conifers and Casuarina.

Cypsela: a dry, indehiscent, one-seeded fruit formed from an inferior ovary.

Drupe: a succulent fruit formed from one carpel; the single seed is enclosed by a stony layer of the fruit wall; kernel: peaches, olives.

Drupelet: a drupe, usually small, formed from one of the carpels in an apocarpous flower. Drupelets usually form a compound fruit, as in raspberries and strawberries.

Multiple fruit: are clusters of fruits produced from more than one flower appearing as a single fruit, often on a swollen axis.

Exocarp: the outer layer of the pericarp, often the skin of fleshy fruits.

Fruit: seed-bearing structure in angiosperms formed from the ovary, and sometimes associated floral parts, after flowering.

Hip: This is a term referring to the fruit of a Rose.

Mast: This refers to edible fruit and nuts produced by woody species of plants.

Mesocarp: is the the fleshy portion of the wall of a succulent fruit inside the skin and outside the stony layer surrounding the seed.

Nut: is a hard, dry, indehiscent fruit, containing only one seed.

Parthenocarpy: refers to the development or production of fruit without fertilization.

Pericarp: the wall of a fruit, developed from the ovary wall.

Pod: is the fruit of a leguminous plant, a dry fruit of a single carpel, splitting along two sutures.

Pome: is a fruit that has developed partly from the ovary wall as in apples.

Pyrene: is the stone of a drupe, consisting of the seed surrounded by the hardened endocarp.

Male Reproductive Structures

Anther: Pollen-bearing part of the stamen. Anthers have 2–4 hollow lobes containing pollen grains.

Anthesis: Period during which pollen is presented and/or the stigma is receptive.

Filament: The male reproductive system known as the stamen consists of filaments bearing the anthers.

Micro strobilus/Macro strobilus: Gymnosperms produce two types of cones. The smaller one is the male or micro strobilus and the larger one is the female or macro strobilus.

Pollen: are powdery mass shed from anthers (of angiosperms) or microsporangia (of gymnosperms).

Pollination: is the transfer of pollen from the male organ (anther) to the receptive region of a female organ (stigma).

Stamen: male organ of a flower in angiosperms, consisting of a stalk (filament) and a pollen bearing portion (anther). Staminate flowers are male flowers wheras pistillate flowers are female flowers.

Staminode: is a sterile stamen, often rudimentary, sometimes petal-like.

Female reproductive system: ovary and ovules

Carpel: is the basic female reproductive organ in angiosperms.

Funicle (funiculus): is the stalk that attaches the ovule to the ovary.

Gynoecium: refers to female parts of flower.

Hermaphrodite: Bisexual flowers with both male and female parts.

Ovule: The seed before fertilization; a structure in a seed plant within which one or more megaspores are formed.

Inferior: An ovary which is at least partly below the level of attachment of other floral parts; A superior ovary is one where the ovary is above.

Integument: refers in general to any covering, but especially the covering of an ovule.

Ovary: is the basal portion of a carpel or group of fused carpels, enclosing the ovule(s).

Pendulous: hanging, for example an ovule attached to a placenta on the top of the ovary.

Placenta: the tissue within an ovary to which the ovules are attached

Pistil: is a single carpel when the carpels are free or a group of carpels when the carpels are united by the superior ovary.

Stigma: is the pollen-receptive surface of a carpel or group of fused carpels, usually sticky, usually a point or small head at the summit of the style.

Style: is an elongated part of a carpel, or group of fused carpels, between the ovary and the stigma.

Seeds

Alate: seeds having a wing or wings: Seeds of Drumstick plant

Albuminous: those Seeds containing endosperm

Aril: is a membranous or fleshy appendage, which partly or wholly covers a seed.

Cotyledon: is the primary leaf or leaves of an embryo, becoming the seed leaf or leaves.

Pericarp: is the outer layer of the wall of a fruit namely the 'skin.'

Epicotyl: the part of the plant axis or stem between the cotyledonory node and first foliage leaves.

Embryo: young plant contained by a seed.

Endocarp: Is the innermost layer of the wall of a fruit, in a drupe, the stony layer surrounding the seed.

Endosperm: a nutritive tissue surrounding the embryo of the seed, usually triploid, originating from the fusion of both polar nuclei with one gamete after the fertilization of the egg.

Germination: refers to the physical and physiological changes that occur when the seed imbibes water and takes the path of development towards a plant.

Glutinous: refers to sticky seeds because of the presence of gluten. Rice seeds may be glutinous (Japanese varieties) or not.

Hilum: is the scar on a seed coat where it separates from its stalk.

Hypocotyl: is the region that marks the transition from root to stem development in the embryo and germinating seed.

Nucellus: is the tissue of the ovule of a seed plant that surrounds the female gametophyte. It is enclosed by integuments.

Palea: The upper of two bracts enclosing a grass flower, major contributors to chaff in harvested grain.

Paleaceous: appears chaff-like in texture. Wheat, rice and other grains have chaff.

Plumule: is the part of an embryo that gives rise to the shoot system of a plant.

Radicle: is the part of an embryo-giving rise to the root system of a plant.

Seed: A fertilized ovule made of a protective seed coat enclosing an embryo and food reserves.

Tegmen: is the inner layer of the testa (seed coat). It develops from the inner integument of the ovule.

Testa: is the seed coat.

Viviparous: are Seeds or fruits that germinate before being shed from the parent plant.

Genetics

Genotype/Phenotype: the genetic make-up of an individual is called the genotype and the physical appearance of the plants (morphology) is called phenotype. 2n = 14 is genotype of wheat, 2n = 46 is the genotype of humans. The physical description of the plant is called the phenotype. In the case of wheat, the phenotype is that it is a monocot, has grass-like features, parallel leaf veins, grains in an ear, grains contain carbohydrates, protein etc.

Cell: basic microscopic unit of plant structure, generally consisting of compartments in a viscous fluid surrounded by a wall.

Chimera: an individual composed of two or more genetically different tissues, most commonly because of a graft and sometimes within the individual, by mutations and irregularities that occur during cell division.

Coenocyte: A single cell with multiple nuclei, formed when nuclear division was not followed by cell division.

Haploid/Diploid/Tetraploid/Polyploids: Haploid: Cells contain one copy of each chromosome. For example the haploid chromosome number of Humans is n = 23, in wheat it is n = 7etc. This is the case in the gametes of all organisms irrespective of sex. In diploids represented by the human body (somatic) it is 2n = 46, in wheat it is, 2n = 14. Higher than diploids in humans is not viable. However, in plants, triploids (3n), tetraploid (4 n) and polyploids etc are common. Polyploidy: refers to any organism with more than two of the basic sets of chromosomes in the nucleus, any sporophyte with cells containing three or more complete sets of chromosomes. Various combinations of words or numbers with '-ploid' indicate the number of haploid sets of chromosomes; e.g. triploid = three sets, tetraploid = four sets, pentaploid = five sets, hexaploid = six sets, and so on.

Hybrid: a plant produced by the crossing of parents belonging to two different named groups, e.g. genera, species, varieties, subspecies, forma and so on; i.e. the progeny resulting within and between the crossings of two different species, varieties, cultivars etc of plants are called hybrids. An F1 hybrid is the primary product of such a cross. F1 hybrids of intergeneric crosses are inviable and they have to undergo doubling of the chromosomes before they can become fertile. Thus, F1 hybrid are the result of a repeatable cross between two pure bred lines of an organism. An F2 hybrid is a plant arising from a cross between two F1 hybrids (or from the self-pollination of an F1 hybrid).

Mutation: an abrupt and inexplicable variation from the norm, such as the doubleness in flowers, changes in colour, or habit of growth. Mutations can result sporadically due to genetic mistakes during DNA replication or because of exposure to irradiation or chemicals.

Reproduction

Apomixes: Reproduction, where viable seed or spores are produced without fertilization A plant produced in this way is an apomict.

Double fertilization: In angiosperms, the pollen generates two gametic nuclei; one nucleus fertilizes the egg and other fuses with the two polar nuclei in the embryo sac forming a triploid nucleus that multiplies by mitosis to generate the nutrient rich endosperm.

Embryo sac: a sac containing the egg nucleus that is fertilized by the male gamete released from the pollen tube when the pollen germinates on the stigma. Most embryo sacs contain 4–8 haploid nuclei of which one is the egg nucleus and others are involved in endosperm formation or other functions.

Parthenocarpy: refers to the production of fruit without pollination. Thus, these fruits are seedless. Parthenocarpy can be produced naturally or through chemical stimulation by plant hormones like gibberellic acid.

Propagules: structures capable of producing a new plant; includes seeds, spores, bulbils, etc.

Zygote: is a fertilized cell, the diploid product of fusion of two haploid gametes.

Anatomy and Cell Biology

Casparian strip: a continuous band of suberin in the radial primary cell walls of the endodermis in vascular plant stems and roots that forms a permeability barrier to the passive diffusion of external water and solutes into the vascular tissue.

Chlorophyll/Anthocyanin: Chlorophylls are green pigments in chloroplasts, essential for photosynthesis. Anthocyanins are pigments in flowers, ageing leaves and in some other organs such as roots of carrots, beets and turnips.

Chloroplast: organelle present in plant cells that contains chlorophyll.

Chlorosis: refers to abnormal lack or paleness of color in a normally green organ.

Collenchyma: A specialized tissue consisting of living cells with unevenly thickened cellulose and pectin cell walls that performs a support function in organs such as leaves and young stems that are composed of primary plant tissues.

Cuticle: a waterproofing layer covering the epidermis of aerial plant surfaces, composed of the polymers cutin, and/or cutan and waxes.

Endodermis: the innermost layer of the cortex of vascular plant roots, also present in the stems of Pteridophytes. The radial walls are impregnated with suberin to form a permeability barrier known as the Casparian strip.

Epicuticular wax: a layer of crystalline or amorphous wax deposited on the surface of the plant cuticle.

Epidermis: is an organ's outermost layer of cells, usually only one cell thick.

Fiber: Fibers may be soluble in water or may be insoluble as in cellulose fibers. Both types of fibers are important for good gastrointestinal and cardiovascular health.

Guard cells: are two special cells that surround the stoma and control gas exchange between the plant cells/tissue and the external air. The opening and closing of stomata by the swelling or shrinking of guard cells controls transpiration (evaporation of water) of the plant.

Lenticel: is typically a lens-shaped porous tissue in bark with large intercellular spaces that allows direct exchange of gases between the internal tissues and atmosphere through the bark.

Lignin: complex organic polymers deposited on woody tissue as well as in some seed coats.

Mesophyll tissue: photosynthetic tissue of a leaf, located between the upper and lower epidermis.

Parenchyma: a versatile ground tissue composed of living primary cells that performs a wide variety of structural and biochemical functions in plants.

Vascular tissue: The conducting xylem and phloem elements.

Phloem: is a specialized conducting tissue in vascular plants that transports sucrose and other metabolites from the leaves to other plant organs.

Pith: is the central region of a stem, inside the vascular cylinder; the spongy parenchymatous central tissue in some stems and roots.

Turgid: swollen with liquid; firm; compare flaccid.

Vascular bundle: a bundle of vascular tissue in the primary stems of vascular plants, consisting of specialized conducting cells for the transport of water, minerals (xylem) and assimilate (phloem).

Vessel: a capillary tube formed from a series of open-ended cells in the water-conducting tissue (Xylem) of a plant.

Xylem: a specialized water-conducting tissue in vascular plants.

General Description of Plant Kingdom and All Plants

Plants are classified into non vascular plants that have no specialized conductive tissue for distributing water and nutrients and Vascular plants that have special conductive tissue known as Xylem and Phloem through which water and nutrients are transported in a manner similar to arteries and veins in animals. The nonvascular plants include the hornworts – Anthoceratophyta, liverworts – Hepatophyta and mosses – Bryophytes.

The vascular plants are divided into two groups namely the spore producing non-seed plants and seed plants. The latter are further divided into Gymnosperms and Angiosperms. The spore producing vascular plants are composed of the whisk ferns – Psilophyta, Club Mosses – Lycopodophyta, Horsetails – Equisetophyta and the

Ferns-Pteridophytes. The seed producing plants are further divided into plants that produce naked seeds without flowers (Gymnosperms) and the flowering plants with enclosed seeds (Angiosperms).

The naked seed producers are the Gymnosperms consisting of the Conifers-Pinophyta, Cycads – Cycadophyta, Ginkgo –Ginkgophyta, the gnetophytes – Gnetophyta. The Angiosperms are plants that produce flowers and seeds that are enclosed. The flowering Angiosperms are further divided into Mesoangiosperms and the more primitive basal angiosperms. The more evolved Mesoangiosperms contain three clades namely the Eudicots, Monocots and the Magnoliids. The broad classification of plants is summarized below:

Kingdom: Plantae

1. Non vascular plants: hornworts – Anthoceratophyta; liverworts-Hepatophyta and mosses – Bryophytes/Bryophyta.

2. Vascular plants:

    a. Spore producing plants: whisk ferns – Psilophyta; Club Mosses – Lycopodophyta; Horsetails – Equisetophyta and the Ferns – Pteridophytes or Pteropsida.

    b. Seed plants with naked seed (Gymnosperms): Conifers-Pinophyta; Cycads-Cycadophyta; Ginkgo-Ginkgophyta; the gnetophytes – Gnetophyta.

    c. Seed plants with enclosed seeds: Angiosperms: These are further divided into the more primitive basal angiosperms and the more advanced Mesoangiosperms consisting of Monocots (Monocotyledonae, with one cotyledon); Eudicots (true dicots (dicotyledonae) with two cotyledons and Magnoliids with multiple spirally arranged flower parts.

Non Vascular moss-like plants: The hornworts – Anthocerotae, liverworts-Hepaticae and mosses – bryophyte/Musci are spore producing lower forms of plants which have no special vascular tissues but can photosynthesize and live mostly in moist environments growing on rocks, soil, trunk of trees, wet roof of homes and other substrates. They have a leafy appearance and do not have true roots, stems and leaves but have root like structures known as rhizoids, stem like and leaf like appearance. The plant body is referred to as a thallus. The green photosynthetic leafy structure known as the gametophyte produces sperms in antheridia and eggs in archegonia. Fusion of the sperms with the eggs produces a stalk like structure known as the sporophyte that produces haploid spores. Based on the Doctrine of Signatures the liverworts were used in ancient times for treatment of liver diseases hence the name liverwort but no real medicinal benefits have been reported.

The hornworts e.g. Anthoceros are so named because of their horn like sporophytes. The gametophyte looks similar to the Liverworts but the sporophytes have the capacity for indefinite growth, often reaching a height of 20 cm making them the tallest members of the bryophytes. There are no known medicinal applications for these plants but they are ecologically significant in being able to grow on many types of moist solid and semi-solid surfaces including trunks of higher plants. They also have the additional ability to harbor nitrogen-fixing cyanobacteria and thus enhance the nitrogenous supply of the substrate where they grow.

The mosses that represent the group Musci contain about 12,000 species including peat/bog moss – *Sphagnum*, fire moss – *Ceratodon purpureus*, step moss – *Hylocomium splendens* and others. Sphagnum or Bog moss was used in the preparation of surgical dressings because of the high moisture absorbing properties, which enable discharges from wounds to be absorbed during ancient times and much later during World War I and II. Dressings made of Sphagnum moss soaked in garlic were used as a germicidal dressing. Moss Bioreactors are used currently to grow various biopharmaceuticals through recombinant DNA technology. The moss *Physcomitrella patens* is being tried in molecular farming for production of potential drugs.

Tracheophyta: The Seedless Vascular Plants, Whisk ferns, Club Mosses, Horsetails and Ferns: These plants have been recorded from the Paleozoic Silurian era about 400 million years ago. This is a very large and diverse group of terrestrial/semi terrestrial plants growing in swamps and solid land-masses characterized by the presence of a special group of cells known as tracheids for transport of water and minerals in the plant. The development of tracheid enable the plants to move from an essentially aquatic environment to a dry land mass where water has to be absorbed from the soil and transported to the various above ground parts of the plant. Here also, there is an alternation of generations involving a gametophyte that is very small often only a few centimeters in length and a very large significant sporophyte that may reach a height of 15–20 meters. The gametophyte produces the male sperm in antheridia and female archegonia that contain eggs. The fusion of the sperms and eggs produce the sporophyte that grows into large structures with root like organs, stem and leaves. Instead of seeds, the plant leaves produce thousands of spores in special spore producing structures known as sporangia. The spores germinate to produce the few celled gametophyte generation. There are four major classes of Tracheophyta namely: Psylopsida, Lycopsida, Sphenopsida and Pteropsida.

Psylopsida: These were the first vascular plants that evolved in the Silurian period of the Paleozoic era about 450 million years ago. These plants are currently extinct except for two genera namely Psilotum and Tsemesipteris but many plants of this group are preserved in the form of fossils. The plants of this group share many characteristics of the bryophytes (mosses) but have conducting tissue in the form of tracheid and phloem so that water and minerals could be distributed. The plants lack true roots but have root-like structures known as rhizoids. They also lack true leaves but have either dichotomously branching green stem like structures or have minute scales or primitive leaf-like flattened photosynthetic organs.

Lycopsida: These are the club mosses. These plants have true roots and have leaves. Both Gametophytes and Sporophytes are independent of each other where the gametophytes produce the sex organs and the sporophytes produce the seedless sporangia with spores. These plants were the dominant vegetation in the carboniferous period about 350 million years ago and certain types of coal called cannel coal were the fossilized remains of the lycopsid known as Lepidodendron. The spores of the club mosses are used to promote healing by drying excess moisture that can cause skin irritation and itching in eczema much like cornstarch or colloidal oatmeal. These spores are nontoxic with biocide properties unlike the leaves and stems of the plant that contain two poisonous alkaloids lycopodine and clavadine. Club moss was used in Chinese Herbal medicine.

The club mosses contain many alkaloids of the quinolizidine group that may have some potential for drug development. Club moss is used in homeopathy for treatments of aneurisms, constipation, chronic lung and ear and bronchial disorders, fevers. Further, if the powdered spores are applied on the skin, it reduces skin irritation and itching. Lycopodium is used to treat various mental conditions like anxiety, forgetfulness, and relief from tiredness and chronic fatigue.

Sphenopsida: Most members of this group are extinct but one genus namely *Equisetum* continues to live in boggy environments. Known as horsetails, these plants appeared during the Devonian period. The Sphenopsida are classified now as a special group of the typical ferns rather than as a separate class. The plants have photosynthesizing hollow stems that are segmented producing scaly leaves from the nodes. More advanced conducting tissue known as Xylem characteristic of higher plants are found. The growth of the plants is mediated by intercalary meristems unlike higher plants that have apical meristems. The plants produce sporangia in clusters arranged in cones similar to those of pine. Because of its high silica content, horsetail plants are used as scouring agents and as folk medicinal herbs for treatment of osteoporosis and to stop bleeding and treating skin ulcers.

Pteropsida: The Pteropsida contain the spore bearing ferns and the seed bearing gymnosperms and Angiosperms. Older plant classifications regarded the ferns as a separate group known as the Pteridophytes. Currently, the Pteropsida is classified to include three groups of plants namely, Filicineae-Ferns, Gymnospermae-naked seed bearing non flowering plants and Angiospermae – Flowering plants.

Filicineae: Members of this class known as Ferns numbering about 12000 species first appeared in the Devonian period. The fern plant has large leaves known as fronds and underground stems known as Rhizomes. They have true roots through which they absorb water and minerals from the moist soil. They inhabit shaded moist woodlands and swampy regions away from directly exposed regions. Since they lack strong woody stems they cannot withstand strong winds. Most ferns are about 12 meters/2.5 Ft. in height but some like the tree ferns can reach heights of 20 meters/6.6 Ft. Some fern species live on other plants e.g. trunk of trees in an epiphytic mode. The fern frond contains several sporangia on the undersurface from which thousands of spores are released. These spores germinate on most surfaces to produce the diminutive haploid gametophyte known as the prothallus. The prothallus that is only about one cell thick produces numerous female sex organs known as Archegonia and male antheridia that produce sperms. Union of the sperms with the eggs in the archegonia results in the generation of the sporophyte generation that grows into the fern plant. Examples of ferns include: *Osmunda regalis* (Royal fern), *Osmunda Cinnamomina* (Cinnamon fern), *Microsorum pteropus* (Java fern), *Polypodium glyrrhiza* (Licorice fern), *Pteris vittatta* (brake fern), *Adiantum pedatum* and *A. Capillusveneris* (Maiden hair fern), *Nephrolepis exaltata cv. Bostoniensis* (Boston Fern) and *Azolla* (Water fern).

Gymnospermae (Gymnosperms): Gymnosperms include the cycads, junipers, cedar, pine, spruce, fir, hemlock, redwood, sequoia, Ginkgo and other evergreen plants. The plants are characterized by the production of "naked seeds" or seeds that are not inside the ovary Gymno = naked. The plants are grouped into four classes namely:

the cycads which are palm like plants, the ginkgos which were common in the Mesozoic era but represented by only one living genus namely *Gingko biloba*, the Gnetales made of three genera *Gnetum, Ephedra* and *welwitchia* and the coniferales which are the largest group consisting of Pine, Fir, Spruce, Juniper etc.

All living gymnosperms grow in width through secondary growth. Except for the Gnetales the rest of the gymnosperms conduct their water and mineral supplies through the more primitive water conducting elements known as the tracheid and yet they grow to enormous heights as exemplified by the redwoods of California that grow over 100 meters/ 350 ft with the tallest being about 115 meters/375 ft tall. The wood of the gymnosperms particularly the confers are the mainstay of the building and lumber industry.

The Gymnosperms do not produce flowers but instead produce cones that are organized into male and female cones either on the same plant (monoecious) or on separate male and female plants (dioecious). The male cones produce pollen that is carried by wind or pollinating insects onto the female cones that contain the ovules. Fertilization of the ovules by the pollen results in the "naked seeds" which eventually germinate to give rise to seedlings that eventually grow into the mature plants. The germination and growth of the seedlings apparently depend on a symbiotic relationship with certain fungi in the soil known as Mycorrhiza.

The following is a brief description of the different groups of gymnosperms.

Cycadophyta (Cycads): There are three families in this class: Cycadaceae, Stangeriaceae and Zamiaceae. The plants have a non-branching woody trunk topped by a crown of large evergreen leaves which grow in a rosette form and look like palm leaves. The leaves are very large and feather like pinnate. The plants are either male or female trees producing female cones or male cones as the case may be. Pollination occurs through the media of specific pollinators usually beetles. Cycads grow in many different habitats and are found in Asia, Africa, Australia and both South and North America. Cycad seeds contain the neurotoxins cycasin, alkaloids macrozamin or methylazoxymethanol and Beta methyl amino L alanine (BMMA) and yet, the starch of the cycad seeds is used to prepare various food preparations usually by drying the seeds or soaking the seeds to remove most if not all of the toxin. Different parts of the plant are said to have various medicinal qualities. A paste of Cycad seeds and coconut oil is used for skin complaints. Cycads are also used as an astringent to regulate energy flow for pain relief and as a kidney tonic to treat hypertension, for rheumatic pain or colds and to cure hepatomegaly/liver cancer and stomach trouble. However, ethno medical investigations show that the use of cycad preparations from seed or leaf can be tied to neurological diseases such as Guam disease that are highly prevalent in certain pacific island cultures which use the cycads for food or other purposes.

Ginkgophyta (Gingko): Gingko plants first appeared about 275 million years ago. Only one species namely *Ginkgo biloba* has survived. Gingko is a large tree growing to a height of 50 meters. The trees are sparsely branched. The leaves have two lobes hence the species name biloba. The plants are highly resistant to disease and apparently to high levels of radiation. The plants are dioecious (separate male and female plants) wherein, the males produce microsporophyll and the females two ovules at the end of a stalk.

Extracts of the plant are used to treat various medical conditions especially relating to blood flow to the brain, correcting leg pain by increasing blood flow and as a memory enhancer.

Coniferophyta (Conifers): The conifers are the largest group of gymnosperms including such plants as the giant sequoias, redwoods, Colorado spruce, Douglas fir, Junipers, pines, araucaria, taxus, yews and cedar. They are also referred to as evergreens or softwood trees. Conifers have separate male and female cones that carry the pollen and ovules respectively.

Gnetales: Gnetaceae Welwitschiaceae and Ephedraceae: The group consists of three genera namely: 1. Gnetum that is a small tree found mostly in the Indian sub-continent, Malay Archipelago and Indonesian islands. 2. Welwitchia found mostly in Africa and, 3. Ephedra that occurs in semiarid regions of Asia, Africa and South and North America. All members have vessel like elements as in Angiosperms through which they transfer water.

Gnetom gnemon is a small tree with shiny glabrous leaves similar to those of angiosperms. Other species of Gnetom are shrubs. The seeds of Gnetum are used to prepare many different types of foods including fried chips. Gnetum plants are cultivated in Indonesia and parts of Malaysia as an agricultural crop. The plant contains many potentially useful phytochemicals such as Resveratrol that has gained prominence due to its purported anti-ageing properties. Many other phytochemicals have been obtained from this plant.

Welwitchia mirabilis the only living member of Welwitschiaceae are small shrub-like plants with just two leaves that arise from the basal region of the plant and grow continuously with the result that the circumference of the plant exceeds their height. The plants are dioecious (separate male and female plants). The seeds of the plant are infected by the fungus Aspergillus that eventually kills the seeds with the result that it is difficult to get uninfected seeds for propagation. The plants are endemic to Namibia and Angola in Africa. There are no reports of any specific medicinal property that is attributed to this genus.

The Ephedra known commonly as Mormon tea, Brigham Tea, Somalata in Sanskrit and Ma huáng in Chinese are leafless desert shrubs with jointed green stems forming in whorls at nodes along the stalk. Unlike other naked seeds, the ephedra lack resin canals. The male cones have 2 to 8 anthers. The female cones have bracts covering the two maturing seeds. Worldwide there is 1 genus and 40 species. The plants contain ephedrine that is a very powerful stimulant and decongestant. Ephedrine extracts have been used by many cultures for medicinal purposes, narcotic properties and even for spiritual religious purposes. Historians have suggested that Ephedra is the plant known as Soma that was used in Indo-Iranian religious ceremonies. It has been in use for a long time for treatment of Asthma, weight reduction and as a performance enhancer by athletes but is now banned because of its highly toxic qualities.

The Angiosperms (seed plants with enclosed seeds): The Angiosperms are the most dominant species of plants growing wild as well as cultivated for food, fiber, medicinal and floricultural purposes. The plants belonging to this group may be herbs, shrubs or trees growing on land, swamps and aquatic environments. They may be annuals completing their life cycle in one season (peas, all beans, corn, rice, wheat) or biennials like carrots, beets, cabbage, turnips, or perennials like oak, ash, rosewood, teak, asparagus, most fruit trees, many vegetable plants. They are characterized by the development of true flowers that may be unisexual or bisexual, and have transport elements phloem and Xylem vessels and tracheid arranged in bundles known as vascular bundles, flowers with stamens having two pairs of pollen sacs, ovules with an 8 nucleate embryo sac and seeds enclosed in an ovary that becomes organized into fruits. All members undergo a process known as double fertilization wherein, one of the two nuclei of the pollen fertilizes the egg in the ovule and the other male nucleus fertilizes two female nuclei in the ovule. This process results in the development of the seed that contains the embryo and the nutrient part of the seed known as the endosperm.

A typical Angiosperm has three types of distinct tissues namely the structural tissue that forms the main body of the plant, the meristematic tissue, which is like the stem cells of animals capable of indeterminate growth and development into cell types, and vascular tissue that carries and distributes water, minerals, vitamins, sugars and all metabolites. The Vascular tissue consist of two main types of cells known as Xylem for conducting water and other dissolved substances including minerals and phloem tissue which transports food manufactured in the leaves.

The Angiosperms were classified until recently into two broad groups the Monocotyledonae, (corn, rice, wheat, all cereals, all grasses, bamboo, sugarcane, coconut, date palm) and the Diciotyledonae (Beans peas, soybeans, all legumes, cotton etc). However, Plant taxonomists have reclassified the original Angiosperms based on the APG III system (Angiosperm Phylogeny Group III) system of flowering plant classification into 12 clades that has been broken down further into orders and families. For purposes of simplicity, we will follow the classification of Angiosperms into Basal angiosperms, Mesoangiosperms consisting of Magnoliids, Monocots (Monocotyledonae) and true dicots (dicotyledonae) or Eudicots.

Basal Angiosperms: This small diverse group branched off from the Angiosperms before the true dicots evolved. They share characteristics of both true dicots as well as certain characters of Monocots. They have numerous flattened laminar stamens with wide filaments; numerous tepals; many separate carpels; aromatic oils and alternate spirally arranged leaves. Most also share the microscopic characteristic of monosulcate or monoaperturate pollen also seen in monocots. Phyllotaxis that is not always readily observable except during early development was probably spiral in the flowers of the ancestor of all angiosperms. A transition to developing floral organs in whorls of three most likely occurred early. The plants in this group include the angiosperm order containing Water Lilies, Nymphaeales and Amborella all of which seem to lack vessel elements homologous to those seen in practically all other angiosperms.

Magnoliids: This group includes the Magnoliales, Laurales, Piperales and Canellales. The plants within this clade are characterized by having flowers with numerous spirally arranged flower parts (sepals, petals, stamens and ovules). The leaves in this group have oil cells with aromatic oils. Thus, plants like pepper (*Piper nigrum*) and nutmeg (Myristica *fragrans*), belong to this clade. The plants are natives of the Australasian, Southern hemisphere region and have been introduced into other regions later.

Monocotyledonae: This clade consists of the grasses that include rice, wheat, corn, barley, and oats, millets, turf grass, lawn grass, bamboos, sugarcane, coconuts and various palms. After the plant undergoes double fertilization, they produce a single cotyledon that is a storehouse of food for the germinating plant until it produces leaves that can undergo photosynthesis. The majority of Monocots are herbaceous except for the bamboo, coconut and other palms that are woody and grow to several feet high. The vascular bundles in stem of the monocots are arranged in a scattered fashion unlike those of the dicots where the Vascular bundles without cambium are organized into a central cylinder surrounding pith. The leaf blade is tapered and long and the veins that supply water minerals and food run parallel to one another. Monocot flowers are arranged in groups of three (three sepals, three petals, 3 stamens,). The leaves have plastids containing protein granules/inclusions.

Eudicots: This is a monophyletic group. Generally, these plants have broad leaves that may be simple or compound having veins that spread from a midrib. They have two cotyledons and have distinct vascular bundles, which are arranged in a cylinder around a pith and main taproot from which branches arise. Members of the group have tricolpate pollen wherein these pollens have three or more pores set in furrows called colpi. In contrast, most of the other seed plants gymnosperms, monocots and the paleodicots produce monosulcate pollen with a single pore set in a differently oriented groove called the sulcus. The name "tricolpates" is preferred by some botanists to avoid confusion with the dicots that are a nonmonophyletic group. Giant oak trees, teak, rosewood, apple, oranges and other orchard plants as well as agriculturally important plants like soybeans, peas, sun flower, chili pepper, eggplant, squash, garden plants like roses, salvia, Delphinium, dahlia, chrysanthemum, carnation etc are all dicotyledonous plants. Plants in this group may be herbs, shrubs, vines, climbers, trees and even parasites or epiphytes. They grow both on land as well as in water and marshy swampy areas. The plants are classified into several families the number and order depending on the system of classification being followed.

The various characteristics of the angiosperms are given below:

Flowers: may be unisexual or bisexual. The different floral parts are arranged in whorls carried on a stalk with a pedestal like structure. A typical angiosperm flower consists of an outer layer of sepals known as calyx, an inner row of petals collectively referred to as corolla, a next layer of stamens made of the pollen containing anthers held on thin filaments and the innermost constituent known as the pistil consisting of the ovary with ovules and style topped by the stigma. In monocots, the sepals, petals and stamens are generally in groups of three whereas in the dicots the floral parts are in groups of four, five, six etc. In unisexual flowers, either the stamens or the pistil is absent. Further, a single plant may carry separate male and female flowers in the same plant in which case the plants are said to be monoecious or there may be separate male and female plants in which case they are said to be dioecious. Flowers may be individual as in roses, hibiscus, petunia, apple, cherry blossom, or clustered together in an inflorescence as in delphinium, gladiolus, canna, many legumes etc.

The initiation of flowering of plants depends on temperature and the length of day light/night they receive. This phenomenon is called photoperiodism. Thus, some plants like tomato are day neutral and flower irrespective of day length. Whereas, long day plants require a longer period of sunlight before flowering and some require a shorter day length for flowering as in Chrysanthemums. The exact length of day/night for each species is different. Some of the long or short day plants are highly specific and follow the day length rules strictly and these are obligate long or short day plants whereas there are others who may generally be short or long day but will flower nevertheless at some time and these are facultative short or long day plants. In general, long day plants flower in the Northern hemisphere in late spring or early summer as daylight is longer and short day plants flower usually after June 21 when the day light gets shorter until December 21. In the Southern hemisphere, the longest day starts on Dec 21 and ends on June 21. Some long day obligate plants are carnation, dianthus, henbane, hyoscyamus, oat – avena, ryegrass, lolium, and clover. Some long day facultative plants are pea, barley, lettuce spring wheat cultivars, turnips. Short day plants flower when the day length is below a certain predefined critical period but will not flower under long day conditions or even if a strong pulse of light is shone at them to interrupt their night cycle but moon light and lawn lights are not of sufficient brilliance to disturb this cycle. Some short-day facultative plants are hemp – cannabis, cotton – gossypium, rice and sugarcane. Day neutral plants such as cucumbers, roses and tomatoes do not initiate flowering based on photoperiodism at all, they flower regardless of the night length. They may initiate flowering after attaining a certain overall developmental stage or age or in response to alternative environmental stimuli such as Vernilization (a period of low temperature) rather than in response to photoperiods.

Reproduction: The anther on the stamen representing the male sex organ contains 2–4 segments or cavities that hold many pollen grains. These pollen grains are the equivalent of the microsporangia of the gymnosperms and the Tracheophyta. The developing pollen grain contains two haploid male sperms and a haploid tube nucleus that plays a role in the germination of the pollen. Small sticky spinal projections are decorated on the pollen grains.

The ovary may contain one or more ovules. Within the ovules, a single cell develops into the embryo sac and repeated meiosis results generally in eight haploid nuclei but in some cases, it may be 4 or 16 haploid nuclei. Only one of the nuclei becomes the egg; two others become the endosperm nuclei and the rest usually degenerate.

Pollination occurs by self-pollination, wind pollination, insect pollination, birds, animals and even humans. When the pollen lands on the stigmatic surface, they germinate and produce a germination tube through which they enter the ovule/s in the ovary and deposit their two sperms therein. One of the two sperms unites with the two-endosperm nuclei in the ovule and the other with female nucleus. This process known as double fertilization is unique to angiosperms. The resulting fusion of the sperm with the two-endosperm nuclei triggers the development of nutritious tissue known as the endosperm and the other fusion product resulting from fusion of the egg nucleus and one sperm gives rise to the embryo. This double fertilization sets the development of the seed.

Fruit and Seed: The process of fertilization sets off several developmental events wherein, the swollen part of the flower stalks including the sepals and petals develop into fruits enclosing the developing seeds inside. If the flower was one with a single ovule that was fertilized then, the fruit will contain one seed as in Mango or if it contained more fertilized ovules then, they develop as many seeds inside the fruit as in strawberries, raspberries and tomatoes. If flowers had developed on inflorescences then, clusters of fruits would be formed as in grapes. Generally, herbaceous plants that are annuals produce many small seeds from a single flower whereas; shrubs, trees and perennials tend to produce fewer but larger seeds from a flower.

True seeds are the products of fertilization but sometimes, the term seed is used to refer to any plant part such as a tuber, which is an underground stem that develops into a plant (Seed potato). True seeds are of four types namely embryonic naked seeds in gymnosperms, endospermic monocotyledonous, endospermic dicotyledonous and nonendospermic dicotyledonous. All seeds contain an outer layer of lignified or thick-celled seed coat enclosing the nutritive endosperm and the embryo. In gymnosperms, there is no true endosperm but the nutritive tissue is haploid made of cells derived from the female mother cells.

Gymnosperm seeds: The seed is composed of the outer seed coat enclosing the haploid nutritive tissue derived from the mother plant-mega gametophyte that surrounds the diploid embryo. The seed is said to be naked since the seed is not enclosed in an ovary and fruit or other similar structure but is exposed since it is located on the scales or leafy sporophylls.

Endospermous Monocotyledon: There are three layers in the seed, namely the outer hardy seed coat composed of several layers of cells enclosing an inner multicellular tissue of nutritive cells called the aleuronic layer rich in proteins and vitamins followed by the multicellular endosperm containing mostly carbohydrates with some protein, lipids and other nutrients. Embedded in the endosperm is the fertilized zygote that develops into the embryo with a single cotyledon that eventually develops into the first leaf of the plant when it germinates. Generally, the seed is mostly made of the endosperm with the embryo located at the bottom of the seed. Examples are rice, wheat, corn and all true cereals.

Endospermous Diciotyledonae: The seed is similar to that of the monocot, except that the embryo contains two thin papery cotyledons that absorb the nutrition from the endosperm within the seed and later become the first two leaves of the seedling. Examples are castor bean, brazil nuts.

Non-endospermic Diciotyledonae: Same as in Endospermous dicots except that the cotyledons are fleshy and are the main source of nutrition. Most of the seed is made of the embryo with the two cotyledons. Examples are peas and all bean species and legumes.

Physiology and Biochemistry

Plant Hormones: The entire life cycle of plants is under the influence of the external environment of temperature, light, water, minerals, etc and by the internal environment by the timely switching on of various developmental genes including hormones. Plant hormones, which are present in low concentrations in the plant, are responsible for the control of the growth of plants including flowering, fruit setting, and seed development. Plant hormones consist of Auxins, Gibberellins, cytokinins, ethylene and abscissic acid.

Auxins are found in growing parts of the plant such as shoot, root tips, and are responsible for controlling cell division and elongation and in development of buds and branching. Along with the cytokinins, they control the ageing process. Synthetic Auxins like 2, 4-dichlorophenoxy acetic acid (2, 4-d) are common components of many weed killers.

Gibberellins are another class of hormones that play a vital role in plant development. They are important in stem elongation, seed germination, induction of flowering and seed setting. Spraying optimal concentrations of Gibberellins will initiate fruit setting without pollination and thus seedless fruits can be developed.

The third class namely the cytokinins induces cell division and delay the onset of senescence of the plant. Thus, for example green parts of the plant contain cytokinins in optimal amounts whereas ageing parts do not. Spraying plants with cytokinins, (Kinetin) will delay the yellowing of leaves and are useful for maintaining green lawns.

Ethylene is a gas in cells but being rather insoluble, it escapes by diffusion from the plant. Ethylene is produced at a rapid rate in dividing cells in the dark but in light, the production slows down allowing greater growth. Further, ethylene is involved in the process by which plants respond to gravity as well as to twine around objects. Ethylene is involved in fruit ripening whereby ripening is promoted by greater production of Ethylene. Inhibitors of ethylene can delay the ripening of fruits and so it is often added in packages of fruits being shipped.

The fifth class, namely abscissic acid previously known as abscissin or dormin plays important roles in maintaining the dormancy of seeds so that the seeds do not germinate at inappropriate times or within the fruits. Abscissic acid accumulates in the winter in the bud regions so that growth remains suspended and when ABA levels drop down during spring, the buds can be induced to grow. Water stress also leads to production of ABA and closure of stoma so that transpiration loss is controlled.

Although each of the above has a specific role in plant life cycle, controlled development of the plant is the coordinated effect of all these hormones. Thus, the ratio of Auxins to Cytokinins and the production of abscissic acid with concurrent absence of Auxins and cytokinins lead to dormancy.

Artificial Hormones: Since the structure of these major plant hormones is known, it has been possible to produce them in industrial quantities. For example, spraying of synthetic Auxins like 2, 4 Dichlorophenoxy acetic acid (2,4-D), Naphthalene acetic acid (NAA) etc will kill many plants because they enhance respiration and growth without regard to food and so plants die. Similarly, cytokinins are used to keep lawn grasses green. Gibberellins are used to induce flowering and produce seedless fruits. Similarly, ethylene gas in warehouses is used to induce controlled ripening of fruits or by flushing out ethylene from storage areas so that fruits and vegetables can be kept in un-ripened form during storage and transport.

Flowering: The flowering of plants is controlled by the phenomenon known as photoperiodism. This is defined as the flowering response of plants to relative lengths of dark and night periods to which they are exposed. All Angiosperms contain photosensitive chemicals known as phytochromes and cytochromes. These chemicals sense seasonal changes in light and dark periods during growth. Based on their responses, plants are broadly classified as short day plants, long day plants and day neutral plants. Although initially it was thought that, the length of daylight was the critical factor.

Long day plants flower in the Northern hemisphere during late spring or summer since days are longer and consequently shorter nights. Carnation *(Dianthus)*, Henbane *(Hyoscyamus)*, Oat (Avena), Pea (*Pisum sativum*), Barley (*Hordeum vulgare*), Lettuce (*Lactuca sativa*), and Wheat (*Triticum aestivum*) are examples.

Short-day plants flower when the night lengths exceed their critical photoperiod (long nights). They cannot flower under short nights or if a pulse of artificial light is shone on the plant for several minutes during the night. They require a continuous period of darkness before floral development can begin. Natural nighttime light, such as moonlight or lightning, is not of sufficient brightness or duration to interrupt flowering. Short-day plants generally flower after June 21 in the Northern hemisphere. Examples are Hemp (*Cannabis*), Cotton (Gossypium), Rice (Oriza sativa), and Mung bean (*Phaseolus mungo*).

Day-neutral plants are not affected by photoperiods but respond to temperature and developmental stage. Examples include tomato, green and hot peppers, cucumber, squash, pumpkin, various bean species.

Vernilization: This is a process whereby flowering of plants is promoted by exposure of the seeds and young plants to cold temperatures for a period. Thus, winter wheat, barley, oats and rye will flower and set seeds in spring only if the seeds were planted just before onset of winter so that the plants go through cold treatment. Seeds of such winter varieties will also flower if they are artificially exposed to a pre-determined cold temperature and then planted in spring. This process of the need for cold exposure appears to be an evolutionary trait in plants like wheat that originated in countries with very cold winters. This phenomenon was originally demonstrated by the Russian scientist T.D. Lysenko who deliberately exposed winter wheat to cold temperatures artificially and planted the seeds in spring. The process of Vernilization has now been shown to be applicable to many other plants that evolved in cold climes.

References

Hammer, K.C.; Bonner, J. (1938): "Photoperiodism in relation to hormones as factors in floral initiation and development" Botanical Gazette 100 (2): 388–431 Doi: 10.1086/334793, JSTOR 2471641

Hamner, K.C. (1940):"Interrelation of light and darkness in photoperiodic induction." Botanical Gazette 101 (3): 658–687. Doi: 10.1086/334903, JSTOR 2472399.

Mader, S.S. (1998): Biology, fifth edition, WCB/McGraw Hill Pp. 944

Mauseth, James D. (2003). Botany: An Introduction to Plant Biology (third Ed.), Sudbury, MA: Jones and Bartlett Learning, Pp, 422–427, ISBN 0-7637-2134-4

Peter H. Raven, P.H., (2013): Biology of Plants – 8th edition, W.H. Freeman ISBN13: 978-1429219617

Purves, W.K., Orians, G.H., & Heller, H.C. (1994): Life, the science of biology, Sunderland, Mass: Sinauer Associates.

Shain-dow Kung, Arntzen, C.J. (2014): In Plant Biotechnology – 2nd edition, Elsevier. ISBN13: 978-0199282616

Tippo, O. and Stern, W.L. (1977): Humanistic Botany, W.W. Norton and Company, New York, Pp 605

Chapter 3

Plants for Nutrition: Nutritional Components and Deficiency Diseases

Research has revealed that a substantial number of all deaths in the world irrespective of economic status of the countries are diet related. Apart from hunger, cancer, cardiovascular diseases, diabetes, digestive disorders, many kidney diseases, arthritis, neurological and other conditions all have a dietary/nutritional component. As per the American cancer society, "At present we have overwhelming evidence that none of the risk factors for cancer is…more significant than diet and nutrition." Plants are the ultimate source for food for all animals and humans. They provide carbohydrates, proteins, fats, vitamins and minerals needed for balanced healthy diet. The plants that provide nutrition can be broadly divided into cereals and pseudocereals, legumes, oil seeds, tubers, nuts, sugar, vegetables, fruits, beverage and spices and condiments.

The major Cereal plants are Rice, Wheat, Corn, Barley, Rye, Oats, Millets and Sorghum as well as the Pseudocereals namely Amaranth, Buckwheat, Chia and Quinoa and other not so common cereals and Pseudocereals. The cereals are the main source of carbohydrates but they also provide smaller amounts of protein, fiber, minerals and vitamins. The legumes represented by the various types of beans, lentils, peas, peanuts, soybeans, Vigna and other legumes often referred as pulses are the major sources of plant proteins in the diet. They also provide carbohydrates, fats, minerals, vitamins and other nutrients. Plant based fats are derived from canola, coconuts, corn, cotton, mustard, oil palm, peanuts, safflower, sesame, soybeans and sunflower. These plants also contain substantial amounts of protein and carbohydrates. Vegetables and fruits provide lower levels of energy from fats, carbohydrates and proteins but they supply dietary fiber, minerals and vitamins phytochemicals and anti-oxidants needed for a healthy body. Likewise, spices and condiments provide phytochemicals and add medicinal value to the foods being consumed.

Glycemic Index

The glycemic index (GI) of various seeds particularly of cereals is often used as a guide to develop nutritional foods for diabetics as well as those with health concerns. This is because; the GI indicates the foods effect on blood glucose level of the person eating the food. A value of 100 is assigned as the standard equivalent of pure glucose. Thus, the GI represents the total rise in blood sugar levels after a meal. A low-GI food will release glucose more slowly and steadily, which leads to more suitable postprandial (after meal) blood glucose readings. A high-GI food causes a more rapid rise in blood glucose levels and is suitable for energy recovery after exercise or for a person experiencing hypoglycemia. Foods with carbohydrates that break down quickly during digestion and release glucose rapidly into the bloodstream tend to have a high GI whereas, foods with carbohydrates that break down more slowly, releasing glucose more gradually into the bloodstream, tend to have a low GI.

Low GI of 55 or less are: Fructose (fruit sugar); beans (white, black, pink, kidney, lentil, soy), almond, peanut, walnut, chickpea; small seeds (sunflower, flax, pumpkin, poppy, sesame, hemp); most whole grains (durum/spelt wheat, millet, oat, rye, black/red rice, barley, quinoa, chia, amaranth); most vegetables, most fruits (peaches, strawberries, mangos); tomatoes; mushrooms; chillies.

Medium GI of 56–69 are: white sugar or sucrose, wheat flour, pita bread, basmati rice, unpeeled boiled potato, grape juice, raisins, prunes, pumpernickel bread, cranberry juice and banana.

High GI 70 and above are: glucose (dextrose, grape sugar), high fructose corn syrup, white bread, most white rice, corn flakes, extruded breakfast cereals, maltose, maltodextrins, sweet potato, white potato, pretzels and bagels.

A database showing the GI of different foods is maintained and updated by the University of Sydney, Australia. All foods tested as per strict standardized methods are certified and given a GI symbol with the GI number. However, these numbers are given for a particular food without taking into account the particular stage of the food. Thus, real GI for apple will depend on the ripeness of the fruit and so a standardized value may not apply correctly.

Further, a meal consumed by an individual is not composed only of carbohydrates but could include legumes, vegetables, meat, fats and other components and hence rather than just GI, the glycemic load (GL) of the meal should be considered. The glycemic load takes into account the total GI of the entire meal. Glycemic load of a serving of food can be calculated as its carbohydrate content measured in grams (g), multiplied by the food's GI, and divided by 100.

Both GI and GL are used in designing foods for lowering triglycerides, serum cholesterol and hence control of diabetes, adult macular degeneration and cardiovascular disease. The American diabetic association recommends the use of GI but also suggests that the use of GL is a better indicator for designing foods for Diabetic control.

Nutrition from Plants

Plants and animals and to a limited extent algae and fungi provide nutrition for growth and development. Plants and algae are autotrophic since they are able to convert and use CO_2, H_2O, and minerals using sun light to synthesize simple and complex carbohydrates, amino acids, proteins, fats, vitamins except B12, phytochemicals and other compounds. Animals depend on plants or other animals for their food. At the bottom level, bacteria are either saprophytic converting organic waste into food or are parasitic. Likewise, fungi are either saprophytic or parasitic. Therefore, whether a person is a vegetarian or is carnivorous, plants are the main source of food. Edible plant parts used as food contain macronutrients like carbohydrates, proteins and fats as well as micronutrients –vitamins, minerals and useful or even toxic phytochemicals. Thus, in general, cereals, pulses (legumes), root, and stem tubers are rich in carbohydrates, protein and in some cases fats. Legumes are the main providers of protein along with carbohydrates and oil plants are the main source of fats. Vegetables, fruits and nuts provide smaller amounts of the macronutrients along with vitamins and minerals as well as several phytochemicals. The individual food components in each plant food vary in quantity and quality. In the following paragraphs, brief descriptions of nutrients are given. Additionally, condensed descriptions of several common sources of food as well as uncommon and potential sources of plant based food and the plants that provide these foods are given.

Carbohydrates

Carbohydrates are molecules containing Carbon, hydrogen and oxygen conforming to the general formula $Cn (H_2O) n$. N (n) is a number based on whether it is a simple sugar like glucose (n = 6) or a disaccharide like sucrose or lactose (n = 12), a tri-saccharide (n = 18), a polysaccharide like starch, glycogen, cellulose (n = many) or a hetero-polysaccharide like many glycoproteins and glycolipids. The latter are molecules of carbohydrates linked to a non-carbohydrate like a protein or fat. Many storage proteins in legumes are glycoproteins. Likewise, glycolipids are molecules of sugar attached to lipid molecules and are components of cell membranes, nerve sheaths etc. Dietary fibers are also complex carbohydrates which are not digested but which are helpful and needed to promote the passage and emptying of the digested food.

Irrespective of structure, carbohydrates other than dietary fiber and cellulose are enzymatically cleaved to release glucose that is the final product for generating energy for growth, maintenance and functioning of the body.

The main source of carbohydrates is from plant sources. Simple sugars like glucose or disaccharides like sucrose provide immediate needs of the body but an excess of these can lead to diabetes, weight gain and resultant health issues. Even those foods that are rich in starch that is a polysaccharide are digested quickly. However, other complex carbohydrates are digested slowly releasing the glucose in a prolonged fashion and thereby providing energy as needed in a sustained fashion. Research data clearly show that foods rich in complex carbohydrates help to ward off cardiovascular disease. Complex carbohydrates are found in: 1. Legumes: Lentils, Chick peas, Split peas, Soy beans, Vicia type beans (cowpea) , Phaseolus beans (common bean, navy bean, black bean, mungo beans, black gram) Pigeon pea and many other legumes. 2. Nuts: almonds, Pistachio, Walnut etc., 3. Whole Grain Breads and Pastas: Breads and pastas made with the whole grains listed below provide more fiber resulting in feeling full sooner, and longer. They are: buckwheat, brown, red and black rice, corn, wheat, barley, oats, sorghum, millets, quinoa, amaranth, chia, 4. Fruits and Vegetables: tomatoes, onions, okra, carrots, yams, tapioca, strawberries, pea pods, vegetable beans, broccoli, spinach, leaf vegetables, green beans, zucchini, apples, pears, cucumbers, asparagus, grapefruit, dates, prunes and others.

Dietary fibers are carbohydrates that the body cannot digest. They pass through the body without being broken down into sugars. Even though the body does not get energy from fiber, fiber is still needed to stay healthy. Fiber helps get rid of excess fats in the intestine, which helps prevent heart disease. Fiber also helps push food through the intestines, which helps prevent constipation. Foods high in fiber include fruits, vegetables, beans, peas, nuts, seeds, and whole-grain foods (such as whole-wheat bread, oatmeal, and brown rice).

In general, it is advisable to limit carbohydrates that increase blood glucose levels. If blood glucose stays high for too long, one can develop type-2 diabetes. Potato starch and white rice are easily digested. However, they should find limited use since they can raise blood glucose levels quickly. Foods with a high glycemic index (white rice, potato starch, yams, and tubers) are not conducive to good health and low glycemic index foods such as whole grains, legumes, vegetables and certain fruits should be included in the diet.

Carbohydrate Deficiency

Hypoglycemia: Hypoglycemia is also known as low blood sugar or low blood glucose. It occurs when the glucose levels in the blood drop below normal. Hypoglycemia occurs when blood glucose level drops below 70 mg./dL. It can be caused by a lack of carbohydrates in healthy people. Symptoms of hypoglycemia are: shakiness, nervousness, or anxiety, sweating, chills and clamminess, irritability or impatience, confusion, including delirium, rapid/fast heartbeat, lightheadedness or dizziness, nausea, sleepiness, blurred/impaired vision, tingling or numbness in the lips or tongue, headaches, weakness or fatigue, anger, stubbornness, or sadness, lack of coordination, nightmares or crying out during sleep, seizures, unconsciousness, tiredness, weakness, confusion and hunger. Carbohydrates are the main source of glucose because they are broken down into simple sugars during digestion and enter the cells with the help of insulin, providing energy. Very often, many people have blood glucose readings below 70 mg/dL without feeling discernible symptoms. This is called hypoglycemia unawareness. People with hypoglycemia unawareness are also less likely to be awakened from sleep when hypoglycemia occurs at night. Hypoglycemia unawareness occurs more frequently in those who frequently have low blood glucose episodes that can cause you to stop sensing the early warning signs of hypoglycemia.

Ketosis

Ketosis is the name given when urine analysis shows excessive levels of ketones which result when the body turns to fats as a source of energy when eating less than 130 grams of carbohydrates a day. It breaks down stored fat, producing ketones. Mild ketosis can cause mental fatigue, bad breath, nausea and a headache, but severe ketosis can lead to painful swelling of the joints and kidney stones. Thus, it is important to maintain proper carbohydrate intake.

Weight Gain: People who are on severe non-physician based weight reduction programs by exempting carbohydrates may eventually go on a binge, eat more fats, and actually gain weight. As per the American diabetic association and the Mayo clinic, eating low calorie carbohydrates (fiber + complex carbohydrates) would help reduce weight rather than a total absence of carbohydrates from food. Thus, eating whole grain products and legumes are good choices for good health.

Protein

Proteins are made up of several essential amino acids attached to each other by peptide bonds. Proteins may be dipeptides with two amino acids, or tri peptides with three amino acids or oligopeptides and polypeptides with multiple amino acids. Di or tri peptides in humans are Carnosine, Anserine, Ophthalmic acid, Thyrotropin-releasing hormone (TRH)) and glutathione.

Oligo and polypeptides are abundant forms of protein found in all muscles, blood, lymph, skin and other body parts. Collagen and hemoglobin are major proteins in the body. Immunogobulins, all enzymes and membranes are proteins or have a protein moiety. Thus, the importance of protein for growth, development and optimal functioning cannot be overemphasized.

The main source of proteins for the human and animal body comes from animal or plant foods. In the case of plants, legumes, cereals, nuts, vegetables and fruits provide the essential requirements. However, plant proteins often lack or are poor in certain essential amino acids such as tryptophan, methionine, lysine and cysteine. Modern scientific methods have created lysine rich corn and other crops do contain sufficient amounts of most essential amino acids. Tryptophan is still an amino acid that is lacking in plant sources. However, this is overcome to some extent by consuming fermented plant proteins such as soy tofu, lentil and bean and supplementing with milk products.

Lack of protein in the diet can cause muscle soreness, weakness and cramping. Protein supports muscle growth and strength. Body fat is lost because protein provides structure for adipose tissues. The wasting away of muscle and fat tissue is known as cachexia.

Kwashiorkor – Kwashiorkor is a life-threatening and debilitating form of malnutrition. It is caused by a lack of protein in the diet. Kwashiorkor is commonly seen in low – and lower-middle-income regions facing famine. Kwashiorkor is easily treated with a change in diet and those who are treated early usually have a full recovery. Kwashiorkor can be prevented by eating a balanced diet with enough carbohydrates, fat, and protein. People suffering from kwashiorkor typically have an extremely emaciated appearance. They have liver that swell with fluid and hence have a swollen abdomen. In addition, they exhibit change in skin and hair color (to a rust color) and texture, fatigue, diarrhea, loss of muscle mass, failure to grow or gain weight, edema (swelling) of ankles, feet, and belly, damaged immune system, which can lead to more frequent and severe infections, irritability and flaky rash. Prevention is by taking adequate amounts of protein.

Edema: Edema causes fluid to accumulate in the tissues and cavities of the body. Edema most often affects the abdomen, hands, ankles and feet. Protein helps regulate and maintain a proper fluid and electrolyte balance within the body. Not getting enough dietary protein can affect the body's fluid and electrolyte balance, causing swelling and edema.

Skin and Nail Alterations: A lack of protein in the diet can cause changes in skin and nails. Protein enables cell regeneration, produces new cells and replaces dead ones. Therefore, if adequate amounts of protein are not consumed then, skin may become very light and burn easily when exposed to sunlight. Cracking, flaking, dryness and rashes of the skin are common. Delayed wound healing and ulcers are signs of low protein intake. Protein aids nail formation. Protein deficiency can cause white bands or brownish spots on the nails.

Hair Loss: Dry, sparse hair that falls out easily or changes color or texture is a sign of low protein intake. Hair contains 90 percent protein. Protein deficiency results in thinning hair or hair loss.

Infections: The immune system needs protein to protect the body and defend against foreign substances such as bacteria and viruses. The risk of infection increases with low and inadequate protein intake.

Gastrointestinal Distress: Low protein intake causes lethargy, fatigue, weakness, tiredness, headaches, nausea, diarrhea, soreness of the stomach and even fainting.

Fats, Fatty Acids and Lipids

Fats along with carbohydrates and protein form the building blocks for energy for growth and sustenance of the body. Fats are also commonly lumped as lipids, fatty acids and triglycerides. The following terms are used in describing various fats. They are saturated fat, unsaturated fat, monounsaturated fat, polyunsaturated fat, Trans fat and Omega fats numbering, ω–3, ω–6, ω–7, ω–9. Excess intake of all types of fatty acids in particular saturated fats will enhance the formation of adipose tissue and hence obesity.

Lipids: The term lipid includes fatty acids, triglycerides, sterols like cholesterol, vitamins A, D and E and various phospholipids found in the cell membranes.

Fatty acids: Fatty acids are molecules that are long chains of lipid-carboxylic acid found in fats and oils and in cell membranes as a component of phospholipids and glycolipids. Carboxylic acids are organic acids containing the functional group – COOH. Fatty acids come from animal and vegetable fats and oils. An essential fatty acid is a polyunsaturated fatty acid needed by the body that is synthesized by plants but not by the human body and is therefore a dietary requirement. Free fatty acids are by-products of the metabolism of fat in adipose tissues.

Saturated and unsaturated fats: Fats may be saturated or unsaturated. Saturated fats are hydrogenated at all sites possible and do not have double bonds between the carbon atoms. Thus, a fatty acid is classified as saturated when the bonds between carbon atoms are all single bonds. It is unsaturated when any of these bonds is a double bond. Saturated fats remain coagulated or solid at low temperatures and have to be melted by heat. Palm oil, coconut oil are rich in saturated fats, others contain smaller levels of saturated fats. Consumption of non-optimal (excess) of saturated fats can lead to arteriosclerosis and other cardiovascular issues as well as obesity.

Unsaturated fats may be mono unsaturated or polyunsaturated. Polyunsaturated fats are lipids in which the constituent hydrocarbon chain possesses two or more carbon–carbon double bonds, whereas monounsaturated fats contain one double bond and rest are single bonds. Polyunsaturated fats become rancid whereas monounsaturated are less likely to denature. All fatty acids have two ends, the carboxylic acid (-COOH) end, and the methyl (CH3) end. The way in which a fatty acid is named as omega – 3 or 6 or 9 is determined by the location of the first double bond, counted from the methyl end, that is, the omega (ω-) or the n – end.

Omega-3-fatty acids: These are polyunsaturated fats wherein there is a double bond at the third carbon atom. Alpha linoleic acid (ALA), eicosapentaenoic acid (EPA) and docosahexaenoic acid (DHA) are examples of omega 3 fatty acids. While ALA is found in plant sources of oil, EPA and DHA are available only from animal sources like fish oil. Omega – 3 ALA fatty acids are found in walnut, hazelnuts, pecans, sunflower oil, Canola oil, flaxseed oil, hemp oil, kiwifruit seed oil,

Chinese gooseberry and chia seed. Omega-3 fatty acids are important for normal metabolism. Since mammals are unable to synthesize omega-3 fatty acids, they have to obtain the shorter-chain omega-3 fatty acid ALA which have 18 carbons and 3 double bonds through diet and use it to form the more important long-chain omega-3 fatty acids, EPA with 20 carbons and 5 double bonds and then from EPA to DHA with 22 carbons and 6 double bonds. The ability to make the longer-chain omega-3 fatty acids from ALA may be impaired in aging.

Evidence suggests that omega-3 fatty acids modestly lower blood pressure in people with hypertension and in people with normal blood pressure. Some evidence suggests that people with certain circulatory problems, such as varicose veins, may benefit from the consumption of EPA and DHA, which may stimulate blood circulation and increase the breakdown of fibrin; a protein involved in blood clotting and scar formation. Omega-3 fatty acids reduce blood triglyceride levels. There is some evidence that consumption of omega 3 oils reduce rheumatoid arthritis and inflammation.

Omega-6-fatty acids: Omega-6 fatty acids (also referred to as ω-6 fatty acids or n-6 fatty acids) are a family of pro-inflammatory and anti-inflammatory polyunsaturated fatty acids that have carbon-carbon double bond in the n-6 position, that is, the sixth bond, counting from the methyl end. Some medical research suggests that excessive levels of certain omega–6 fatty acids relative to certain omega-3 fatty acids may increase the probability of a number of diseases. It is thought that a low ratio of Omega6: **Omega** 3 is conducive to good health whereas, an excess of Omega6 with low intakes of Omega 3 oils can promote bad health. Omega 6 oils are found in many plant sources: All nuts, cereals, wheat, avocado, canola oil, rapeseed oil, cottonseed, sunflower, pumpkin oil, corn oil, coconut oil and sesame oil.

Trans-fatty acids: Trans – fats are chemically and industrially derived unsaturated fats that have been converted into a saturated state by hydrogenation into the trans configuration from the normal cis configuration found in unsaturated fats. Thus, vegetable oils rich in cis configuration unsaturated fats are converted to trans configuration as in margarine, and for use in snack food industry and bakery products. Intake of trans fats cause increased risk of heart disease raises low-density lipoproteins and lowers the good high-density lipoproteins. It is important to know the trans-fat content of all edible oils used in cooking.

Omega – 9 – fatty acids: Omega 9 fatty acids are mono unsaturated fatty acids with a single double bond at the ninth carbon from the end. These are not essential fatty acids since they can be synthesized by the human body from other unsaturated fatty acids and hence are not essential from diet. This fatty acid is found in rape, mustard, canola, olive, sunflower, macadamia and other vegetable oils. Oleic acid from olives and other seeds mentioned above contain Omega 9 fatty acids in the ester form. Erucic acid found in members of the Brassicaceae (Mustard family) is also an omega 9 fatty acid. However, many studies have indicated that erucic acid could have adverse health repercussions for proper functioning of cardio vascular system if consumed at a high rate. Nevertheless, it must be pointed out that mustard oil which is rich in erucic acid is the main cooking oil used by large sections of the population in Indian sub-continent as well as in other regions of middle east and Asia and there is no clear evidence that these populations have higher incidence of cardiovascular disease.

Minerals

The human and animal bodies need many minerals for growth, development and function. These essential minerals are broadly divided into macro elements and microelements. The macro elements are Calcium, Magnesium, Phosphorus, Potassium, Sodium, Sulfur, nitrogen and Chlorine. The minor or trace dietary elements are Boron, Bromine, Cobalt, Chromium, Copper, Iodine, Iron, Manganese, Molybdenum and Zinc. The macro elements are required in larger doses since they are needed for body structure development and maintenance. For example, Calcium is needed for bone development and cardiovascular functions; Phosphorous is needed for synthesis of nucleotides/nucleic acids, phosphorylation reactions and many enzyme reactions. The microelements or trace elements are needed in smaller doses since they act as catalysts for various reactions or part of important functional molecules as in the case of iron in hemoglobin. The following reference terms define the various terms used by nutritionists:

(DRIs): Dietary Reference Intakes

EAR: (Estimated Average Requirement): the intake that meets the estimated nutrient need of 50 percent of the individuals in that group.

RDA: (Recommended Dietary Allowance): refers to the intake that meets the nutrient need of almost all (97 to 98 percent) individuals in that group.

AI: (Adequate Intake): observed or experimentally derived intake by a defined population or subgroup that, in the judgment of the DRI Committee, appears to sustain a defined nutritional state, such as normal circulating nutrient values, growth, or other functional indicators of health.

UL: the highest level of daily nutrient intake that is likely to pose no risk of adverse health effects to almost all individuals in the general population. As intake increases above the UL, the risk of adverse effects increases.

The following is a brief description of the role and function of various macro and microelements and best sources from plants for these elements.

Macro Elements

Calcium: Calcium is a major component of bones and teeth and is needed for functioning of muscles, heart and nerves. Inadequate calcium intake will lead to brittle bones and osteoporosis, rickets and tetany. Calcium is needed for muscle contractions and in functioning of the heart muscles. The recommended dietary allowance (RDA) is about 1000–1200mg per day. Although, dairy products are the best source for calcium, most seeds and vegetables supply substantial amounts of this mineral. The following are important plant sources: Blackberries, Blackcurrants, Dates, Grapefruit, Mulberries, Orange, Pomegranate, Prickly Pears, Amaranth leaves, Bok Choy, Brussels Sprouts, Butternut squash, Celery, Chinese Broccoli, French Beans, Kale, Okra, Parsnip, Swiss Chard, Turnip, Almonds, Brazil Nuts, Filberts/Hazelnuts, Pistachios, Sesame Seeds, Wheat – Durum, Wheat – Hard White, soya beans, Oats, Edamame, Navy Beans, White Beans, Winged Beans.

Chlorine: Chlorine is present mainly in table salt. Chlorine is necessary to ensure the regulation of water balance throughout the body. Chlorine stimulates the production of gastric acid and in turn helps to create hydrochloric acid needed for digestion. Since the exact RDA is not established, the AI is used to recommend intake. It is: 0 to 6 months old: 0.18 grams per day (g/day), 7 to 12 months old: 0.57 g/day, Children (AI), 1 to 3 years: 1.5 g/day, 4 to 8 years: 1.9 g/day, 9 to 13 years: 2.3 g/day; Adolescents and Adults (AI) Males and females, age 14 to 50: 2.3 g/day, Males and females, age 51 to 70: 2.0 g/day, Males and females, age 71 and over: 1.8 g/day and for

Pregnant and lactating females of all ages it is 2.3 g/day.

Magnesium: Magnesium is involved in maintaining heart rhythms, muscle function and immune reactions. Deficiency may result in fatigue, nervousness, insomnia, heart problems, high blood pressure, osteoporosis, muscle weakness and cramps. Magnesium is rich in Avocado, Banana, Blackberries, Blackcurrants, Breadfruit, Cherimoya, Dates, Guava, Kiwi, Loganberries, Mulberries, Passion Fruit, Pomegranate, Prickly Pear, Raspberries and Watermelon. Vegetable sources include Amaranth leaves, Artichoke, Butternut squash, French Beans, Lima Beans, Okra, Peas, and Swiss Chard. Nut/Grain sources are:: Almonds, Amaranth,

Brazil Nuts, Buckwheat, Cashews, Oats, Peanuts, Pine Nuts/Pignolias, Pumpkin Seeds, Quinoa, Rye, Wheat – Durum, Wheat – Hard Red, wheat – Hard White. Most legumes are a good source of Magnesium but these are the highest: Adzuki beans, Black beans, and Black Eye Peas.

Nitrogen: Nitrogen is required for the growth of plants. Nitrogen is part of free aminoacids as well as in proteins and is a component of nucleic acids and nucleotides and in lipids. The nitrogen is derived from the degradation of organic matter in soil as well as from nitrates, nitrites and ammoniacal compounds in soil. Further, many plants particularly legumes fix atmospheric nitrogen. All types of food contain nitrogen mostly in the form of protein and free aminoacids.

Phosphorus: Phosphorus is a part of the Nucleic acid molecules as well as nucleotides like ATP. It is needed for bone formation and development of strong teeth. RDA is about 2 grams. Avocados, Blackcurrants, Breadfruit, Dates, Guava, Kiwi, Lychee, Mulberries, Passion fruit, Pomegranate are sources of phosphorus from fruits. Vegetable Sources are: Amaranth leaves, Artichoke, Brussels Sprouts, Celery, Corn, French Beans, Lima Beans, Parsnip, Peas, Potatoes, Pumpkin and, Taro. Nut/Grain Sources include: Brazil Nuts, Buckwheat, Cashews, Oats, Pine, Nuts/Pignolias, Pumpkin Seeds, Quinoa, Rye, Spelt, Sunflower Seeds and wheat. Most legumes are good source of Phosphorous but the following have the highest amounts of phosphorus: Adzuki Beans, Black Beans, Black Eye Peas, Fava Beans, Edamame, Garbanzo Beans, Kidney Beans, Lima Beans, Navy Beans, Pigeon Beans, Pinto Beans, Soy Beans, White Beans and Winged Beans.

Potassium: Potassium is an essential electrolyte critical for heart, muscle and nerve functions. RDA is 4700 mg. Deficiency causes muscle cramps, irregular heartbeats. Fruit Sources: Avocado, Bananas, Blackcurrants, Breadfruit, Cherimoya, Cherries, Dates, Grapefruit, Guava, Kiwi, Lychee, Papaya, Passion fruit, Pomegranate, Prickly pear, Watermelon. Vegetable Sources: Amaranth leaves, Bamboo Shoots, Bok Choy, Butternut squash, French Beans, Lima Beans, Parsnips,

Potatoes, Pumpkin, Sweet Potatoes, Swiss Chard, Nut/Grain Sources: Almonds, Buckwheat, Chestnuts, Coconut, Oats, Pistachios, Pumpkin Seeds, Rye, Sunflower Seeds, Wheat – Durum, Wheat – Hard Red, Wheat – Hard White. Legume Sources: Most legumes are a great source of Potassium but, Adzuki Beans, Edamame, Kidney Beans, Lima Beans, Pinto Beans, Soy Beans and White Beans are major sources of potassium.

Sodium: Sodium is required by the body to regulate blood pressure and blood volume. It helps regulate the fluid balance in the body. Sodium also helps in the proper functioning of muscles and nerves. Excess sodium causes fluid retention and hypertension. Loss of Sodium due to excessive perspiration, urination can cause brain damage, dizziness, coma and death. The American Heart Association recommends a daily intake of no more than 1.5 g/day in order to maintain sodium requirement without causing hypertension. Fruit Sources: Sodium occurs naturally in almost all fresh, whole fruits but passion fruit has a significant amount. Vegetable Sources: Sodium occurs naturally in almost all fresh, whole vegetables, but, these have significant amounts: Amaranth leaves, Artichoke, Broccoli, Beetroot, Bok Choy, Brussels Sprouts, Celery, Fennel, Kale, Spaghetti squash, Sweet Potatoes, Swiss Chard. Nut/ Grain Sources: Most seeds, nuts and grains have some sodium, these have more than others do: Amaranth seeds, Coconut, Pumpkin Seeds, Quinoa, Spelt, legume Sources: Most legumes are not a good source of Sodium. Winged Beans have more than most other legumes.

Sulfur: Sulfur is a constituent of many enzymes and of aminoacids. It is present as amino acids in many vegetables, grains and nuts.

Trace Elements: These minerals are Needed in Very Small Amounts.

Boron: Boron is an essential trace element that protects against calcium loss by helping to maximize the activity of both estrogen and vitamin D in bone. Boron is present in apples, pears and grapes. Leafy greens, legumes and nuts are also good sources of this mineral.

Cobalt: Cobalt is an essential trace element for red blood cell formation that is a component of Cyanacobalamin (Vitamin B-12). Most authorities do not consider cobalt as a direct requirement but only as a part of vitamin B12. Cobalt is not directly absorbed by the intestine. Excess of cobalt can lead to enlarged heart.

Chromium: Chromium is considered an essential trace element involved in regulation of sugar metabolism. It is supplied as chromium picolinate for improving blood sugar control for people with pre-diabetic condition. It is found naturally in broccoli, whole grains and red grape juice.

Copper: Copper is involved in the absorption, storage and metabolism of iron and the formation of red blood cells. It also helps supply oxygen to the body. Copper is a cofactor or part of some enzymes. The symptoms of a copper deficiency are similar to iron-deficiency anemia. The RDA is 1.5 – 3.0 mg/day. Plant sources of copper are: Avocado, Blackberries, Dates, Guava, Kiwi Fruit, Lychee, Mango, Passionfruit, Pomegranate. Vegetable Sources: Lima Beans, Amaranth leaves, Artichoke, French Beans, Kale, Parsnip, Peas, Potatoes, Pumpkin, Spirulina, Squash – Winter, Sweet Potato, Swiss Chard, Taro, Nut/ Grain Sources: Brazil Nuts, Buckwheat, Cashews, Chestnuts, Filberts/ Hazelnuts, Oats, Sunflower Seeds, Walnuts, wheat. Legume Sources: Adzuki Beans, Black Beans, Black Eye Peas, Fava Beans, Edamame, Garbanzo Beans, Kidney Beans, Lima Beans, Navy Beans, Pigeon Beans, Pinto Beans, Soy Beans, Winged Beans.

Fluorine: Fluoride is useful in preventing dental cavities. There appears to be no metabolic role.

Iron: iron is a component of hemoglobin that transports oxygen to cells via blood. It is also needed for proper muscle function and some enzymatic reactions. The lack of Iron leads to anemia. The required daily allowance (RDA) ranges from 8 mg to 18 mg depending on sex and age.

Iodine: Iodine helps regulate the rate of energy production and body weight and promotes proper growth. It also promotes healthy hair, nails, skin and teeth. Iodine is needed for functioning of thyroid. Inadequate intake of iodine causes Goiter and thyroid malfunctioning resulting in hypothyroidism. RDA is 70 – 150 micrograms. Fruits, Vegetables, nuts and grains raised in soil that have iodine can supply the minimum requirements. Plant sources are: Avocado, Blackberries, Blackcurrant, Boysenberries, Breadfruit, Cherries, Dates, Figs, Grapes, Kiwi, Lemon, Loganberries, Lychee, Mulberries, Passion Fruit, Persimmon, Pomegranate, Raspberries, Strawberry, Watermelon, Vegetable Sources: Amaranth leaves, Bok Choy, Brussels Sprouts, Butternut squash, French Beans, Kale, Leeks, Lima Beans, Peas, Potatoes, Pumpkin, Swiss Chard, Nut/Grain Sources: Amaranth Buckwheat, Cashews, Coconut, Oats, Pine Nuts/Pignolias, Pumpkin Seeds, Rye, Spelt and Wheat.

Manganese: Manganese is an essential nutrient involved in many chemical processes in the body, including processing of cholesterol, carbohydrates, and protein. It might also be involved in bone formation. It is found in nuts, legumes, seeds, tea, whole grains, and leafy green vegetables. A maximum RDA of 11 mg is suggested. Excess Manganese could be toxic.

Molybdenum: This metal is required for activities of oxidases like xanthine oxidase, aldehyde oxidase, and sulfite oxidase. Higher concentrations result in molybdenum toxicity. There is no need to supplement this mineral since trace amounts are found in legumes, whole grains and nuts.

Selenium: Selenium is an anti-oxidant that helps maintain the immune system and regulate thyroid function. Deficiency of selenium causes Keshan disease that result in congestive cardiac myopathy. Reduced selenium levels have been noted in individuals diagnosed with Kashin-Bek disease also known as endemic osteoarthritis. RDA is 55 micrograms. Fruit Sources: Most fruits contain a small amount of selenium, but dates have a significant amount. Examples are

Bananas, Breadfruit, Guava, Lychee, Mango, Passion fruit, Pomegranate and Watermelon. Vegetable Sources: are Asparagus, Brussels Sprouts, French Beans, Lima Beans, Parsnip, and Peas. Most nuts and grains contain selenium, but the following have a significant amount, they are Amaranth, Barley, Brazil Nuts, Buckwheat, Cashews, Coconut, Rye, Wheat – Durum, Hard Red Wheat. Legume seeds are a good source of Selenium examples are Black Eye Peas, Fava Beans, Garbanzo Beans, Lima Beans, Mung Beans, Navy Beans, Pigeon Beans, Pinto Beans, Soy Beans, and Winged Beans.

Zinc: Zinc is needed for normal growth, regulation of appetite and reducing stress. Zinc nasal sprays control or prevent colds. Zinc is essential for certain enzyme activities. Severe deficiency can contribute to stunted growth. Deficiency can sometimes be seen in white spots on the fingernails. Fruit Sources: Most fruits contain a small amount of zinc. Vegetable Sources are: Leaf vegetables, Asparagus, Bamboo Shoots, Brussels Sprouts, Corn, Beans, Okra, Peas, Potatoes, Pumpkin, Swiss Chard. Nut/Grain Sources: Most nuts have some zinc, but these have a significant amount: Buckwheat, Cashews, Oats, Pine Nuts/Pignolias, Pumpkin Seeds, Rye, Sunflower Seeds, and Wheat – Durum, Wheat – Hard Red, Wheat – Hard White. Legume Sources: Most legumes are a good source of Zinc but these are the highest: Adzuki Beans, Black Beans, Black Eye Peas, Fava Beans, Edamame, Garbanzo Beans, Kidney Beans, Navy Beans, Soy Beans, Split Peas, White Beans, and Winged Beans.

Ultra Trace or Questionable Trace Elements

The necessity of these is not fully established but may be needed in ultra-trace amounts. These include Bromine, Lithium, Nickel, and Vanadium.

Vitamins

Vitamins are needed in order to carry out various metabolic functions in the body. They act as catalysts and co-factors for various enzymatic reactions. Inadequate intake of vitamins can lead to disease and poor health. Vitamins are classified into those that are fat-soluble and those that are water-soluble. Vitamins A, D and E are fat-soluble vitamins whereas; Vitamins of the B-complex group, vitamin C, Folic acid and B-12 are water-soluble vitamins. Brief descriptions of various vitamins and their potential role in health are given below.

Fat-Soluble Vitamins (Vitamins A, D, E and K)

Vitamin A: This fat-soluble vitamin is available in many animal fat sources such as fish oil. However, plants do not supply vitamin A but many plant foods contain beta-carotene that can be converted by the body into vitamin A. This vitamin is important for proper vision, bone and tissue growth, regulation of the immune system, preventing scaly skin, brittle nails and possibly in cancer prevention. Plant sources of carotene are: carrots, sweet potato, broccoli, spinach, mango, pumpkin, yellow zucchini, red/yellow/colored chili pepper, tomato, oatmeal, apricot, peach, peas, papaya and almost all colored leafy vegetables(most amaranths), all colored fruits and vegetables. Over eating of carotene-containing foods will result in yellowing of skin which will revert to normalcy upon reducing carotene to normal levels. Excess vitamin A causes hypervitaminosis A that causes blurred vision, drowsiness, irritability, sensitivity to light and many other symptoms.

Vitamin D: Vitamin D3 or cholecalciferol is the natural form of Vitamin D used by the body. The other form D2 (calciferol) may also be used. Vitamin D helps the body absorb calcium, a mineral that is responsible for the normal development and maintenance of healthy teeth and bones. This vitamin also helps maintain proper blood levels of calcium and phosphorus. Vitamin D is often called the sunshine vitamin because the body skin produces it after being exposed to ultraviolet rays from the sun. People with dark skin are often low in this vitamin from sunshine since the melanin acts as a shield against UV light from sunlight. Getting adequate amounts of vitamin D and calcium can prevent or slow osteoporosis and reduce bone fractures. A growing body of research also suggests that maintaining healthy levels of vitamin D may reduce the risk of developing muscle pain and weakness, autoimmune diseases, cardiovascular disease and certain cancers. Vitamin D is found in animal foods such as fish oils. Plant sources of Vitamin D are very few. However, Soybean Tofu, orange juice and fortified cereals and other foods can be the sources to meet minimum needs. Excess vitamin D causes hypervitaminosis D whose symptoms include dehydration, vomiting, constipation, calcium deposition in blood vessels, fatigue, irritability and depletion of vitamin K.

Vitamin E: Vitamin E (tocopheral) is an antioxidant that helps prevent oxidative stress, protects red blood cells, and may play a role in immune function, DNA repair and other metabolic functions. It has long been thought that diets rich in antioxidants, such as vitamin E, could help lower the risk of some cancers and other conditions, such as heart disease. However, recent studies suggest that vitamin E supplements do not provide the same health benefits as dietary sources do, and may even be harmful to health. In fact, some research indicates that vitamin E supplementation in high doses may increase the risk of heart failure or death. If vitamin E is taken with certain other supplements, it may slow the progression of early age-related macular degeneration. Nevertheless, it is best not to use vitamin E for this purpose until after discussion of the pros and cons, and safe dosages, with a physician. Hypervitaminosis E results from excess intake of vitamin E whose symptoms include increase in blood triglycerides, bleeding, blotchy skin and decreased thyroid activity.

Leafy vegetables like spinach, mustard greens, kale, seeds like Almonds, Sun flower seeds, fruits like Avacados, Olives, Rice and wheat germ oil, canola oil, corn oil, most veg oils, and certain vegetables like Broccoli are good sources.

Vitamin K: Vitamin K 1 and Vitamin K 2 play key roles in formation of blood clots so that bleeding can be stopped. Low levels of vitamin K can raise the risk of uncontrolled bleeding. Vitamin K1 is obtained from leafy greens and some other vegetables. Vitamin K2 is a group of compounds largely obtained from meats, cheeses, and eggs, or synthesized by bacteria in the gut.

Water-Soluble Vitamins

Vitamin B1: Vitamin B1 also known as Thiamin, or Thiamine, is an essential nutrient required by the body for maintaining cellular function and consequently a wide array of organ functions. Deficiency of vitamin B1 leads to wholesale degeneration of the body, particularly the nervous and circulatory systems, and eventually death. Further, deficiency of vitamin B1 can lead to development of beriberi and/or Wernicke-Korsakoff syndrome. Symptoms of both include severe fatigue, and degeneration of cardiovascular, nervous, muscular, and gastrointestinal systems. Over-consumption of vitamin B1 is unknown and studies show that amounts taken well in excess of the daily value (DV) can actually enhance brain functioning. Sunflower seeds, Macadamia and other nuts, Wheat bread, Peas, Acorn squash, Asparagus, Edamame (Soy), Navy beans, pink beans, Green gram and Black beans are good sources of vitamin B1.

Vitamin B2, or Riboflavin: This, is an essential vitamin required for proper energy metabolism and a wide variety of cellular processes. A deficiency of riboflavin can lead to cracking and reddening of the lips, inflammation of the mouth, mouth ulcers, sore throat, and even iron deficiency anemia. Riboflavin, is well regulated by the body, thus overdose is rare, and usually only occurs with vitamin B2 injections or supplements. Plant sources are Almonds, other nuts, Sesame seeds, and Sunflower seeds, Spinach, Beet Greens (24%), Asparagus (14%), Drumstick Leaves (13%), Collard Greens (12%), Dandelion Greens (11%), and Chinese Broccoli (8%).

Vitamin B-3 (Niacin): Niacin is one of the eight B complex vitamins that help the body to convert food to energy. It also helps improve blood circulation, cholesterol levels and regulate blood sugar. In high doses, niacin can reduce low-density lipoprotein (LDL, or "bad") cholesterol and triglycerides and raise high-density lipoprotein (HDL, or "good") cholesterol. Studies show niacin may also slow the development of atherosclerosis when used with other cholesterol lowering drugs, diet and exercise. However, in the doses needed for these effects (usually greater than 1,000 mg/day), niacin can cause liver damage. A deficiency of niacin leads to pellagra, a condition characterized by diarrhea, dermatitis, dementia, inflammation of the mouth, amnesia, delirium, and if left untreated, death. Even a slight deficiency of niacin can lead to irritability, poor concentration, anxiety, fatigue, restlessness, apathy, and depression. Overdose of niacin results in skin rashes, flushing, dry skin, various digestive maladies. A long-term overdose can lead to liver damage, elevated blood sugar levels and type II diabetes, as well as increased risk of birth defects. The following are good sources of this vitamin: Brown and red rice, whole wheat, barley, Peanuts, Peas, Sunflower seeds, Avacados and Tomatoes. A modified form of Niacin namely Nicotinamide riboside has been reported to delay the ageing process and is marketed by the supplements industry.

Vitamin B-5 or Pantothenic Acid: This is an essential vitamin required by the body for cellular processes and optimal maintenance of fat. A deficiency of vitamin B5 is rare. However, when it does occur it is usually in the form of irritability, fatigue, apathy, numbness, and muscle cramps. It can also lead to increased sensitivity to insulin, or hypoglycemia. Plant Sources of this vitamin are Avacados, Sunflower seeds, Flax seeds and Sweet potato

Vitamin B-6 (Pyridoxine): Vitamin B-6 is necessary for the proper maintenance of red blood cell metabolism, the nervous system, the immune system, and many other bodily functions. Serious deficiencies of vitamin B-6 are rare, but they can increase the level of homocysteine, and potentially boost the risk of heart disease and stroke. A deficiency in vitamin B-6 can lead to skin inflammation (dermatitis) depression, confusion, convulsions, and even anemia. Recent studies also suggest that a diet low in vitamin B6 increases risk of heart attack. High doses of vitamin B-6 have been touted as a treatment for carpal tunnel syndrome and premenstrual syndrome but studies have generally not supported the effectiveness of this treatment in relieving these conditions. In addition, large daily doses of the vitamin have been associated with neurological problems, such as numbness in the hands and feet (peripheral neuropathy), and skin lesions. Conversely, too much vitamin B6 taken from supplements can lead to nerve damage in the arms and legs. Sources from plants are Sunflower, Pistachio, dry Prunes, apricots, raisins, banana, spinach, and avocado.

Biotin or Vitamin B7: This vitamin was formerly known as Vitamin H or coenzyme R. Biotin is a co factor for the activity of many carboxylase enzymes involved in digestion and metabolism of fats and carbohydrates. The average requirement of this vitamin as per FDA is about 30 micrograms but the value as set by the European food safety authority ranges from 25–30 micro grams for children to an average of 40 micro grams for adults and for pregnant women. Many anecdotal reports suggest that biotin intake helps growth of nails and hair and as such, even though scientific evidence is not clear, biotin is added to many cosmetic preparations.

Vitamin B-9 (Folates/folic acid): Vitamin B-9, also called folate, is important in red blood cell formation and for healthy cell growth and function. It is also important for the developing fetus during pregnancy. Folic acid is the synthetic form of folate. Folic acid has been shown to work together with vitamins B-6 and B-12 to control elevated blood levels of homocysteine, which is associated with an increased risk of heart disease. However, there is no clear evidence that folic acid can prevent or treat heart disease. Studies do indicate that folate or folic acid can help prevent anemia during pregnancy and reduce the risk of neural tube defects, such as spina bifida. A deficiency of folate can lead to anemia in adults, and slower development in children. For pregnant women, folate is especially important for proper fetal development. There are also some reports that show that adequate intake of folic acid protects the body from developing colon cancers. Plants that are good sources are:

Black eyed peas, lentils, Spinach, Mung Beans, Pinto Beans, Chickpeas, Pink Beans, Lima Beans, Black Beans, Navy Beans, and Kidney Beans, Turnip Greens, Pak Choi (Chinese Cabbage), Savoy Cabbage, Collard Greens, Asparagus, Chinese Broccoli, Cauliflower, Lettuce, Endive, Butterhead, Salad Cress, Chicory, Pomegranate, Papaya, Guava, Kiwi, Banana, Mango and Oranges.

Vitamin B-12/Cyanacobalamin: Vitamin B-12 (Cobalamin) is the largest and most complex vitamin currently known to man. It plays essential roles in red blood cell formation, cell metabolism and nerve function. Plants cannot supply this vitamin but fermented plant foods like soy, fermented rice, fermented rice/pulse dough used to make rice dumplings contain this vitamin. Yogurt is also a good source for those who eat dairy products. For vegetarians, particularly those above the age of 50, supplementation of Vitamin B12 may be required. Likewise, supplementation is necessary for those who have had surgery of the duodenum/small intestine since these individuals cannot absorb this vitamin adequately. Vitamin B-12 deficiency can cause permanent nerve damage, resulting in numbness and tingling in the hands and feet, and balance problems. Deficiency can also cause anemia, depression, confusion, poor memory and dementia. Concerns have also been raised about the apparent link between low levels of B-12 and an increase in homocysteine, an amino acid that can cause problems within your coronary arteries. Vitamin B12 can be consumed in large doses because excess is excreted by the body or stored in the liver for use when supplies are scarce. Stores of B12 can last for up to a year.

Vitamin C (ascorbic acid): Vitamin C is an anti-oxidant, which maintains healthy tissue and helps the body absorb iron. Lack of vitamin C can cause a disease known as scurvy whose symptoms include poor gums, bleeding of skin, tiredness and formation of curly hair. This vitamin also plays a role in wound healing. Studies have shown that eating foods high in vitamin C can lower rates of cancer. All Citrus fruits, Sweet yellow, red and green peppers, Cayenne pepper, Guava, Kiwi fruit, Broccoli, Strawberries, tomatoes, papaya, most leaf vegetables particularly drumstick, Indian gooseberry and all fruits contain this vitamin.

Choline: Choline is listed sometimes as vitamin B3 but it is not currently listed as a vitamin but as a required nutrient. Choline is important for synthesis of cell membranes, the important neuro transmitter acetylcholine and for methylation reactions in the cell. Although animal foods like eggs, shrimp are the main suppliers of choline, plant sources include Asparagus, Brussel sprouts, Swiss Chard, cauliflower, spinach, beans, squash and many leafy vegetables.

Fiber

There are two types of fiber namely soluble fiber and insoluble fiber. Both types are carbohydrates obtained from plants. Fibers cannot be digested. Fiber not only helps bowel movements but also helps to lower cholesterol and regulate blood sugar. Foods rich in soluble fiber are oatmeal, grains, nuts, all bean types, most fruits and vegetables.

Insoluble fiber is found in skins and peels of fruits, vegetables and grain. It consists of cellulose and pectin. Insoluble fiber helps bowel movements through roughage and prevents indirect weight gain by reducing hunger pangs.

Other Nutrients

Lutein: Lutein is an important nutrient needed to maintain good eye health. It controls photophobia, cataract development and reduces macular degeneration. Lutein is found in leafy vegetables like Kale, carrots and other xanthophyll –carotenoid fruits and vegetables.

Zeaxanthan: This is another nutrient originally found in yellow corn (Zea mays), saffron, wolfberries, and green leafy vegetables including spinach, kale, and turnip and mustard greens. It is believed to control age related macular degeneration (AMD) although this claim has not been approved.

Table 1   Nutrient requirements for infants and children recorded as AI or as RDA (*)

NUTRIENT	Age	Age	Age	Age	NUTRIENT	Male, age	Male, age	Female, age	Female, age
	0-6 mths	7-12mths	1-3 yrs	4-8 yrs		9-13 Yrs	14-18 Yrs	9-13 Yrs	14-18 Yrs
vitamin A – retinol	400* µg	500* µg	300 µg	400 µg	vitamin A – retinol	600 µg	900 µg	600 µg	700 µg
vitamin C – ascorbic acid	40* mg	50* mg	15 mg	25 mg	vitamin C – ascorbic acid	45 mg	75 mg	45 mg	65 mg
vitamin D #1	5* µg	5* µg	5* µg	5* µg	vitamin D #1	5* µg	5* µg	5* µg	5* µg
vitamin E	4* mg	5* mg	6 mg	7 mg	vitamin E	11 mg	15 mg	11 mg	15 mg
vitamin K	2.0* µg	2.5* µg	30* µg	55* µg	vitamin K	60* µg	75* µg	60* µg	75* µg
vitamin B1 – thiamin	0.2* mg	0.3* mg	0.5 mg	0.6 mg	vitamin B1 – thiamin	0.9 mg	1.2 mg	0.9 mg	1.0 mg
vitamin B2 – riboflavin	0.3* mg	0.4* mg	0.5 mg	0.6 mg	vitamin B2 – riboflavin	0.9 mg	1.3 mg	0.9 mg	1.0 mg
vitamin B3 – niacin	2* mg	4* mg	6 mg	8 mg	vitamin B3 – niacin	12 mg	16 mg	12 mg	14 mg
vitamin B5 – pantothenic acid	1.7* mg	1.8* mg	2* mg	3* mg	vitamin B5 – pantothenic acid	4* mg	5* mg	4* mg	5* mg
vitamin B6 – pyridoxine	0.1* mg	0.3* mg	0.5 mg	0.6 mg	vitamin B6 – pyridoxine	1.0 mg	1.3 mg	1.0 mg	1.2 mg
vitamin B12 – Cyanacobalamin	0.4* µg	0.5* µg	0.9 µg	1.2 µg	vitamin B12 – Cyanacobalamin	1.8 µg	2.4 µg	1.8 µg	2.4 µg
biotin	5* µg	6* µg	8* µg	12* µg	biotin	20* µg	25* µg	20* µg	25* µg
choline	125* mg	150* mg	200* mg	250* mg	choline	375* mg	550* mg	375* mg	400* mg
folate – folic acid	65* µg	80* µg	150 µg	200 µg	folate – folic acid #3	300 µg	400 µg	300 µg	400 µg

Recommended Daily Allowances for Minerals

calcium	210* mg	270* mg	500* mg	800* mg
chromium	0.2* µg	5.5* µg	11* µg	15* µg
copper	200* µg	220* µg	340 µg	440 µg
fluoride	>0.01* mg	0.5* mg	0.7* mg	1* mg
iodine	110* µg	130* µg	90 µg	90 µg
iron	0.27* mg	11 mg	7 mg	10 mg
magnesium	30* mg	75* mg	80 mg	130 mg
manganese	0.003* mg	0.6* mg	1.2* mg	1.5* mg
molybdenum	2* µg	3* µg	17 µg	22 µg
phosphorus	100* mg	275* mg	460 mg	500 mg
selenium	15* µg	20* µg	20 µg	30 µg
zinc	2* mg	3 mg	3 mg	5 mg
potassium	0.4* g	0.7* g	3.0* g	3.8* g
sodium	0.12* g	0.37* g	1.0* g	1.2* g
chloride	0.18* g	0.57* g	1.5* g	1.9* g

Recommended Daily Allowances for Minerals

calcium	1300* mg	1300* mg	1300* mg	1300* mg
chromium	25* µg	35* µg	21* µg	24* µg
copper	700 µg	890 µg	700 µg	890 µg
fluoride	2* mg	3* mg	2* mg	3* mg
iodine	120 µg	150 µg	120 µg	150 µg
iron	8 mg	11 mg	8 mg	15 mg
magnesium	240 mg	410 mg	240 mg	360 mg
manganese	1.9* mg	2.2* mg	1.6* mg	1.6* mg
molybdenum	34 µg	43 µg	34 µg	43 µg
phosphorus	1250 mg	1250 mg	1250 mg	1250 mg
selenium	40 µg	55 µg	40 µg	55 µg
zinc	8 mg	11 mg	8 mg	9 mg
potassium	4.5* g	4.7* g	4.5* g	4.7* g
sodium	1.5* g	1.5* g	1.5* g	1.5* g
chloride	2.3* g	2.3* g	2.3* g	2.3* g

Over Dosing

Most processed foods and even processed water contain vitamins and as such, additional supplementation of minerals and vitamins can cause some health issues. These mild symptoms may include difficulty sleeping or concentrating, nerve problems such as numbness or tingling, or feeling more irritable.

Table 2 Nutrient requirements for adults and pregnant women recorded as AI or as RDA (*).

RDA Chart NUTRIENT	Male 19-50 Yrs	Male >50 Yrs	Female 19-50 Yrs	Female >50 Yrs	Pregnancy 14-18 Yrs	Pregnancy 19-50 Yrs	Lactation 14-18 Yrs	Lactation 19-50 Yrs
RDA Vitamins (Per Day)								
vitamin A -	900 μg	900 μg	700 μg	700 μg	750 μg	770 μg	1200 μg	1300 μg
vitamin C -	90 mg	90 mg	75 mg	75 mg	80 mg	85 mg	115 mg	120 mg
vitamin D	5* μg	10* μg	5* μg	10* μg	5* μg	5* μg	5* μg	5* μg
vitamin E	15 mg	15 mg	15 mg	15 mg	15 mg	15 mg	19 mg	19 mg
vitamin K	120* μg	120* μg	90* μg	90* μg	75* μg	90* μg	75* μg	90* μg
vitamin B1	1.2 mg	1.2 mg	1.1mg	1.1 mg	1.4 mg	1.4 mg	1.4 mg	1.4 mg
vitamin B2	1.3 mg	1.3 mg	1.1 mg	1.1 mg	1.4 mg	1.4 mg	1.6 mg	1.6 mg
vitamin B3	16 mg	16 mg	14 mg	14 mg	18 mg	18 mg	17 mg	17 mg
vitamin B5	5* mg	5* mg	5* mg	5* mg	6* mg	6* mg	7* mg	7* mg
vitamin B6	1.3 mg	1.7 mg	1.3 mg	1.5 mg	1.9 mg	1.9 mg	2.0 mg	2.0 mg
vitamin B1	2.4 μg	2.4 μg	2.4 μg	2.4 μg	2.6 μg	2.6 μg	2.8 μg	2.8 μg
biotin	30* μg	30* μg	30* μg	30* μg	30* μg	30* μg	35* μg	35* μg
choline	550* mg	550* mg	425* mg	425* mg	450* mg	450* mg	550* mg	550* mg
folate – fo	400 μg	400 μg	400 μg	400 μg	600 μg	600 μg	500 μg	500 μg
Recommended Daily Allowances for Minerals								
calcium	1000* mg	1200* mg	1000* mg	1200* mg	1300* mg	1000* mg	1300* mg	1000* mg
chromium	35* μg	30* μg	25* μg	20* μg	29* μg	30* μg	44* μg	45* μg
copper	900 μg	900 μg	900 μg	900 μg	1000 μg	1000 μg	1300 μg	1300 μg
fluoride	4* mg	4* mg	3* mg	3* mg	3* mg	3* mg	3* mg	3* mg
iodine	150 μg	150 μg	150 μg	150 μg	220 μg	220 μg	290 μg	290 μg
iron	8 mg	8 mg	18 mg	8 mg	27 mg	27 mg	10 mg	9 mg
magnesiur	400/420 m	420 mg	310/320 m	320 mg	400 mg	350/360 m	360 mg	310/320 mg
manganes	2.3* mg	2.3* mg	1.8* mg	1.8* mg	2.0* mg	2.0* mg	2.6* mg	2.6* mg
molybden	45 μg	45 μg	45 μg	45 μg	50 μg	50 μg	50 μg	50 μg
phosphoru	700 mg	700 mg	700 mg	700 mg	1250 mg	700 mg	1250 mg	700 mg
selenium	55 μg	55 μg	55 μg	55 μg	60 μg	60 μg	70 μg	70 μg
zinc	11 mg	11 mg	8 mg	8 mg	12 mg	11 mg	13 mg	12 mg
potassium	4.7* g	4.7* g	4.7* g	4.7* g	4.7* g	4.7* g	5.1* g	5.1* g
sodium #5	1.5* g	1.3* g	1.5* g	1.3* g	1.5* g	1.5* g	1.5* g	1.5* g
chloride #	2.3* g	2.0* g	2.3* g	2.0* g	2.3* g	2.3* g	2.3* g	2.3* g

References

Atkinson, F.S, Foster-Powell K, and Brand-Miller, J.C (2008): "International tables of glycemic index and glycemic load values: 2008." Diabetes Care 31 (12): 2281–3. Doi: 10.2337/dc08–1239, PMC 2584181, PMID 18835944.

Basu, T.K. (1996): Vitamins in human health and disease, Wallingford, Eng., CAB International, 1996, 345 p.

Bays, H.E. (2007): Safety considerations with omega-3 Fatty Acid therapy, Am J Cardiol., 2007, 99(6A): S35–43.

Belluzzi A, Boschi S, Brignola C, Munarini A, Cariani C, Miglio F. (2000): Polyunsaturated fatty acids and inflammatory bowel disease, Am J. Clin Nutr. 2000; 71(suppl): 339S-342S.

Berbert, A.A, Kondo, C.R, Almendra, C.L et al. (2005): Supplementation of fish oil and olive oil in patients with rheumatoid arthritis, Nutrition, 2005; 21: 131–6.

Berson, E.L, Rosner B, Sandberg, M.A, et al. (2004): Clinical trial of docosahexaenoic acid in patients with retinitis pigmentosa receiving vitamin A treatment, Arch Ophthalmol. 122(9): 1297–1305.

Boelsma E, Hendriks H.F. Roza L. (2001): Nutritional skin care: health effects of micronutrients and fatty acids, Am J. Clin Nutr. 2001, 73(5): 853-864.

Brouns F, Bjorck I, Frayn K.N., et al. (June 2005): "Glycaemic index methodology." Nutr Res Rev 18 (1): 145–71. Doi: 10.1079/NRR2005100, PMID 19079901

Combs, G.F. (1998): The vitamins: fundamental aspects in nutrition and health, 2nd ed. San Diego, Academic Press, c1998, 618 pages

Dietary Guidelines for Americans, (2010): U.S. Department of Health and Human Services http://www.cnpp.usda.gov/

Duff, R.L. (2012): American Dietetic Association Complete Food and Nutrition Guide 4th ed. Hoboken, N.J.: John Wiley & Sons, 2012: 55

Eastwood, M. (2013): Principles of Human Nutrition, John Wiley & Sons, Jun 5, 2013 – Medical – 704 pages

Encyclopedia of human nutrition: 2nd ed. Edited by Michele Sadler. v. 3 San Diego, Academic Press, 1999. 1973p.

Freund-Levi Y, Hjorth E, Lindberg C, Cederholm T, Faxen-Irving G, Vedin I, Palmblad J, Wahlund LO, Schultzberg M, and Basun H, Eriksdotter Jönhagen M. (2009): Effects of omega-3 fatty acids on inflammatory markers in cerebrospinal fluid and plasma in Alzheimer's disease: the OmegAD study. Dement Geriatr Cogn Disord. 2009, 27(5): 481–90.

Geerling, B.J, Badart-Smook, A, van Deursen, C, et al. (2000): Nutritional supplementation with N-3 fatty acids and antioxidants in patient's iwth Crohn's disease in remission: effects on antioxidant status and fatty acid profile. Inflamm Bowel Dis. 2000, 6(2): 77–84.

Goldman, I.L. (2003). Recognition of fruits and vegetables as healthful: vitamins and phytonutrients, HortTechnology 13: 1–6 PDF

Goldman, I.L. (2003). Back to the future of food: phytonutrients and quality in vegetable crops for the 21st century, Acta Horticulturae. 637: 353–360.

Goldman, I.L. (2014). The Future of Breeding Fruit and Vegetables with Human Health Functionality: Realities, Challenges, and Opportunities HortScience49: 133–137.

http://www.canolacouncil.org/oil-and-meal/what-is-canola/the-history-of-canola/

http://www.glycemicindex.com/

http://www.loc.gov/rr/scitech/SciRefGuides/veganism.html

http://www.loc.gov/rr/scitech/selected-internet/molecular.html

http://www.loc.gov/rr/scitech/tracer-bullets/vitaminstb.html

http://www.soyatech.com/canola_facts.htm

http://www.the-gi-diet.org/glycemicindexchart/

Institute of Medicine, (1997): Dietary Reference Intakes for Calcium, Phosphorous, Magnesium, Vitamin D, and Fluoride Washington DC: National Academy Press

Institute of Medicine, (1998): Dietary Reference Intakes for Thiamin, Riboflavin, Niacin, Vitamin B6, Folate, Vitamin B12, Pantothenic Acid, Biotin, and Choline. Washington, DC: National Academy Press.

Institute of Medicine, (2000): Dietary Reference Intakes for Vitamin C, Vitamin E, Selenium, and Carotenoids, Washington, DC: National Academy Press.

Institute of Medicine, (2001): Dietary Reference Intakes for Vitamin A, Vitamin K, Arsenic, Boron, Chromium, Copper, Iodine, Iron, Manganese, Molybdenum, Nickel, Silicon, Vanadium, and Zinc, Washington, DC: National Academy Press.

Institute of Medicine, Food and Nutrition Board (2005): Dietary Reference Intakes for Water, Potassium, Sodium, Chloride, and Sulfate, National Academy Press, Washington, DC: 2005, PMID: 101209392, www.ncbi.nlm.nih.gov/nlmcatalog/101209392.

Jenkins D, J, Kendall C, W, and McKeown-Eyssen G, et al. (2008): "Effect of a low-glycemic index or a high-cereal fiber diet on type 2 diabetes: a randomized trial." JAMA 300 (23): 2742–53.

Jing K, Wu T, Lim K. (2013): Omega-3 polyunsaturated fatty acids and cancer. Anticancer Agents Med Chem. 2013, 13(8): 1162–77.

Magness, J.R., G.M. Markle, C.C. Compton, (1971): Food and feed crops of the United States, Interregional Research Project IR-4, IR Bul. 1 (Bul. 828 New Jersey Agr. Expt. Sta.)

Nelson, David. L.; Michael M. Cox (2000–02–15): Lehninger Principles of Biochemistry, Third Edition (3 Har/Com Ed.), W.H. Freeman, p. 1200, ISBN 1-57259-931-6

Nielsen, F.H. (1999): Ultra traces minerals. *In* Modern nutrition in health and disease/editors, Maurice E.S. *et al.*, Baltimore: Williams & Wilkins, p. 283-303

Vaclav, V., Pimentel, M.H., Devine, M.M., 2013: Dimensions of Food: Edition 4, Springer Science & Business Media, 279 pages

World Health Organization: Vitamin and Mineral Requirements in Human Nutrition, World Health Organization, Health and Fitness, Pp 341

Chapter 4

The Cereals – Botanical Descriptions Nutritional Profile and Health Relatedness

Rice – Oriza Sativa

Botany: Kingdom: Plantae Division: Angiospermae; Class: Monocotyledonae; Order: Poales; Family: Poaceae/graminae, Genus and Species: *Oriza sativa* (Asian rice), *O.glabrrema* (African rice). Chromosome Number: 2n = 24.

Rice is ranked as the number 1 cereal based on usage. There are more than 10,000 varieties of rice and about 60% are found in India. Asian rice *Oriza sativa* and African rice *O. glaberrema* are the only two currently cultivated species. Both species may have originated from a wild species *O.longistaminata/O.perennis*.

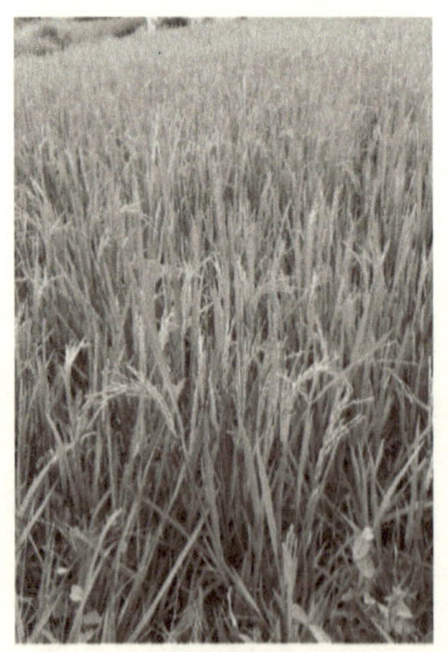

Rice plants

Rice is a cereal belonging to the grass group of Monocotyledonae. The plant is raised in semi-submerged conditions known as paddy in South East Asia and or grown in irrigated land (Lowland rice) and in dryland (upland rice). Currently, rice is also grown with minimal usage of water using underground drip irrigation. Rice plants are able to germinate and grow well under submerged conditions because of their special anatomy wherein, special types of thin walled parenchyma cells known as aerenchyma can transport and hold oxygen from the aerial parts of the plant to the submerged root system. Additionally, they have some negatively geotropic roots that grow on the soil-water inter-surface that allows oxygen supply to the roots.

Oriza sativa or rice consists essentially of three basic types namely the long grained indica varieties, the short grain sticky glutinous japonica varieties and the intermediate sized Javanica/tropical japonica varieties. The indica group comprises all of the cultivated forms of tropical regions of India, Indochina, the Philippines and Southern China while the japonica group includes the cultivated rice varieties of the subtropical regions of Japan and Korea and the intermediate Javanese in Indonesia. However, now, all three varieties are grown in the different rice growing regions based on local needs. The sticky types contain amylopectin as the starch whereas the non-sticky rice contains amylin starch. There are many sub varieties within each group. The rice grain comes in many colors such as white rice, brown rice, red rice, purple rice, golden rice and black rice/forbidden rice. Golden rice is genetically modified rice (GMO) containing high levels of carotene that is a precursor for vitamin A synthesis. It was developed as a means of helping to control blindness in poorer parts of the world.

African rice (*O.glaberrima*) had its origin in West Africa. The quality of the rice is not as good as that of Asian rice and the yield is also poorer. However, African rice has been largely replaced by Asian varieties in Africa and new varieties derived by crossing the African and Asian species have been developed for growth suitability in African environments.

Both Asian and African rice plants are monocots and are annual herbaceous grass plants. The rice plant grows to a height of 3–6 ft, depending on the variety and soil fertility. Plants have long, slender light green to dark green leaves. Flowers are produced in branched pendulous inflorescence. The flowers are wind pollinated. The grains known as caryopsis are produced after pollination. These grains may be long, short or of intermediate size.

The rice grain is covered by the silicified hull/chaff which is not edible but which is used to produce building materials and carbonized for use as tooth powder and as activated carbon in industry. The hull covers the edible rice grain with an outer layer called the bran that contains rice bran oil, antioxidants, vitamins and protein. When the bran is removed, the result is white rice. The embryo also known as germ is embedded in the endosperm. Therefore, depending on the variety, the grain with bran gives the specific color mentioned above.

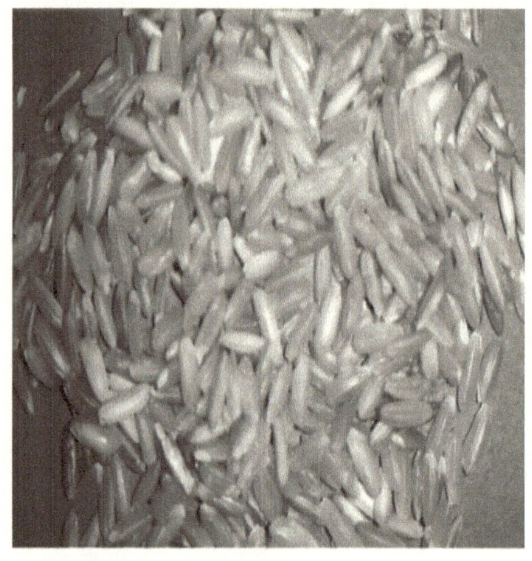

Brown

Brown Rice: This is unpolished rice grain containing the husk/bran after removing the chaff. It is rich in vitamins of the B group, minerals, protein and fats.

White Rice: This is rice after the hull and bran is removed. Most of the nutrients except starch and small amounts of protein are removed in white rice and is the most commonly consumed form of rice.

Parboiled Rice: The entire grain with hull/chaff is steeped in water and steamed prior to removal of both the nonedible hull and edible bran/husk. Essentially, it is like white rice except that the process of steaming allows some of the nutrients to enter the endosperm and so is somewhat more nutritious than white rice.

Red and Black Rice: These are varieties of rice with either a red colored or black colored outer husk/bran and thus very rich in nutrients such as anthocyanin and antioxidants. Black rice in particular is said to be as rich as Blueberries in their antioxidant content.

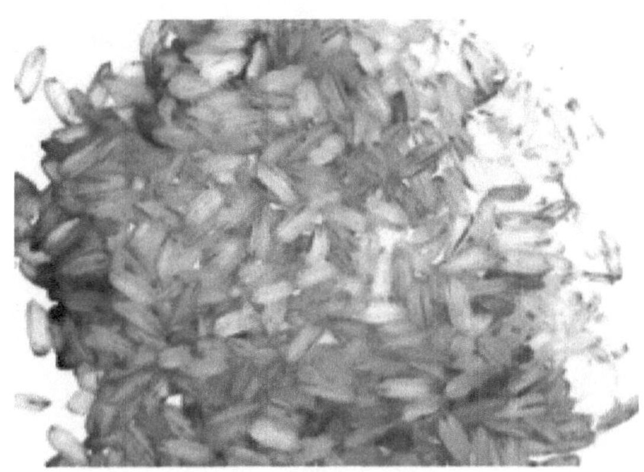

Red

Golden Rice: This is genetically modified GM rice created to enrich the rice grain with carotene a pre-curser of Vitamin A. Rice per se does not have this vitamin. The purpose of developing this rice variety was to help fight blindness caused due to Vitamin A deficiency in poorer countries where the people may not have access to vitamin enriched rice or vitamin supplements.

Wild Rice: This is not true Asian rice *Oriza sativa* but obtained from the grass plant species *Zizania palustris* (Northern/Canadian

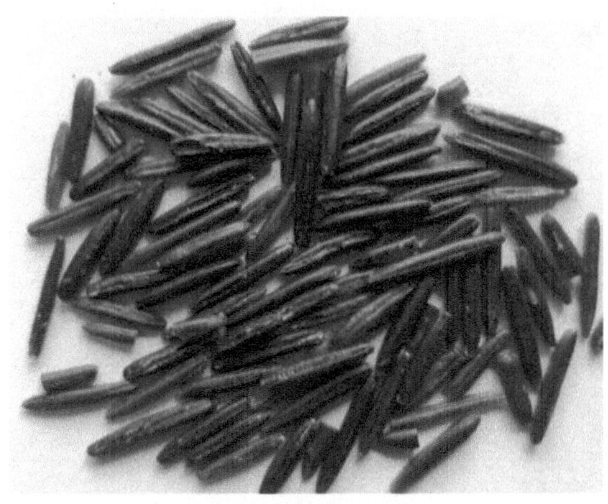

Wild

wild rice), *Z. latifolia* (Manchurian wild rice), *Z.texana* (Texas wild rice), *Z.aquatica* (Wetland Wild rice). The rice grain that is grey/black in color is rich in protein, dietary fiber and B vitamins. It was a staple food among American Indians but is now cultivated and consumed by the public in North America as an exotic health food. It has about the same amount of protein as wheat and is rich in the amino acid lysine. It has no gluten and is rich in dietary fiber.

Rice varieties: There are many different varieties of rice that may be long grained, intermediate sized or short grained or also aromatic as in Jasmine rice and Basmathi. Likewise, there are many varieties of pigmented red and black rice. Rice is now grown in many countries that are both producers and consumers of rice. The table below is a short list of some of the different popular varieties of rice. This list is incomplete. Several other varieties are popular in different rice consumption regions.

Rice Variety	Type	Character
Akitamochi	Short,	Glutinous, good for Sushi,
Ambemohar	Short, japonica	Sticky, India
Arborio	Short, japonica	Round, creamy, Amylopectin, Italy
Aromatic	Medium-long, indica	Aromatic,
Basmati	Long/slender	Non-sticky, amylose, low glycemic index,
Bhutanese red	Medium grain, Japonica	Flavanoids, Bhutan
Black rice	Medium grain, tropical japonica	Anthocyanin/Flavanoids, Longevity,
Bora Saul	Short,	Glutinous, India
Calrose rice	Medium grain	Soft sticky rice, good for Sushi, USA
Camarague red	Red rice, medium grain	Wet land rice, France
Carnaroli	Medium grain,	higher amylose, Risotto, Italy
Champa	Medium grain Indica-Javanica	Non-sticky, South Asia, China
Dubraj	Short-Medium	Amylose, aromatic, India
Glutinous rice	Short, Indica, Japonica and Javanica	Amylopectin, very sticky/waxy, S. Asia
Golden rice	GM rice	High Beta carotene, genetically modified

Japanese rice	Short grain	Translucent, sticky, Japan
Jasmati	Long, hybrid of Basmati and Jasmine	Aromatic, soft and nutty, India
Jasmine/Fragrant	Long grain	Aromatic, slightly sticky, South East Asia
Joha rice	Long grain	Aromatic, Assam-India
Koshihikari	Short, Sticky	Translucent, good for Sushi, Japan
Maratelli	Intermediate semi-fine	High Amylose, less sticky, Italy
Matta rice	Kerala red, Rosematta, Palakkadan	Coarse red rice, carotene, India, Sri Lanka
Molakolukulu	Nellore rice, Long grain	Non-aromatic, India,
Mottaikaruppan	Red-Matta rice, medium grain	Red, Sri Lanka, South India
Rice Variety	**Type**	**Character**
Nàng Thơm Cho	Vietnamese fragrant rice	Aromatic, Viet Nam
Navara	medium grain	Ayurvedic Medicinal massage, India
Nishiki rice	Medium grain	Soft sticky, used for brewing Sake, Japan
Patna rice	Very long grain Non sticky white rice	High amylose, mild aroma, India
Perennial rice	various varieties	Upland/irrigated perennial rice,
Pokkali	Large grains	Salinity resistant rice, high protein, India
Ponni Rice	Opaque, long grain, mild aroma	Par boiled and raw white rice, India

Pusa 1121	Longest rice known	Mild aroma, non-sticky, India
Red rice	many different varieties	High Anthocyanin content
Rakthashali	Type of red rice	Ayurvedic medicinal, India
Red Cargo	Long grain red rice with bran	Non-glutinous, unpolished red rice,
Samba	Small ovular grain, sub varieties, red	not fluffy when cooked, India, Sri Lanka
Sona Masuri	Medium grain	lightweight, aromatic, India
Tulaipanji	Medium long aromatic	Non-Basmati, Bangladesh/India
Vialone Nano	Medium, Japonica	Medium sticky, Risotto rice, Italy
Wehani	Aromatic brown	Aroma similar to peanuts, USA
Yamada Nishiki	Medium, japonica	Used for making Sake, Japan

Medicinal properties: Rice bran oil is rich in monounsaturated and polyunsaturated oils and contains gamma oryzanol, phytosterols and vitamin E. Tests show that consumption of this oil reduces cholesterol and may help in reducing hot flashes and may even have anticancer properties. Apart from starch, polished white rice has no rice bran oil. Apart from its nutritional value, rice flour is used as a poultice. The water obtained during cooking is used to treat dehydration and diahorrea. The Navarra variety known as medicinal rice is mainly raised in kerala, India, and is especially considered useful for treating gastrointestinal disease, for healing ulcers and colitis, peripheral cardiovascular circulation and rheumatoid arthritis. In the main, Navarra is cooked and steeped in milk, oil along with various herbals and the steeped rice bundled in cheese, or homespun cloth is massaged onto affected areas for rheumatic pain and improvement in peripheral circulation. Navarra rice cooked in milk along with special herbs is prescribed by Ayurvedic physicians for protein deficiency, improvement in general health and sexual problems. Some of the prominent medicinal rice varieties include Karibatha, Kalame, Karikalave, Doddabaira nellu, Kari Gajivili and Sannakki that are all grown in southern India. Karibatha is used to cure herpes while Karikalave is usually served to lactating mothers due to its high calcium content. Kalame is used to treat piles while Sannakki, grown in North Karnataka, India, is used to treat diarrhoea in children. Dodda Baira Nellu is also popular for its curative values for various diseases. Another rice variety, The 'Dia anna' ('rice for diabetics'), is an indigenous rice variety from Nagarkoil in Tamil Nadu, India, is rich in fiber, minerals and Vitamin B and E. Originally known as 'Thuruvai Kalangi,' this fiber-rich rice digests slowly and releases sugar in a timed slow fashion thus controlling blood sugar. The black rice (Emperors rice) and the various red varieties such as red samba, Camarague, Bhutanese red in particular are very rich in anthocyanins and antioxidants and hence considered useful for preventing occurrence of cancer and other diseases.

Toxicity: Rice plants can accumulate Arsenic from the soil and this Arsenic can be present in the grain mostly in the bran especially in rice grown in areas subjected to heavy usage of pesticides. In the USA, rice grown in fields where cotton had been grown previously and thus containing arsenic based pesticide residues contain very high levels of Arsenic. The approved level of arsenic in water in the USA is limited to less than 10 ppm. Single helping of rice can exceed this level if the rice is from an area that was sprayed with arsenic based pesticides. Arsenic is a powerful carcinogen. It is very likely that Arsenic may be present in rice grown in other parts of the world also, since use of pesticides and micro-biocides is common in all rice-growing countries. When cooked rice is kept overnight without refrigeration, it attracts growth of toxic bacteria such as *Bacillus cereus*. The toxin from this bacterium is heat stable and so consumption of this 'spoiled rice" can create digestive distress. Rice stored in humid environment attracts growth of molds, which produce various toxic mycotoxins. Yellowed cooked rice kept at room temperature for a few days contains a liver toxin known as cyclochlorotine and luteoskyrin due to growth of a fungus *Penicillium islandicum*. Various species and strains of Aspergillus and Penicillium have been found growing on rice grains and paddy stored in moist environments and in rice mills awaiting milling.

Table 3 Nutrient values per 100 grams of rice. Data excerpted from the USDA National Nutrient Database for Standard Reference Release. Black rice data from www.blackrice.com

Abbreviations: NA = Data not available. G = grams; mg = milligrams, ug = micrograms, sat = saturated; mono = mono unsaturated; poly = polyunsaturated.

Metabolite/100 g	White – L	White – M	White-S	White-G	Brown-L	Brown-M	Bhutan	Black
	Long	Medium	Short	Glutinous	Long	Medium	Red	Forbidden
Protein, g	7.13	6.61	6.5	6.81	7.94	7.5	6.8	7.5
Total lipid, g	0.66	0.58	0.52	0.55	2.92	2.68	2.68	
Carbohydrate, g	79.95	79.34	79.15	81.68	77.24	76.17	81.6	76.17
Dietary Fiber, g	1.3	NA		2.8	3.5	3.4	5.1	3.4
Sugar, g	0.22	NA	NA	NA	0.85	NA	NA	
Calcium, mg	28	9	3	11	23	33	NA	33
Iron, mg	0.8	0.8	0.8	1.6	1.47	1.8	NA	1.8
Magnesium, mg	25	35	23	23	143	143	NA	143
Phosphorus, mg	115	108	95	71	333	264	NA	264
Potassium, mg	115	56	76	77	223	268	NA	268
Sodium, mg	5	1	1	7	7	4	NA	4
Copper, Mg	NA	NA	NA	NA	NA	NA	NA	0.277
Zinc, mg	1.09	1.16	1.1	1.2	2.02	2.02	NA	2.02
Vitamin C, mg	0	0	0	0.18	0	0	NA	NA
Thiamin, mg	0.07	0.07	0.18	0.055	0.401	0.413	NA	0.413

Riboflavin, mg	0.049	0.048	0.055	2.145	0.093	0.043	NA	NA
Niacin, mg	1.6	1.6	2.145	0.107	5.091	4.308	NA	4.308
Vitamin B-6, mg	0.164	0.145	0.107	7	0.509	0.509	NA	0.509
Folate, µg	8	NA	7	0	20	20	NA	20
Vitamin B-12, µg	0	0	0	0	0	0	NA	NA
Vitamin A, µg	0	NA	0	0	0	0	0	NA
Vitamin E, mg	0.11	NA	0	0	0.59	0	NA	NA
Vitamin D (D2 + D3), µg	0	0	0	0	0	0	NA	NA
Vitamin K µg	0.1	NA	0	0	1.9	NA	NA	NA
Fatty acids, sat, G	0.18	0.158	0.14	0.111	0.584	0.536	0	0.536
Fatty acids, mono, g	0,206	0.181	0.161	0.2	1.056	0.971	0	0.971
Fatty acids, poly, g	0.177	0.155	0.138	0.198	1.044	0.959	0	0.959
Cholesterol, mg	0	0	0	0	0	0	NA	NA
Anti-oxidants	+	+	++	++				

Triticeae: Wheat, Barley, Rye and certain grasses

Wheat, Barley and Rye are the major edible members of this tribe within the Pooideae subfamily as shown below.

Kingdom: Plantae; Division: Angiospermae, Class: Monocotyledonae; Order: Poales; Family: Poaceae, Sub family: Po-oidae; Genera: *Triticum* (Wheat); *Hordeum* (Barley), *Secale* (Rye), Triticale *(Triticale hexaploide Lart)*. Each of these genera has several species and subspecies associated with them.

General introduction to Triticeae: All three genera grow in temperate/sub-temperate climates and share all features common to monocotyledonous grasslike plants.

Seeds: The seeds of the Triticeae conform to the basic structural features of all cereals described earlier.

Human Health: All three-plant grains are the staple diet of many people in the world and provide their main nutritional needs. The seeds in all these cases and in particular wheat contain variable amounts of gliadin and gluten protein which is linked to the autoimmune celiac disease, colitis. Exposure to this protein even if it is denatured, induces an inflammatory reaction in the intestine. This reaction can be severe, leading to surgery and of use of steroids to curb inflammation. Tolerance to these products appears to have developed in populations that have a long history of consuming these grain products and yet between 0.5%-1percent of the population in wheat consuming countries develop this disease. It is possible, that individuals switching to a wheat/barley/rye based diets from other cereal-based diets are likely to develop intolerance to an even greater degree. Wheat is very rich in phytates that are a complex class of phosphorus compounds. Phytic acid has a strong binding affinity for multivalent cations and proteins and as such, the absorption of essential elements like iron would be impaired in diets based on wheat. Thus, people suffering from Iron deficient anemia would not get the needed iron through oral supplementation of iron if they consume iron tablets along with a wheat-based diet. The iron supplement should be consumed before the meal or a few hours after a wheat based diet.

Wheat and other triticae can be infected by the fungus *Fusarium graminearum* and *F. Culmorum* and this fungus produces a toxin known as Vomitoxin. Ingestion of contaminated grain can cause gastrointestinal distress and loss of appetite. Likewise, another major health problem is due to consumption of contaminated grain particularly Rye infected by the fungus *Claviceps purpurea* which causes Saint Antonys fire and gangrene.

Barley *(Hordeum vulgare*, Chromosome # 2n = 14):

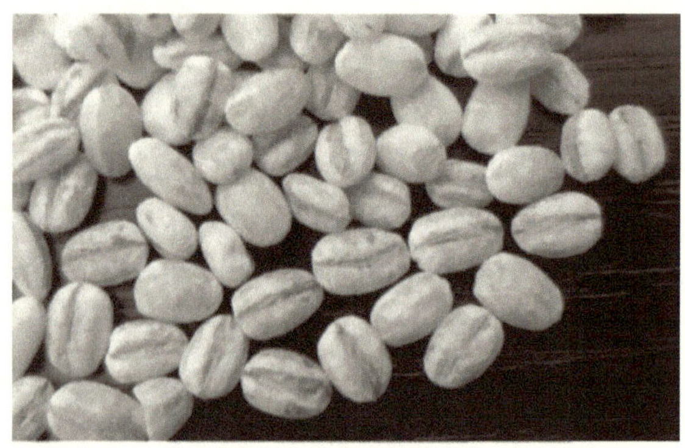
Barley

Barley is grown in the summer in the temperate countries and in the winter in the tropical countries. Like Wheat, it is essentially grown under milder temperatures. It is a diploid plant with 14 chromosomes. The flowers are formed in spikes wherein, the spikelets are arranged in triplets. In old world and certain cultivars only, the central spikelet is fertile whereas the other two are infertile. These are called two row barley (*Hordeum vulgare* var. distichum) and are lower in protein and used for brewing English style ale and German beer and Scotch whiskey. Certain other varieties of barley known as six row barley (*Hordeum vulgare* var. hexastichum), contain additional lateral spikelets which develop into fertile flowers and these are richer in protein. Barley grain is consumed through barley bread, porridge, broth, and also and as cooked grain in many countries and is the chief cereal food in Tibet. **Health:** Barley water is a nonalcoholic drink made by boiling the barley in water. Similarly, barley porridge and broth are prescribed in Islamic, Greco-Roman and Ayurveda alternative medicine as a panacea for ameliorating gastrointestinal distress such as irritable bowel syndrome. Barley water is also said to have diuretic properties and as a substitute for wheat and rice for diabetic patients because of a lower glycemic index.

Rye *(Secale cerale*, Chromosome # 2n = 14):

Rye is grown in East Central and Northern Europe as well as in parts of North America, South America and cooler regions in Asia. The grain is used for making bread/bakery items, rye beer, and whiskey and rye flour. The plants share all features of the Triticeae. It is the most winter hardy plant of all cereals and can withstand temperatures as low as 33 degrees F. Rye seeds contain about: 80% Carbohydrate, 12–15% protein, 23% fat and various amounts of B vitamins. It is less nutritious than wheat. Since Rye is a cross-pollinated plant, it was possible to cross wheat and Rye to produce the hybrid Triticale that has some of the winter hardiness properties of Rye and the nutritive value of Wheat. Rye is highly susceptible to infection by the ergot fungus *Claviceps purpurea* and as such, the seeds could easily be contaminated with this mycotoxin producing fungus

Triticale – (TriticumXsecale, 2n = 42, 56): This is a second-generation artificial hybrid of Wheat (Triticum) and rye (Secale). This hybrid cereal combines the nutritional qualities of wheat and environmental tolerance of rye. Although originally considered as a forage crop, it is now grown more extensively as a breakfast cereal. **Health:** Triticale contains gluten and hence not suitable for those suffering from gluten sensitivity.

Wheat *(Triticum sp)*: Chromosome Number: 2n = 14: 4n = 28; 6n = 42.

There are diploid, tetraploid and hexaploid wheat varieties with **Chromosome** Numbers: 2n = 14; 4n = 28; 6n = 42 respectively. Wheat is grown mainly in Europe including Russia, North and South America, China, many temperate and semi-temperate regions of Asia, Pakistan,

Ukraine, North India, Australia and New Zealand. Cultivated wheat can be classified into three groups namely: Einkorn, Emmer and Vulgare

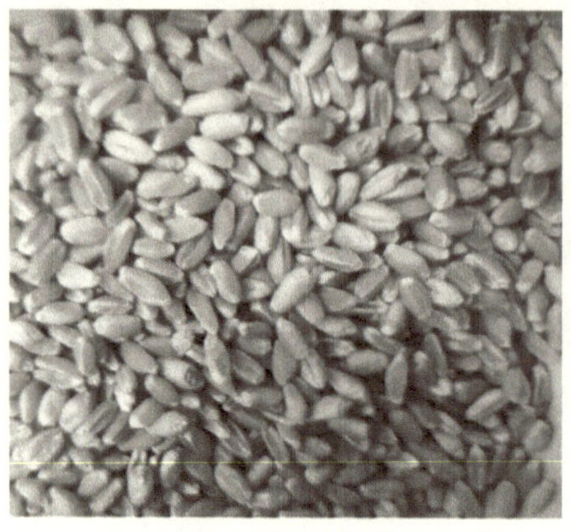

Wheat

groups. The Einkorn group consists of the wild form *T.boeoticum* and the cultivated form *T. monococcum*. Both are diploid with 7 pairs of chromosomes (2n = 14). The Emmer group which is a tetraploid with 14 pairs of chromosomes (4n = 28) is a cross of the wild form T. dicoccoides and the cultivated forms. *T. dicococcum, T. timopheevi, T. durum, T. turgidum, T. polonicum, T. carthlicum, T. turanicum/T. orientale,* The vulgare group (common wheat) which are hexaploid with 21 pairs of chromosomes (6n = 42) consists of *T.aestivum* sub sp. Speltoides, *T. aestivum* subsp Vavilov, *T.aestivum* sub sp.macha, *T.aestivum* sub sp. Vulgare, *T.Aestivum* sub sp. Compactum, and *T.aestivum* subsp. Sphaerococcum.

The Einkorn wheat is used mostly as fodder and is not grown widely. Common wheat (*Triticum aestivum*), sometimes called "bread wheat," is the most widely grown species, and yields the flour ingredient in commercial foods, such as loaf and raised breads, tortillas, doughnuts, cakes, and East Asian noodles. Durum wheat (*Triticum turgidum* ssp. durum) is used in most dried pasta and couscous, for raised and flat breads in parts of Europe and the Middle East, and, less often, in the United States. Although higher quality pasta is made from durum wheat flour, it can also be made using common wheat flour.

Wheat (*Triticum aestivum L.*) can be classified as winter or spring wheat based on flowering responses to cold temperatures. Winter wheat development is promoted by exposure of the seedlings to temperatures in the 38 degrees to 46 degrees F (3 degrees to 8 degrees C) range. Such types are usually planted in the fall which exposes the seedlings to cold temperatures during late fall and winter. This type of cold exposure is called Vernilization. Spring-types of wheat can be planted in spring, as they do not require exposure to cold temperatures for normal development.

Poaceae: Corn, Oats, Millets and Sorghum

Corn/Maize *(Zea mays):* Kingdom: Plantae; Division: Angiosperms, Class Monocotyledonae, Order: Poales, Family: Poaceae, Subfamily: Panicoideae Tribe: andropogoneae Genus: *Zea* species: *mays.* Subspecies: *Z. mays* subsp., Mays, Chromosome Number = 2n = 20.

Although considered often as a cereal, it is not a member of the Triticeae family but belongs to the poaceae and has some characters that are different from the Triticeae. Corn is the most important cereal in

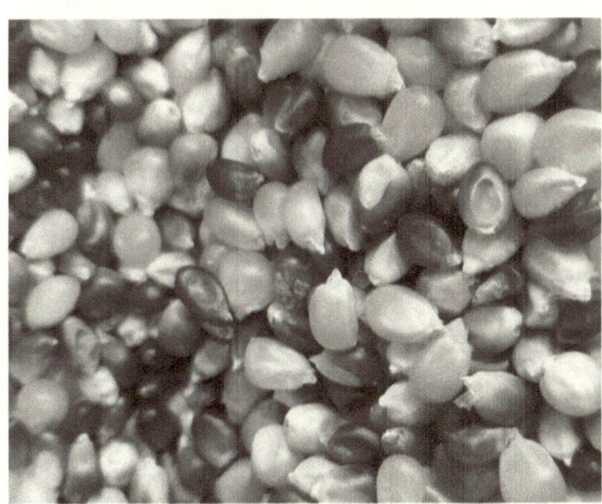

South and North America and in Africa although it is now grown for food, fiber and ethanol production in many countries. Corn is a native of Central South America having originated in southern Mexico. Corn seeds are white, yellow, red, blue or multiple colored. Yellow corn derives its color from the

Multi-color Corn grains

phytochemicals lutein and zeaxanthin wheras, red and blue corn get their color from anthocyanins. Overall, corn has been bred for specific uses such as flour corn for making corn flour (Z.mays var amylacea), sweet corn which has a sugary taste and consumed as corn on the cob (Z.mays var saccharata and *Z. mays* rugosa), multi colored flint corn used for making Hominy and popcorn (Z. *mays* var indurate), yellow or white Dent corn which has a dent with high starch and is used for corn meal, corn bread, chips and tacos. *Zea mays* var indentata, (Popcorn) which has moisture sealed in the hull allowing the trapped water inside to pop when heated. *Zea mays* everta) and waxy corn (Z. mays var ceratina) are rich in amylopectin giving them a sticky glutinous nature and are used for animal feed, adhesives and gelatinous food. Waxy corn is also popular in China as a food source. Blue corn is used for making corn chips and has a low glycemic index with more protein. Baby corn that is consumed as a vegetable is young corncob that has been harvested along with stalk at an early stage. The young corn is eaten along with the cob.

The bulk of the corn grown in the USA (>86%) is genetically modified to contain genes for glyphosate weedicide resistance as well as resistance to corn borer through incorporation of the insecticidal thuringin genes from *Bacillus thuringensis*. The insecticidal thuringin is not toxic to humans. Throughout the world, 35% of corn grown is the GM hybrid.

Cultivated corn is about 8 ft-12 ft tall with a bamboo-like stem from which long leaves with parallel veins arise from about 12 internodes. The mature plant produces female flowers from the axils of the leaves in an inflorescence known as the ear wherein the long styles with stigma silk arises. The male inflorescence known as the tassel arises at the terminal end of the plant. The male flowers produce large numbers of heavy pollen that fall down toward the female flowers. These are caught by the silk stigma resulting in fertilization. The entire ear then becomes the grain-bearing cob containing kernels or seeds. The cob can be harvested before full maturity and consumed as corn on the cob. When fully mature, usually at the end of summer, the seeds are dry. Young ears can be consumed raw with the cob and silk but as the plant matures usually during the summer months, the cob becomes tougher and the silk dries to inedible. By the end of the growing season, the kernels dry out and become difficult to chew without cooking them. Corn seeds are rich in carbohydrates but rather low in protein compared to the Triticiae. It is rich in oil and hence is a great source for cooking oil. The seeds are also poor in the content of the essential amino acids methionine and lysine. Lysine rich hybrid seeds have been produced through genetic techniques.

Health: Other than nutritional value, there is no other known medicinal use for corn although corn silk has been used to produce surgical sutures. It is important to dry the seeds before storage, since moisture enhances postharvest infection of seeds. Blue corn has a lower glycemic index and is rich in flavonoids and hence a good nutritional source.

Oats-cultivated *(Avena sativa)*: Kingdom: Plantae, Division: Angiospermae, Class: Monocotyledonae, Order: Poales Family: Poaceae Genus: Avena Species: sativa, Chromosome number: 6n = 42. Other species not generally cultivated are *A. byzantina, A. sterilis, A. fatua, A. ludoviciana, and A. occidentalis.*

Common oats known as *Avena sativa* is a hexaploid with 42 chromosomes. It is grown in temperate regions even in poor soils and is capable of withstanding greater moistures as compared to wheat and barley. The plant is an annual grass growing to a height of 1.5 meters. The plant bears the stipulated characters of monocots. The flowers are set in inflorescences called panicles with 23 bisexual florets and undergo self-pollination. Each grain is tightly enclosed by the lemma and palea. The grain proper has a seed coat enclosing the outer layer of bran and starchy endosperm with the embryonic germ. Two other species *A. byzantina* and *A. strigosa* are adapted to warmer subtropical conditions and low summer temperatures respectively. Oat grains have approximately 65% carbohydrate, 16% protein, 7% lipids-fats, 10% dietary fiber including beta glucans that are soluble fiber and B vitamins, plus minerals Iron, Magnesium, Manganese, Phosphorus and zinc. After de-hulling, the seed is called groats and is made up of the bran, endosperm and germ. After the whole groat is separated, the rest is then processed by cutting with steel blades into coarse regular and fine steel cut oats. These different classes are used for preparing different nutritional cooking needs. **Health:** Oats are recommended in diets to lower LDL cholesterol due to the presence of high levels of soluble fiber in the seeds. It is used as a component in soaps, skin lotions and other cosmetics as it is believed to help maintain healthy skin. Recently, *Avena* extracts are being marketed as sexual aids similar to Viagra for natural correction of erectile dysfunction. This claim is essentially anecdotal. **Toxicity:** *Avena* is also believed to cause coeliac disease in some individuals, although it is possible that cases of coeliac disease believed to be caused by *Avena* is actually because this grain is often processed in mills that also process wheat products which are known to have proteins that cause coeliac disease.

Other Cereals: Millets and Sorghum

The collective name Millet refers to pearl millet, finger millet, proso millet and foxtail millet. Sorghum on the other hand is a genus of about 30 species. Both Millets and Sorghum grow in warm arid and sub arid regions of Africa and Asia particularly India and Pakistan. Both Millets and Sorghum are free from gluten and since they contain about the same percentage of protein as wheat they are considered as good alternative cereals for those suffering from celiac disease. These grains have a low glycemic index and so are good alternative cereals for diabetic persons. *Sorghum bicolor* is an important crop in West Africa, South America and South Asia and is the fifth most consumed grain cereal in the world. In the USA, it is mainly used as a feed for animals. The seeds are yellow, white, brown or of mixed color. Sorghum flour is used to make various types of porridges, bread and alcoholic beverages as well as sorghum syrup.

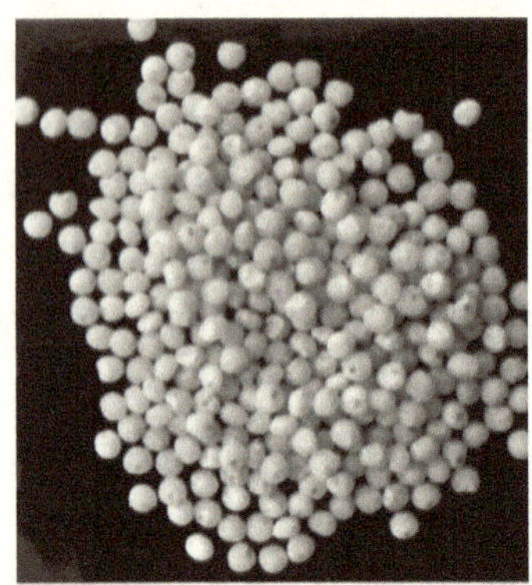

Millet

Millets are a collection of various genera and species: Guinea millet *(Bracharia deflexa), Japanese or* Indian Barnyard Millet *(Echinochloa sp),*

Corn millet/Proso millet *(Panicum miliaceaum)*, Kodo millet *(Paspalum scrobiculatum)*, Pearl millet *(Pennisetum glaucum)*, Foxtail Millett *(Setaria italica) and finger millet (Eleusine coracana)*. Pearl millet ranks number one in acreage grown. Millets are highly nutritious and used for making unleavened bread, gruel and broth. The seed extracts are also used for brewing various indigenous alcoholic beverages in Nepal, Romania, Bulgaria and Sikkim. In India, they are used as flour for making unleavened bread, gruel, porridge, noodles and other local culinary preparations.

Sorghum contains about 30 species of which the most commonly cultivated species is *S. bicolor/S.vulgare*.

Finger millet/Ragi/(*Eleusine coracana*, Kingdom: Plantae; Division: Angiospermae, Class: Monocotyledonae Order: Poales Family: Poaceae. Chromosome number; 4n = 36

Finger millet known as Ragi/nagli/telabun/marua/korakan/ Kezhvaragu is a high protein cereal grown mainly in India and Africa (Ethiopia). It is grown in smaller acreages in Nepal, Sri Lanka and Viet Nam. The cereals are rich in the amino acid methionine that is lacking or present only in low concentrations in the major cereals. Finger millet seeds are smaller than those of pearl millet are and can be white, orange, red, purple or black.

Fox tail millet/Thinai/Kakum (*Setaria italica,*) Kingdom: Plantae, Division: Angiospermae, Class: Monocotyledonae, Order: Poales Family: Poaceae. Chromosome number 2n = 18.

Foxtail millet is also known as Siberian millet, German millet or Hungarian millet. It is a popular cereal grown especially in Southern India and in Semi-arid regions of Asia and Africa. Foxtail millet is an annual grass that produces seeds in a panicle. Seeds are round and small. They are rich in protein.

Pearl Millets/Baja/Bajra/Kambu *(Pennisetum glaucum)*: Kingdom: Plantae; Division: Angiospermae, Class: Monocotyledonae, Order: Poales Family: Poaceae. Chromosome number: 2n = 14

Pearl millets grow to a height of about 0.54 meters (1.5 ft 12 ft). The seeds are small in comparison to corn and may be white, pale yellow, brown, slate blue or purple.

Japanese Barnyard millet *(Echinochloa utilis)*: **Kingdom: Plantae; Division: Angiospermae, Class: Monocotyledonae, Order: Poales Family: Poaceae. Chromosome number 6n = 54**

The seeds of this millet are used for preparing porridge in Japan. In most countries, it is a forage plant.

Kodo millet/Varagu *(Paspalum scrobiculatum)*: **Kingdom: Plantae; Division: Angiospermae, Class: Monocotyledonae, Order: Poales Family: Poaceae. Chromosome number 4n = 40.**

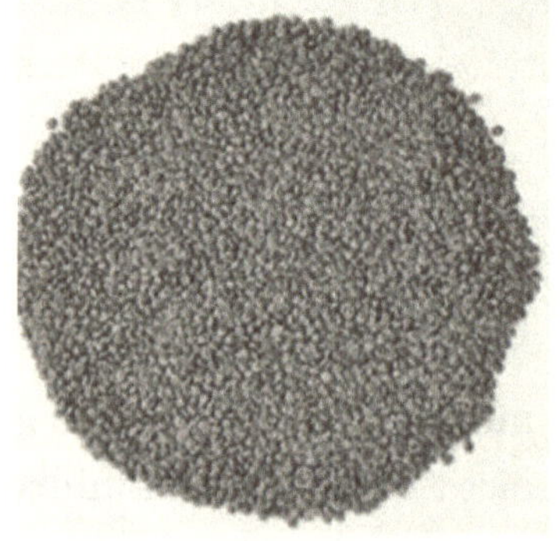

Kodo Millet

Kodo millet also known as cow grass, rice grass, ditch millet or Native Paspalum is a high protein cereal containing about 11% protein. It is also a rich source of fiber. The plants are perennial grasses but cultivated as annuals in Southern India where it is an important cereal grain. The seeds are rich in protein and are an important source of cereal food consumed after cooking or made into gruel or as a kind of bread.

Corn millet/Proso millet *(Panicum miliaceaum)*: **Kingdom: Plantae; Division: Angiospermae, Class: Monocotyledonae Order: Poales Family: Poaceae. Chromosome number: 2n = 36, 3n = 54, 4n = 72.**

Plants are annuals grown in Russia, India, Egypt, Japan, China and Mediterranean countries. It grows well in arid regions. The seeds are mostly used for livestock in Europe and in North America but in other countries it is used as a component of breads, porridge and breakfast cereals.

Sorghum/Jowar/Milo *(Sorghum bicolor/S.vulgare):* **Kingdom: Plantae; Division: Angiospermae, Class: Monocotyledonae, Order: Poales Family: Andropogoneae. Chromosome number: 2n = 20.**

Sorghum is the fifth most important cereal after Rice, Wheat, Corn and Barley. Sorghum seeds are used for making unleavened bread known

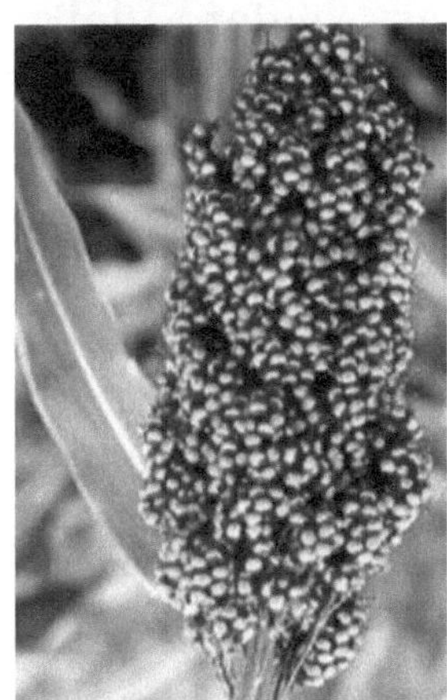

Sorghum

as Jowar bread, which is the common food in semi-arid areas of Southern and western India. It is similarly used in Egypt, Sudan, other arid regions of Africa and Asia. The ground seeds are also used for making pancakes and other food preparations. The seeds are protein-rich (>10%). **Health:** Millets and Sorghum contain high protein, are rich in fiber and many have antioxidants. Sorghum and Millets also contain certain anti-nutrient factors such as phytate, which impair the assimilation of iron. They also have tannins that affect digestibility and goitrogens that cause goiter. In addition, like most cereals, millets and sorghum are good substrates for infestation by fungi like *Aspergillus sp. Penicillium sp,* and *Fusarium* sp,-.causing mycotoxicoses.

White fonio/fonio/Hungry rice or acha rice *(Digitaria exilis):* **Kingdom: Plantae; Division: Angiospermae, Class: Monocotyledonae; Order: Poales, Family: Poaceae. India, Africa. Chromosome numbers are inconsistent: 2n = 34, 36 and 54**

Fonio or hungry rice is popular names of *Digitaria exilis* grown in West Africa and India. Diploid, tetraploid and hexaploid varieties of *Digitaria* exist. It grows in arid and semi-arid regions reaching maturity and setting seeds in six to eight weeks after sowing which makes it one of the fastest growing plants. The seeds are nutritious with high protein content and a low glycemic index and are used for making bread, porridge and beer. Many nutritionists point out that this cereal could be even more important as a protein rich food especially since it grows in semi-arid (water poor) regions. Black fonio (*D. iburua*) is a related species grown in Africa. *Digitaria compacta* known as raishan is another edible millet grown in the Kasi Hills region of India-Myanmar region and in parts of Cambodia, Viet Nam and other regions of South Asia.

Indian barnyard millet/sawa millet, or billion dollar grass *(Echinochloa frumentacea)*: Kingdom: Plantae; Division: Angiospermae, Class: Monocotyledonae; Order: Poales, Family: Poaceae. India, Africa. Chromosome number 6n = 54

Echinochloa frumentacea is widely grown as a cereal in India, Pakistan, and Nepal. The seeds are cooked like rice or boiled in milk to make porridge and is often the only means of nutrition when people in certain regions of India go on a semi-fasting routine during specific religious days.

White French millet, red French millet/hog millet/brown corn millet/broomcorn millet/*(Panicum sumatrense)* Kingdom: Plantae; Division: Angiospermae, Class: Monocotyledonae; Order: Poales, Family: Poaceae. India, Africa India, Australia. Chromosome number: 2n = 36.

This millet is similar in habit to the proso millet except that it is smaller. It is an annual herbaceous plant, which grows straight or with folded blades to a height of 30 cm to 1 m. The grain is round and smooth, 1.8 to 1.9 mm long. The millet is a common person's food in many parts of India and is called Kutki in Hindi, Sama in Bengali, Suan in Odissa, Sava in Marathi, Samai in Tamil, and Samalu in Telugu. It is cooked like rice, made into porridge (Kanji) or made into a kind of unleavened bread. The seeds have a content of over 7% protein.

Table 4: Nutritional value per 100 grams (g) of uncooked grain

All values in grams (g), milligrams (mg) or micrograms (u).

Nutrition/100g	Wheat White	Wheat Red	Wheat Red Winter	Corn Yellow	Corn White	Barley	Rye	Sorghum	Millets
Protein, g	13.68	15.4	12.61	9.42	9.42	9.91	10.34	10.62	11.02
Total lipid (fat), g	2.47	1.92	1.54	4.74	4.74	1.16	1.63	3.46	4.22
Carbohydrate, g	71.13	68.03	71.18	74.26	74.26	77.72	75.86	72.09	72.85
Fiber, g	NA	12.2	12.2	7.3	NA	15.6	15.1	6.7	8.5
Sugars, g	NA	0.41	0.41	0.64	NA	0.8	0.98	2.53	
Calcium, Ca, mg	34	25	29	7	7	29	24	13	8
Iron, Fe, mg	3.52	3.6	3.19	2.71	2.71	2.5	2.63	3.36	3.01
Magnesium, Mg, mg	144	124	126	127	127	79	110	165	114
Phosphorus, P, mg	508	332	288	210	210	221	332	289	285
Potassium, K, mg	431	340	363	287	287	280	510	363	195
Sodium, Na, mg	2	2	2	35	35	9	2	2	5
Zinc, Zn, mg	4.16	2.78	2.65	2.21	2.21	2.13	2.65	1.67	1.68
Vitamin C, mg	0	0	0	0	0	0	0	0	0
Thiamin, mg	0.419	0.504	0.383	0.385	0.385	0.191	0.316	0.332	0.421
Riboflavin, mg	0.121	0.11	0.115	0.201	0.201	0.114	0.251	0.096	0.29
Niacin, mg	6.738	5.71	5.464	3.627	3.627	4.604	4.27	3.688	4.72
Vitamin B-6, mg	0.419	0.336	0.3	0.622	0.622	0.26	0.294	0.443	0.384

Nutrition/100, g	Wheat White	Wheat Red	Wheat Red Winter	Corn Yellow	Corn White	Barley	Rye	Sorghum	Millets
Folate, DFE, µg	43	43	38	19	0	23	38	20	85
Vitamin B-12, µg	0	0	0	0	0	0	0	0	0
Vitamin A, RAE, µg	0	0	0	11	0	1	1	0	0
Vitamin A, IU	0	9	9	214	0	22	11	0	0
Vitamin E, mg		1.01	1.01	0.49	0	0.02	0.85	0.5	0.05
Vitamin D (D2 + D3), µg	0	0	0	0	0	0	0	0	0
Vitamin D, ug	0	0	0	0	NA	0	0	0	0
Vitamin K, ug	NA	1.9	1.9	0.3	NA	2.2	5.9	0	0.9
Fatty acids, saturated, g	0.454	0.314	0.269	0.667	0.667	0.244	0.197	0.61	0.723
Fatty acids, mono, g	0.344	0.303	0.2	1.251	1.251	0.149	0.208	1.131	0.773
Fatty acids, poly, g	0.978	0.765	0.627	2.163	2.163	0.56	0.767	1.558	2.134
Cholesterol, mg		0	0	0	0	0	0	0.005	0
Other	Phytate	Phytate	Phytate						

References

Rice

Abdel-aal El-Sayed M.; Young J.C. and I. Rabalski (2006): "Anthocyanin composition in black, blue, pink, purple, and red cereal grains," Journal of agricultural and food chemistry, 2006, vol. 54: 13, p. 4696–4704.

Champagne, E.T. (2004): RICE: Chemistry and Technology, Third Edition, Editor: Elaine T. Champagne, U.S. Department of Agriculture, Agricultural Research Service, Southern Regional Research Center, New Orleans, Louisiana. ISBN: 978-1-891127-34-2

Deshpande, S.S., Sing, B. and U. Singh (1991): Cereals, in Foods of Plant origin; Production, Technology and Human Nutrition, Eds. Salunkhe, D.K.M and Deshpande, S.S., Pp. 6–136., Van Nostrand, Reinhold, New York. Pp499.

Garris, A.J, Tai, T.H, Coburn, J., Kresovich, S., McCouch, S. (2005): Genetic structure and diversity in Oryza sativa L. Genetics 169(3): 1631–1638.

Heun M., Pregal-Schafer R., Klawan D., Castagan R., Accesbi M., Borghi B., Salomini F. (1997): Site of einkorn wheat domestication identified by DNA fingerprinting, Science, 278: 1312-1314

http://irri.org,

http://irri.org/

http://irri.org/almanac-references

http://ricepedia.org/about-ricepedia/selected-references-and-other-information-sources

http://ricepedia.org/index.php/china;

http://world-crops.com/rice/, https://hort.purdue.edu/newcrop/Crops/Rice.html

http://www.theplantlist.org/

https://www.hort.purdue.edu/newcrop/afcm/millet.html

https://www.hort.purdue.edu/newcrop/projects.html.

Jena, K.K., (2010): The species of the genus Oryza and transfer of useful genes from wild species into cultivated rice, O. sativa. Breed. Sci. 60: 518-523.

Nayar, N.M., (2014): In Origins and Phylogeny of rices, Academic Press, Elsevier, Amsterdam/New York. Pp324.

Singh, R.K.; Baghel, S.S. (2003): "Aromatic Rices of Manipur" (PDF), a Treatise on the Scented Rices of India (1st. ed.), New Delhi: Kalyani Publishers, pp. 347–354, ISBN 8127210315

Vaughan DA, Ge S, Kaga A, Tomooka N. (2008): Phylogeny and biogeography of the genus Oryza, In: Hirano HY, Hirai A, Sano Y, Sasaki T, editors, Rice biology in the genomics era, Biotechnol. Agric. 62: 219-234.

Vaughan DA, Lu BR, Tomooka N. 2008: The evolving story of rice evolution, Plant Sci. 174: 394-408.

www.blackrice.com

Wheat

Bowden, W.M. (1959): The taxonomy and nomenclature of the wheats, barleys, and ryes and their wild relatives. Canadian Journal of Botany 37: 657-684.

Bowden, W.M. (1966): Chromosome numbers in seven genera of the tribe Triticeae. Canadian Journal of Genetics and Cytolology 8: 130-136.

http://www.whfoods.com/genpage.php?tname = foodspice&dbid = 66

Khalil Khan, and Peter R. Shewry (2009): WHEAT: Chemistry and Technology, Fourth Edition, Editors: Khalil Khan, and Peter R. Shewry, ISBN: 978-1-891127-55-7 (2009).

Shewry, Peter R (2009):" Wheat," Journal of Experimental Botany 60 (6): 1537–1553,

Stallknecht, G.F., K.M. Gilbertson, and J.E. Ranney: (1996); Alternative wheat cereals as food grains: Einkorn, emmer, spelt, kamut, and triticale. p. 156-170. In: J. Janick (ed.), Progress in new crops, ASHS Press, Alexandria, VA.

Oats:

Haboubi, N.Y., Taylor, S. and Jones, S (2006): "Coeliac disease and oats: a systematic review." Postgrad Med J (Review) 82 (972): 672–8, PMC 2653911, PMID 17068278.

http://wholegrainscouncil.org/whole-grains-101/rye-triticale-august-grains-of-the-month

Lasztity, R. (1999): The Chemistry of Cereal Proteins, Akademiai Kiado., ISBN 978-0-8493-2763-6.

Oelke E.A., Oplinger, E.S., and M.A. Brinkman (1989): Triticale, In Alternative Field Crops Manual, University of Wisconsin Extension and University of Minnesota Extension service

Tovoli, F., Masi C., Guidetti, E., Negrini, G., Paterini, P. and Bolondi L (2015): "Clinical and diagnostic aspects of gluten related disorders." World J Clin Cases 3 (3): 275–84. doi: 10.12998/wjcc.v3.i3.275, PMC 4360499. PMID 25789300

Webster, F.H., and Wood, P.J., (2011): OATS: Chemistry and Technology, Second Edition, Editors: Francis H. Webster, Francis Webster & Associates, Branson, Missouri, U.S.A. and Peter J. Wood, P.J., (2011): Guelph Food Research Centre, Guelph, Ontario, Canada, ISBN: 978-1-891127-64-9 (2011).

Barley and Rye:

Anderson, J.W, Hanna, T.J, and Peng, X, Kryscio, R.J (2000): Whole grain foods and heart disease risk. J Am Coll Nutr 2000 Jun; 19(3 Suppl): 291S-9S. 2000. PMID: 17670.

Behall, K.M, Scholfield, D.J, Hallfrisch, J. (2005): Comparison of hormone and glucose responses of overweight women to barley and oats. J Am Coll Nutr. 2005 Jun 24(3): 182-8. 2005. PMID: 15930484.

Dai, F.; Nevo, E.; Wu, D.; Comadran, J.; Zhou, M.; Qiu, L.; Chen, Z.; Beiles, A.; et al. (2012):"Tibet is one of the centers of domestication of cultivated barley." Proceedings of the National Academy of Sciences 109 (42): 16969–16973. doi: 10.1073/pnas.1215265109.

Reid, D.A. (1985): Morphology and Anatomy of the Barley Plant, doi: 10.2134/agronmonogr26.c4, Agronomy Monograph, Barley, 26: 73-101 (1985)

https://www.hort.purdue.edu/newcrop/duke_energy/Secale_cereale.html

Corn:

"Origin, History and Uses of Corn"(2014): Iowa State University, Department of Agronomy. February 11, 2014.

Carter, P.R., Hicks, D.R., Doll, J.D., Schulte, E.E., Schuler, R. and B. Holmes (1989): Popcorn (Flint corn), https://hort.purdue.edu/newcrop/afcm/popcorn.html

Duke, J.A. (1983): Zea mays. https://www.hort.purdue.edu/newcrop/duke_energy/Zea_mays.html

http://www.ers.usda.gov/topics/crops/corn.aspx

https://www.hort.purdue.edu/newcrop/Crops/Corn.html

Roney, J., (Winter 2009). "The Beginnings of Maize Agriculture," Archaeology Southwest 23 (1): 4.

Sprague, G.F., and J.W. Dudley, eds. Corn and Corn Improvement, 3d ed. Madison, Wis.: American Society of Agronomy, 1988

Millets

Baltensperger, D.D. (1996): "Foxtail and Proso Millet," In Progress in New Crops Edited by Jules Janick…: ASHS Press, 1996, Alexandria, VA, USA…

http://millets.res.in/aicrp_small.php

Kumar, J., Kumar. and V.K. Yadav (2007): Small millet research.G.B. Pant University of Agricultural research, Hill Campus, Ranichuri, Uttarakhand, India Pp58.

National Research Council (1996): "Fonio (Acha)," Grains, Lost Crops of Africa 1, Washington: National Academies Press, ISBN 978-0-309-04990-0.

Oelke, E.A., Oplinger, E.S., Putnam, D.H., Durgan, B.R., Doll, J.D. and D.J. Undersander (1990): Millets, In Alternative Field Crops Manual, University of Wisconsin Extension and University of Minnesota Extension service, https://www.hort.purdue.edu/newcrop/afcm/millet.html

Travis L. Goron and Manish N. Raizada (2015): Genetic diversity and genomic resources available for the small millet crops to accelerate a New Green Revolution, Front Plant Sci. 2015; 6: 157, PMCID: PMC4371761

Chapter 5

Pseudo Cereals: Amaranth, Buckwheat, Chia and Quinoa

Unlike true cereals that are monocots, pseudo cereals are dicots whose grains are consumed as staple diets in South America and now in the United States and other countries. These grains have a lower glycemic index, have high protein, and hence considered suitable in diabetic diets. Amaranth, Quinoa, Chia and Buckwheat are among the most common grains known also as ancient grains that belong to this group. These grains were the main source of nutrition among the Maya, Inca and Aztec populations of Central and South America. These are becoming very popular among health conscious individuals all over the world. Although, these Pseudocereals cannot replace existing conventional cereals, these grains would be of special benefit to diabetics and some with celiac disease. Further, some of these grain plants can grow in nutritionally poor soils and semiarid regions where conventional cereal plants would be difficult to grow.

Amaranth/Kiwicha: Kingdom: Plantae Division: Angiospermae Class: Eudicots, Order: Caryophyllales, Family: Amaranthaceae Genus: and species: *Amaranthus caudatus A. cruentes,* *A. hypochondriacus.* **Chromosome number, 2n = 34.**

Amaranth is one of the most well-known grain plants grown in South America. The Aztecs cultivated Amaranth for centuries but their use subsided after the decline of the Aztec kingdom and the

116

plants were treated as weeds. However, a revival in interest in this ancient grain occurred recently due to the realization of its nutritional value. The low glycemic index and the fact that the plants can grow in conditions adverse to growth of many conventional cereals that require high water and fertilizer requirements is an additional incentive for growing these. The seeds are typical dicotyledonous seeds. They are rich in protein about 14-17% and about 24% fiber. The grains have the amino acids lysine and tryptophan that are low in other cereals. They contain higher levels of Magnesium and iron. In particular, they have no glutens that cause celiac disease and as such are a good alternative cereal for those suffering from this intestinal disease. However, the seeds contain oxalates and saponins that are anti – nutritional factors but these can be removed by soaking in water and decanting the boiled water while cooking. The raw seeds are not digestible. The leaves of *A. Cruentes* along with *A. dubius, A. blitum* and *A. tricolor* are edible after cooking and are rich in folates and vitamin C and form important leafy vegetable components of certain African, Chinese, Indonesian, Fijian, Filipino Sri Lankan, Indian and Mediterranean cuisine.

The plants are annual herbs with thick tough stems similar to sunflower stem and broad palmate leaves. The stem and leaves are colored pink to purple and are rich in flavonoids, anthocyanin and carotene. The inflorescence is a catkin and each catkin produces multiple small white to pale yellow seeds of about 1 mm diameter. Seeds have a tough seed coat enclosing two cotyledons, endosperm and the embryo. The whole seed is consumed after toasting or cooking. Amaranth flour is produced by milling and often mixed with other cereal flours for preparing breads and other baked products. **Medicinal:** Some studies report a lowering of cholesterol by consumption of Amaranth as a nutritional cereal source. There are also studies indicating a lowering of sugar in pre-diabetic individuals. Due to the absence of gluten, the Amaranth seed is considered good for persons with celiac disease.

Buckwheat *(Fagopyrum esculentum, 2n = 16, 4n = 32)*: Kingdom: Plantae, Division: Angiospermae, Class: Eudicots, Order: Caryophyllales, Family: Polygonaceae, Genus and species: *Fagopyrum esculentum.*

Buckwheat is not related to wheat but is a Pseudo cereal that is a dicotyledonous plant. It contains protein of high nutritional value and is relatively rich in lysine and other essential amino acids and it has high levels of iron, chromium, calcium, magnesium, selenium and polyunsaturated fatty acids. It is an annual plant with branched stems and arrow shaped leaves. Flowers arise in panicles from the leaf nodes. Seeds are broad at the base and pointed at the top. They are about 46 mm in width. The seed has an outer hull and inner seed coats enclosing the endosperm and cotyledons. The seeds are rich in protein containing all essential amino acids especially lysine and do not contain gluten.

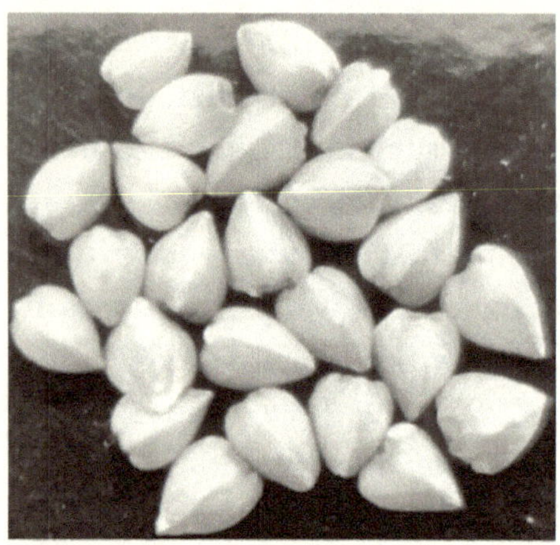

Buckwheat

Buckwheat is a native of Western China but is grown as a staple crop in some areas of Eastern Europe. The de – hulled grain is cooked like rice and is called Kasha. In the USA, it is used to make pancakes and is a component of some breakfast cereals. Noodles made of Buckwheat are popular in Japan, Korea, Tibet and Northern Italy. **Health:** The low content of gluten makes buckwheat a valuable nutritional alternative for people suffering from celiac disease. Further, the glucoside rutin found in the seeds allegedly strengthen capillary walls of blood vessels and may have a role in treating chronic venous insufficiency disease. The grain helps to lower cholesterol and experiments suggest that it is a good alternative cereal for diabetics. The buckwheat honey is a good source for sweeteners. **Toxicity:** Some individuals are susceptible to igE mediated allergic reactions. Others may develop rashes on exposure to light (Fagopyrism) due to the presence of fagopyrin in the seeds.

Canihua/KAÑIWA/ *(Chenopodium pallidicaule)*: Kingdom: Plantae: Division: Angiospermae, Class: Eudicots; Order: Caryophyllales Family: Amaranthaceae Sub Family: Chenopodiaceae.

These plants have similar growth habits that are similar to Amaranth and Quinoa and are grown in the Andes region of South America. The plants are included as plants of the future and listed among ancient grains. It is not yet commercially popular elsewhere in the world. Plants are herbaceous with hermaphrodite flowers. Seeds contain about 16% protein. Both leaves and seeds are used as food. Leaves contain about 30% protein but also toxic saponins and oxalic acid that make them somewhat toxic if consumed in large amounts. However, cooking, removes most of the saponins. Seeds have only minute amounts of saponins and hence a good choice as an alternative protein-rich grain.

Chia *(Salvia hispanica)*: Kingdom: Plantae; Division: Angiospermae, Class: Eudicots; Order: Lamiales; Family: Lamiaceae; Genus and Species: *Salvia hispanica; S. Columbariae*.

The plant belongs to the mint group of plants and produces seeds that were among the staple grains of the Aztecs in Central America. The

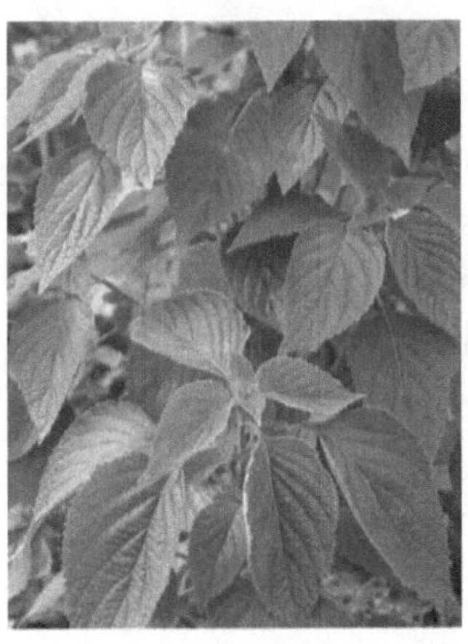

Chia plant

seeds are highly hydrophilic producing a mucilaginous substance that swells by absorbing water, in the GI tract thereby reducing hunger. The plant is a native of Guatemala and Southern Mexico. The seeds are tiny about 1 mm and are dicotyledonous. They are rich in protein, calcium, unsaturated oil, Omega 3 fatty acids – α-linolenic acid and soluble fiber. Seeds can absorb 12 times their weight when soaked in water. Chia plants are annual herbs that grow to about 3 ft similar to basil and have small aromatic leaves. White or pink flowers are produced in spikes at the end of stem branches. **Health:** Because of the hydrophilic properties due to its high soluble fiber, it is considered as a good food for reducing cholesterol levels. Similarly, it is considered useful for reducing blood sugar and hence good for diabetic control. In view of these two properties, it may be considered as a good food supplement and useful in weight control. There are no reports of any toxic reactions due to consumption of Chia seeds or seed products. Chia seeds absorb water resulting in swelling and hence the seeds should not be eaten raw as the seeds may absorb water from the esophagus forming a gel that might obstruct the gastro-intestinal region. It may also promote acid reflux disease if eaten raw.

Quinoa/Kinuva *(Chenopodium quinoa):* **Kingdom: Plantae: Division: Angiospermae, Class: Eudicots, Order: Caryophyllales, Family: Amaranthaceae, Sub Family: Chenopodiaceae, Genus and species:** *Chenopodium quinoa.*

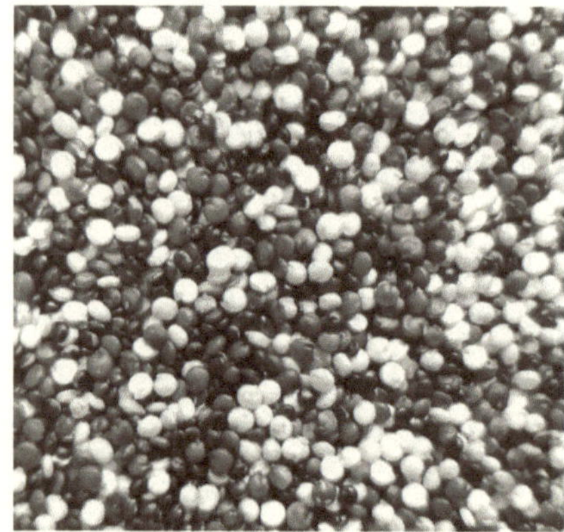

Black, Brown, white Quinoa

The plant is a native of the Andes mountain ranges and has been a major source of food for the people living in the mountainous regions of Chile, Bolivia, Peru and Ecuador. It is commonly referred to as *Inca* rice. The plant is related to the weeds: lambs quarters (*Chenopodium album.*), and *C. pallidicaule* and the medicinal anthelminthic plant *C.ambrosoides L antihelmincum.* It is also related to sugarbeets and spinach. The dicot seeds are small and range in color from beige – black, red, pink, orange, yellow or white in color. The seed color is due to a resinous coating that contains two to six percent saponins. The embryo comprises 60% of the volume within the pericarp and these results in the higher protein content of the seed in comparison to cereal grains. Plants grow to a height of 6 Ft and have a thick erect woody stalk with palmate leaves that look like the webbed feet of geese. The leaves become yellow red or purple as the plant matures with young leaves being green. The leaves are used as a leafy vegetable similar to spinach. The plants are drought resistant like millets. The flowers are produced on a panicle and are normally self-pollinated. **Health**: The seeds are rich in the amino acid Lysine that is low in cereals. The nutritional quality is similar to that of casein. The seed coats are thick and contain the bitter tasting saponins that have to be removed by soaking in water or by mechanical procedures similar to those used for preparing white polished rice. Quinoa seeds have a low glycemic index and so useful for preparing foods for diabetics. The seeds are lower in sodium and have high concentrations of calcium, phosphorus, iron, copper, manganese and zinc as compared to other cereals.

Other Pseudo cereals: The following plants have been in use as pseudo cereals by different ethnic communities but are not in general use as cereals.

1. **Jobs tears *(Coix lacryma-jobi* var. ma-yuen): Kingdom: Plantae, Division: Angiospermae, Class: Monocotyledonae, Order: Poales, Family: Poaceae.**

The seeds are used in Asia as a minor cereal in peninsular Malaysia, Himalayan regions of India, Thailand, Vietnam, South China and Japan, Korea. In the USA, the Cherokee Indians used the seeds as corn beads in religious functions. The seeds are also used in traditional alternative medicine to control diahorrea, and as a diuretic.

2. **Knotweed *(Polygonum erectum)*: Kingdom: Plantae, Division: Angiospermae, Class: Eudicots, Order: Caryophyllales, Family: Polygonaceae**

Plants were cultivated by American Indians in North America. It is a minor cereal.

3. **Lambs quarters huauzontle/** *(Chenopodium berlandieri; C. berlandieri ssp. nuttalliae)* **Kingdom: Plantae, Division: Angiospermae, Class: Eudicots, Order: Caryophyllales, Family: Amaranthaceae.**

Plants grown in continental North America as weeds and were ancient Pseudocereals. It is still cultivated on a minor scale in Mexico as a Broccoli-like flower vegetable.

4. **Sump weeds** *(Iva annua):* **Kingdom: Plantae, Division: Angiospermae, Class: Eudicots, Order: Asterales, Family: Asteraceae.**

This herbaceous annual is native to Mexico and Southern United States and cultivated several hundred years ago as a source of food. The seeds are similar to sun flower and contain over 30% protein and over 40% oil but plants are no longer cultivated. **Health:** similar to Amaranth seeds.

Table 5: Nutritional value of uncooked grain per 100 grams (g)

Values are expressed in grams (g), milligrams (mg) and micrograms (u).

Metabolite	Amaranth	Buckwheat	Chia	Oats	Oat Bran	Quinoa	Triticale
Protein, g	13.56	13.25	16.54	16.89	17.3	14.12	13.05
Total lipid (fat), g	7.02	3.4	30.74	6.9	7.03	6.07	2.09
Carbohydrate, g	65.25	71.5	42.12	66.27	66.22	64.16	72.13
Fiber, total dietary, g	6.7	10	34.4	10.6	15.4	7	
Sugars, total, mg	1.69				1.45		
Calcium, CA, mg	159	18	631	54	58	47	37
Iron, Fe, mg	7.61	2.2	7.72	4.72	5.41	4.57	2.57
Magnesium, mg	248	231	335	177	235	197	130
Phosphorus, mg	557	347	860	523	734	457	358
Potassium, Mg	508	460	407	429	566	563	332
Sodium, mg	4	1	16	2	4	5	5
Zinc, mg	2.87	2.4	4.58	3.97	3.11	3.1	3.45
Vitamin C, mg	4.2	0	1.6	0	0		0
Thiamin, mg	0.116	0.101	0.62	0.763	1.17	0.36	0.416
Riboflavin, mg	0.2	0.425	0.17	0.139	0.22	0.318	0.134
Niacin, mg	0.923	7.02	8.83	0.961	0.934	1.52	1.43
Vitamin B-6, mg	0.591	0.21	0	0.119	0.165	0.487	0.138

Folates, µg	82	30	NA	56	52	184	73
Vitamin B-12, µg	0	0	NA	0	0	0	0
Vitamin A, µg	0	0	54	0	0	1	0
Vitamin A, IU	2	0	NA	0	0	14	0
Vitamin E, mg	1.19	0	0.5	0	0	2.44	0.9
Vitamin D (D2 + D3)	0	0	NA	0	0	0	0
Vitamin D	0	0	NA	NA	0	0	0
Vitamin K, µg	0	0	NA	NA	3.2	0	0
Fatty acids, total satura	1.459	0.741	3.33	1.217	1.328	0.706	0.366
Fatty acids, total mono	1.685	1.04	2.309	2.178	2.376	1.613	0.211
Fatty acids, total polyun	2.778	1.039	23.665	2.535	2.766	3.292	0.913
Cholesterol	NA	0	0.14	0	0	0	0
Other	Oxalates	Phytate					Saponin

References

Arora, R.K., (1977): "Job's tears (Coix lacryma-jobi) – a minor food and fodder crop of northeastern India," Economic Botany, Vol. 31, No. 3, 358–366.

Bonasora, M.G, M.G., Pogo, L.G., and Greizerstein, E.J. (2013): Cytogenetic studies in four cultivated Amaranthus (Amaranthaceae) species. Comp Cytogenet. 2013, 7(1): 53–61. PMCID: PMC3833744

Deshpande, S.S., Sing, Band U.Singh (1991): Cereals, in Foods of Plant origin; Production, Technology and Human Nutrition, Eds. Salunkhe, D.K.M and Deshpande, S.S., Pp. 6-136, Van Nostrand, Reinhold, New York, Pp 499.

Edwardson, Steven (1996): "Buckwheat: Pseudocereal and Nutraceutical," In Progress in New Crops, Edited by Jules Janick, Alexandria, Va.: ASHS Press, 1996.

http://www.encyclopedia.com/doc/1G2-3403400119.html

http://www.n8ture.com/grains.html

https://www.hort.purdue.edu/newcrop/default.html.

Lost Crops of the Incas (1989): Little-Known Plants of the Andes with Promise for Worldwide Cultivation, *In* the National Academies Press, 1989, pp 128-161

Myers, Robert L. (1996): "Amaranth: New Crop Opportunity," *In* Progress in New Crops. Edited by Jules Janick Alexandria, Va.: ASHS Press, 1996

Oelke, A., Putnam, D.H., Teynor, T.M., and E.S. Oplinger (1992): Quinoa, In Alternative Field Crops Manual, University of Wisconsin Extension and University of Minnesota Extension service.

Oplinger, E.S. Oelke, E.A., Brinkman, M.A. and K.A. Kelling (1989): Buckwheat, In Alternative Field Crops Manual, University of Wisconsin Extension and University of Minnesota Extension service.

Putnam, D.H., Oplinger, E.S., Doll, J.D., and E.M. Schulte: (1989) Amaranth, In Alternative Field Crops Manual, University of Wisconsin Extension and University of Minnesota Extension service.

Chapter 6

The Legumes and Hemp

Legumes and Hemp belong to the same taxonomic order but belong to different families. Legumes belong to the Fabaceae but Hemp belongs to the Cannabaceae. Hemp is included here because it is a good source of FDA-approved protein provided it has no or low (4, ppm) psychoactive cannabinoids.

Legumes

Kingdom: Plantae; Division: Angiosperms, Class Eudicots; Order: Fabales, Family: Leguminosae/Fabaceae; Genera and species: Many. Legume Food-Seed and Vegetable genera are: Arachis(Peanut), Cajanus (pigeon pea), Cicer (Garbanzo/Bengal gram), Cyamopsis (Guar), Dolichos (Lab Lab), Glycine (Soybean), Lens (Lentil), Phaseolus (Bean), Pisum (Peas) , Psophocarpus, Sesbania (Sesame), Vigna (Cowpea) , Vicia (fava bean).

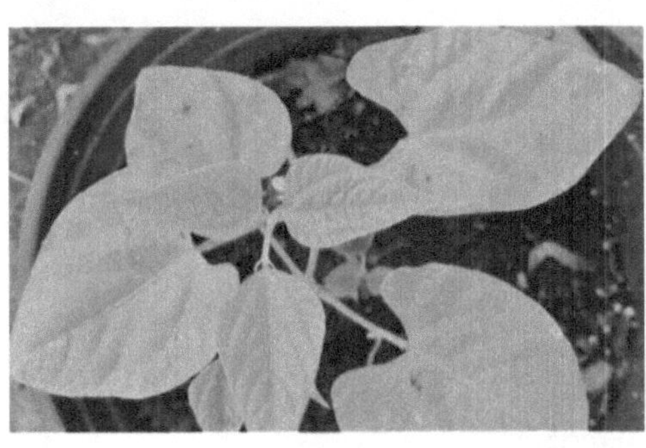

Bean plant

Legumes are plants belonging to the family Fabaceae also known as Leguminosae. This family of plants contains more than 700 genera and about 20,000 species. The plants may be trees e.g., *Tamarindus indica*, (Tamarind), *Cesalpinia pulcherrima* (bird of Paradise); Vines like *Cajanus Cajan* (lentil), *Pisum sativum* – (garden pea) or herbs *Arachis hypogeae* (Peanut). The plants may be annuals or perennials. They are classified into three sub families: Mimosoideae, Caesalpinoideae and Papilinoideae. The leaves of the legumes may be simple or compound. The flowers form a basic pattern but can be differentiated based on the sub families. In the Cesalpinoid family exemplified by *Poinciana regia and cassia* sp., the flowers have five petals of which one is a banner petal with 10 stamens. In the mimosa family, the flowers are arranged in clusters and look like balls with petals that are tiny and fused with elongated stamens e.g. touch me not plant – *Mimosa pudica*. The Flowers of the papilionoid family are arranged in a more elaborate fashion. The flowers have two fused lower petals and 3 upper single petals. The typical legume seed has an outer seed coat consisting of the outer testa and inner tegmen layers enclosing two cotyledons that arise from the two sides of the highly developed embryo. The plumule that grows into the shoot, leaves and stem and the radicle that develops into the root system on germination are found in the seed embryo. The two cotyledons contain stored food materials and supply the germinating plant with nutrients until the seedling establishes itself through photosynthesis and uptake of water and minerals from the soil.

Depending on usage, legumes may be classified as: 1) Forage Legumes: alfalfa, clover, vetch, 2) Grain Legumes: also known as pulses. Peas, Lentils, Cowpea, dry beans of many types, Garbanzo, Peanuts, and Soybeans belong to this group. 3) Garden Bloom Legumes: Laburnum, Acacia, Mimosa. 4) Industrial and Pharmaceutical legumes: Indigo, Guar gum, for food additives and fracking, Acacia for gum; *Derris* for insecticide rotenone, White clover, Sweet clover, and alfalfa for honey and hay. 5) Timber: *Acacia, Dalbergia, Castanospermum.*6) Vegetable legumes: Various beans, peas, Dolichos bean, Guar. Vigna 7). Oil seed legumes: *Sesbania* (Sesame), Soybeans, Peanuts, 8) Medicinal/ spice legumes: There are many legumes whose roots, bark, flowers and seeds are used for treating medically relevant conditions other than as nutritional sources e.g. Fenugreek, Licorice.

This section will focus mainly on the grain and vegetable legumes. The 68th UN General Assembly declared 2016 the International Year of Pulses (IYP) (A/RES/68/231). "The IYP 2016 aims to heighten public awareness of the nutritional benefits of pulses as part of sustainable food production aimed towards food security and nutrition. The Year will create a unique opportunity to encourage connections throughout the food chain that would better utilize pulse-based proteins, further global production of pulses, better utilize crop rotations and address the challenges in the trade of pulses" (Quote from FAO).

Grain Legumes or Pulses

1. Phaseolus Beans *(Phaseolus vulgaris):* **Plantae; Division: Angiosperms, Class Eudicots; Order: Fabales, Family: Leguminosae/ Fabaceae; Chromosome Number: 2n = 22:**

This is a common term covering many different bean varieties. They include Field beans, Kidney bean, Pinto bean, Navy bean, Northern bean, Black bean/Black Turtle bean, Cranberry bean, English bean/French green beans, Molasses face bean, Wax bean. There are more than 2,500 different varieties of *P. vulgaris*. All have trifoliate compound leaves, bilaterally symmetrical, pink, red, white or yellow flowers, and pods that contain from three to a dozen or more usually kidney-shaped seeds. The pods come in

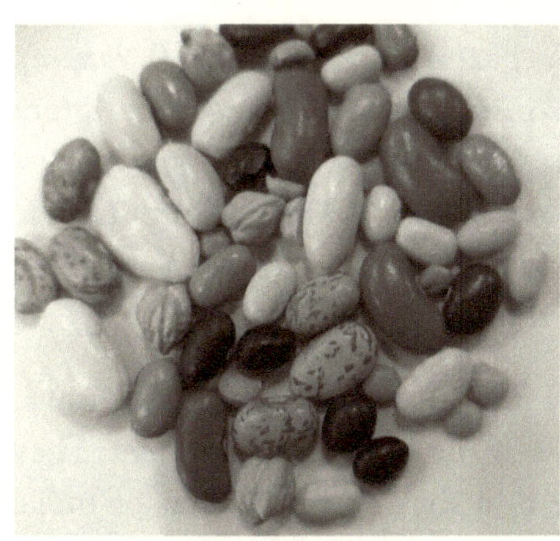

Bean varieties

various shades and combinations of green, purple, and yellow. Wax beans are so named because their pods are waxy and light yellow-green which makes them easy to see amidst the foliage, and purple-podded varieties are popular for the same reason. There are dwarf or bush varieties that support themselves, and trailing or climbing varieties (called pole beans) that need support and may extend 15 ft (4.6 m) or more in length. (Beans climb by twining; they do not have tendrils.) The beans inside the pods come in many colors.

The various types of beans usually are named for their culinary use, especially the stage of development at which they are eaten. Those grown for the immature pods are called snap, string, French or green beans; important cultivars are 'Blue Lake' and 'Kentucky Wonder.' The stringless varieties are usually grown commercially for canning and freezing. 'Romano' and 'Spanish Meralda' are flat-podded stringless snap beans. When the pods swell but have not yet dried, the beans inside are called horticultural or shelly beans; types usually grown for this stage include flageolet, 'Jacob's Cattle' and cranberry beans. When fully dried, the beans are called dry or soup beans and well-known types are navy beans, pinto beans, kidney beans, and black turtle beans. A fourth kind of bean is the popping bean or nuna, grown in the South American Andes and cooked like popcorn. All varieties of *P.vulgaris* can be eaten in any stage of development.

2. **Other Bean species**: Lima beans/butter beans (*P. lunata*), Scarlet runner bean (*Phaseolus coccineus*), Mung bean/Green gram (*Phaselus radiatus/Vigna radiatus*) Black gram/urad bean (*Vigna mungo/ Phaselus mungo*), Tepary bean (*Phaselus acutifolius*) belong to the genus *Phaseolus* but are categorized as different species. Some of these are also listed now as belonging to a different genus namely *Vigna*.

The mung bean (*Vigna radiata*) and urad/black gram (*P. Mungo/ V. Mungo*) are important native plants of the Indian subcontinent. They are both significant sources of protein in the vegetarian diets of India. Both are now grown extensively in South East Asia, Africa and in South and N. America as components of bean sprouts. Both species have pinnate trifoliate leaves with papilionaceous flowers.

Lima beans (*P. Lunatus*) are twining vines or herbaceous bushes. They are perennials, but are usually grown as annuals. The twining pole types can climb more than 12 ft (3.7 m) up a trellis or leaf thatched roof in the tropics. Some of the bush types stay under 2 ft (0.6 m) tall. The leaves have three leaflets, each 2–5 in (5–12.7 cm) long. The flowers are small, white to yellowish. Depending on cultivar, the pods can be 2–6 in (5–15.24 cm) long and an inch or so wide. There are more than a hundred lima bean cultivars.

The Tepary bean (*P. acutifolius*) is a twining annual vine with leaflets in threes, pale purple flowers, and 3–4 in (7–9 cm) pods. The pods are hairy, green when fresh and dry to a light straw color. Each pod usually has five or six small beans that look like little lima beans. Wild Tepary are quite vines, scrambling over desert shrubs and cacti. The cultivated varieties (var. latifolius) are semi-vining or bush types. Tepary beans are grown in desert and semi-desert conditions in Arizona, Mexico and southward to Costa Rica.

Runner beans (*P. coccineus*) are long, twining perennial vines that are usually grown as annuals. Leaves are trifoliate and each leaflet is broad oval and 4–5 in (10–12.7 cm) long. The flowers in most cultivars are bright scarlet red, and shaped like typical bean family flowers with the two lowermost petals united into a "keel." The uppermost petal modified into a hood like "standard," and the lateral petals modified into spreading "wings. The flowers are clustered on many-flowered racemes 10 in (25 cm) long. There can be as many as 20 flowers on a single flowering stalk. The legumes (pods) range from 6–12 in (15–30 cm) in length and the seeds are about an inch long, with 6–10 seeds per pod. The most well-known cultivars are Scarlet Runner, Black Runner, 'White Dutch Runner, Case Knife and tinted Lady. The varieties 'Butler' and Polestar' are stringless cultivars with very long pods to 12 in (30.5 cm). 'Hammond's Dwarf' and 'Pickwick Dwarf' are non-climbing bush types that mature 2–3 weeks earlier than the running kinds.

3. Vicia Beans/Faba bean *(Vicia* sp.): Kingdom: Plantae; Division: Angiosperms, Class Eudicots; Order: Fabales, Family: Leguminosae/ Fabaceae; Chromosome number: 2n = 12.

Broad bean/Field bean (*Vicia faba*), are edible members of a larger group that are commonly referred as vetches. Broad bean plants are essentially bush-like without tendrils or twining properties. They grow to a height of 3–5 ft. They have comparatively large innately compound leaves. Flowers are borne in clusters and are white or pink. Fruits are leathery pods with black/brown seeds. **Health note:** A diet that is based on fava bean causes a hemophilic disease known as favism in certain individuals with a defect in the glucose – 6-phosphate dehydrogenase gene (G6PD) that is prevalent in many Mediterranean countries where fava beans are a staple food.

4. Vigna Beans *(Vigna* sp.). Kingdom: Plantae; Division: Angiosperms, Class Eudicots; Order: Fabales, Family: Leguminosae/ Fabaceae, Chromosome number 2n = 22. There are many important species of Vigna namely: Adzuki beans (*Vigna angularis*), Asparagus/ Snake or yard long beans (*Vigna unguiculata* subsp. Sesquipedalis): Bambara Groundnut/Earth pea (*Vigna subterranea*), cow pea (*Vigna unguiculata*), Rice bean (*Vigna umbellate*), Moth bean (*Vigna aconitifolia*), Mung bean or green gram (V. radiata), Black gram or urad bean (V. mungo), as well as a number of wild species.

a. **Adzuki beans, *(Vigna angularis)*:** Depending on variety, Adzuki beans can be erect herbs or twining vines. The flowers are yellow. The pendent pods are slender, 3–5 in (7–12 cm) long, and contain up to a dozen little red beans with cream-colored seams.

b. **Cowpea/black eyed peas *(Vigna unguiculata)*. Kingdom: Plantae; Division: Angiosperms, Class: Eudicots; Order: Fabales, Family: Leguminosae/Fabaceae**

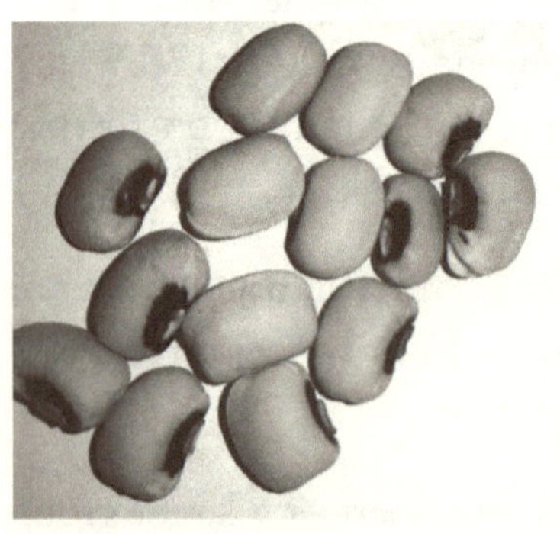

Cowpea

Cowpea includes many kinds of edible legumes. There are three sub species: 1. *Vigna unguiculata* ssp. Unguiculata: This subspecies include cowpeas, field peas, black eyed peas, Crowder peas, white acre, Zipper cream, southern peas. 2. *Vigna unguiculata* ssp. Cylindrical: This subspecies include Marble peas, Catjang peas and

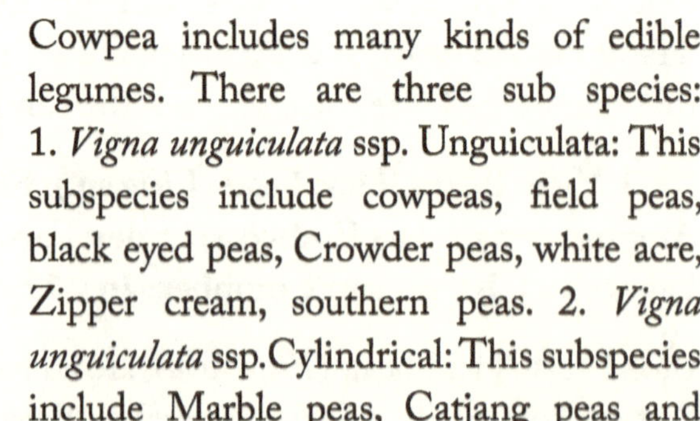

Jerusalem peas. 3. *V. sesquipedalis*: This subspecies include Asparagus peas or Yard long peas.

Plants are sprawling vines that grow on the ground or twine around supports. Most are annuals but the sub species cylindrical is a perennial. Flowers are white/pink and exhibit the typical Ligule features. The pods are long and cylindrical with varying lengths. When mature, the seeds can be felt or seen bulging out from the pods like pearls. The seeds have a colored eye representing the hilum.

    c. **Moth bean *(Vigna aconitifolia)*. Kingdom: Plantae; Division: Angiosperms, Class Eudicots; Order: Fabales, Family: Leguminosae/Fabaceae Chromosome number, 2n = 22.** The pods, sprouts and protein rich seeds of this crop are commonly consumed in India. This bean is an herbaceous creeper. Pods are yellow/brown. Seeds are high in protein.

    d. **Earth beans, *(Vigna subterranean)*:** This is one of the most important legumes of semi-arid West Africa. The seedpods grow underground as in peanuts. The seeds are rich in protein.

    e. **Black gram *(Vigna mungo/Phaselus mungo)*: Kingdom: Plantae; Division: Angiosperms, Class: Eudicots; Order: Fabales, Family: Leguminosae/Fabaceae Chromosome number, 2n = 22**

The plants are natives of India. The plants are erect or semi erect trailing herbaceous bushes. Like most legumes, they have trifoliate leaves and typical legume-type flowers. The seeds are borne in slender pods. Seeds have a black exterior skin. The whole seed along with skin are used in some culinary preparations wheras in most cases, the skin is removed and the beige colored cotyledons known as Urad dhal is cooked, ground into flour and or fermented for preparing

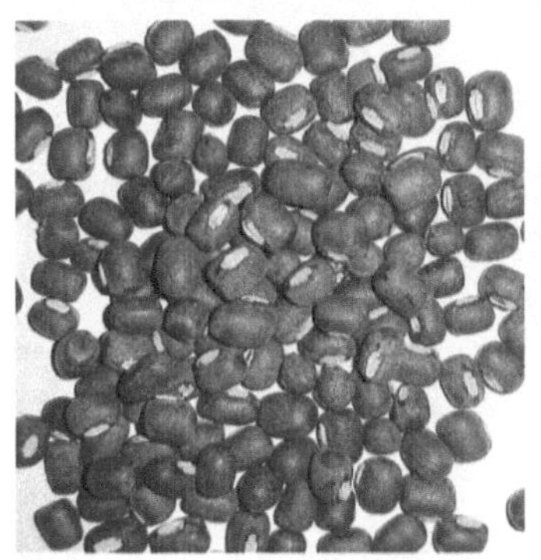

Black gram

food items. The seeds are very nutritious with a protein content of over 25%. The seeds of the urad plant are an important source of protein comparable to soybeans for vegetarians.

f. **Green gram/mung bean** *(Vigna radiata/Phaselus aureus/ P.radiatus):* **Kingdom: Plantae; Division: Angiosperms, Class: Eudicots; Order: Fabales, Family: Leguminosae/ Fabaceae Chromosome number 2n = 22**

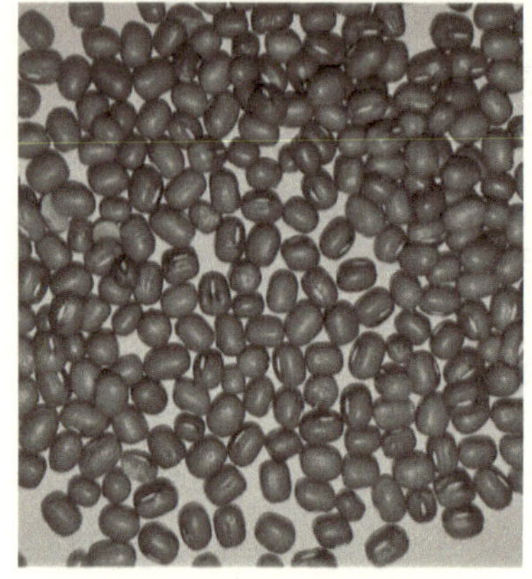
Green gram

The mung bean is widely grown in the Middle East and in particular the Indian sub-continent. The plants are also grown in China, Thailand and other south Asian countries. Plants are climbing runners or small bushes with trifoliate leaves. The seeds have greenish skin that is often removed before cooking although in many cuisines, the whole seed is cooked. The seeds are also sprouted as bean sprouts and consumed in salads and in stir-fried preparations. The seeds are rich in protein (23%) and are rich in various vitamins and minerals.

5. Other dry beans: Horse gram (Dolichos *biflorus)***, Chromosome number: 2n = 20.**

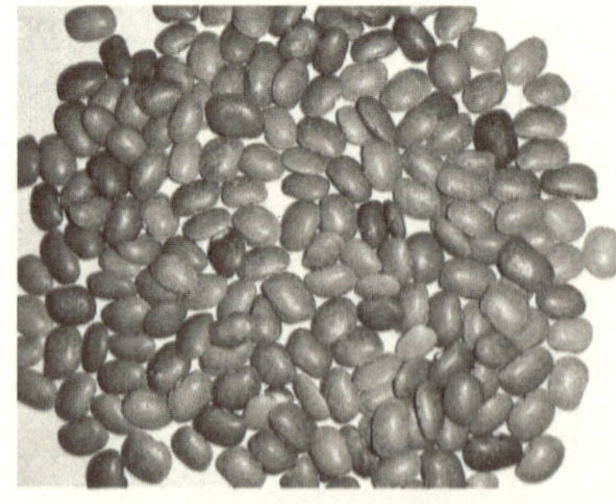
Horse Gram

Horse gram/Madras gram/Kulthi bean/Hurali (Macrotyloma uniflorum syn Dolichos biflorus): Kingdom: Plantae, Division: Angiosperm, Class: Eudicots; Order: Fabales Family: Fabaceae.

Horse gram is an annual herbaceous climbing plant that grows in semi-arid regions mainly in Indian subcontinent, Africa, Malaysia, Indonesia, Australia and Carribean islands. The climbing stems are hairy and bear trifoliate lanceolate leaves. Small yellow flowers grow in clusters from the leaf axils. The flowers are 1.3 cm to 2 cm long. Fruits (pods) with 4–8 seeds are slightly curved. Dry seeds are round and flattened. Seeds are brownish-black. Seeds are cooked, pan fried or powdered along with the seed coat and used in food preparations. Seed sprouts are also either cooked or used in salads. Dry seeds or seeds soaked in water are used as cattle food. Removal of the seed coat reduces the health benefits of this legume. **Health:** Ayurveda uses horse gram to treat a variety of conditions ranging from rheumatism to worm removal, treating conjunctivitis and hemorrhoids/piles. It is also an expectorant for cough relief. Horse gram is also considered good for lowering cholesterol, hyperglycemia and dissolving kidney stones. Horse gram seeds have higher trypsin inhibitor and hemagglutinin activities than most seeds and as such, it could stimulate pancreatic hyperplasia if consumed as a sole source of food.

Pigeon pea/Tuvar/Toor dhal/Arhar dhal, *(Cajanus cajan)*: **Kingdom: Plantae, Division: Angiospermae, Class: Eudicots, Rosids, Order: Fabales, Family: Fabaceae. Chromosome number: 2n = 22**

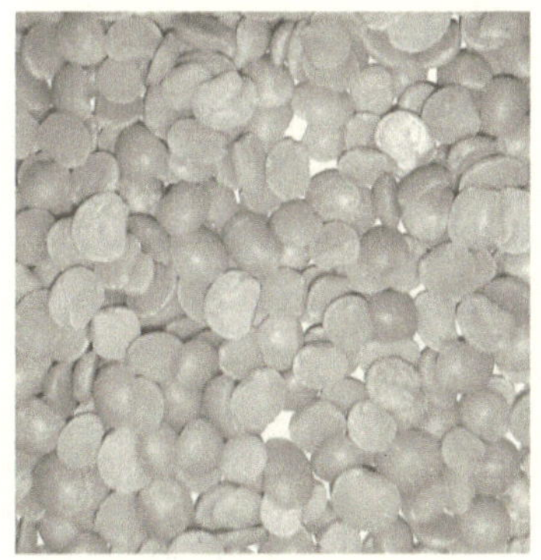

Pigeon pea

Pigeon pea is a very popular source of legume protein along with soybeans and lentils for vegetarians. A perennial plant had been domesticated in India for over three thousand years. It is now an important food grain in Asia, Africa, Latin America and many other tropical and sub-tropical parts of the world. Pigeon pea is a perennial that can grow into a small tree.

Pigeon pea (*Cajanus Cajan*) is a perennial shrub/tree plant that extends up to 10 feet at maturity. Pigeon pea grows well in most climates and requires very little maintenance in moist, nutrient-rich soil. The pigeon pea has an average life span of five years. Seeds are produced in pods. Generally, the seed coat is removed before the nutritious cotyledon is split in two and used as food by cooking or as flour. The seedpods along with the young immature seeds are also edible as vegetables. Sprouted seeds are also a good source of food. **Health:** Pigeon peas are a good source of protein but lacks the essential amino acids methionine and cysteine.

Lentil/Masur dhal *(Lens culinaris):* **Kingdom: Plantae, Division: Angiospermae, Class: Eudicots, Rosids, Order: Fabales, Family: Fabaceae. Chromosome number 2n = 14.** Lentil is an edible pulse whose seeds after removal of skin are red-orange or yellow depending on the variety. The outer skin is either brown or black. The lentil seeds are used as cooked food directly or after removing the seed coat/skin. Seeds are protein rich and contain a high percentage of resistant starch that is digested only slowly and hence is good as a diabetic food.

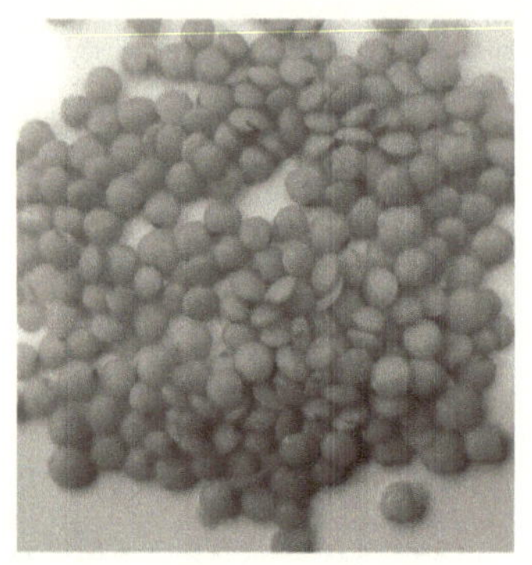

Orange Lentil

Plants are bushy annuals growing to a height of about 1.5–2 ft (40 cm) with two seeds in each pod. The plants are drought resistant and grow in semi-arid regions as well as temperate cold weather regions in Canada. Canada is the world's top producer of lentils followed by India. Lentils are a common food item in Northern India and are a major food source in the Middle East in particular Iran.

Health: Lentils like most legumes contain phytic acid as well as anti-nutrient factors (anti-tripsinases) which lower the absorption of minerals and increase pressure on the pancreas to produce more trypsin to counter the anti-nutrient factors. However, digestibility of lentils is increased by boiling and heat cooking as well as by sprouting the seeds. Lentils remain one of the most important sources of protein especially in the vegetarian diet.

Chickpeas/Garbanzo/Bengal gram *(Cicer arietinum)*: **Kingdom: Plantae, Division: Angiospermae, Class: Eudicots, Rosids, Order: Fabales, Family: Fabaceae. Chromosome number: 2n = 16.**

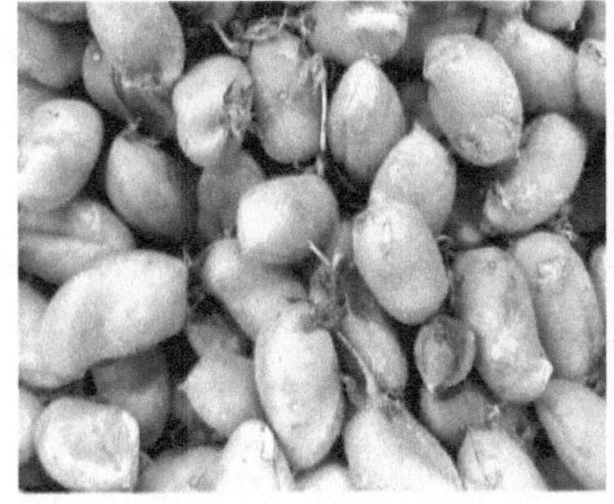

Garbanzo pods

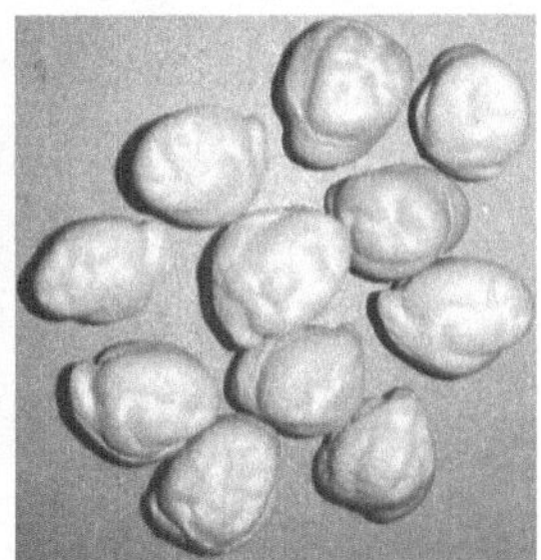

Beige Garbanzo

Chickpeas are also known as Garbanzo, Ceci bean, Chana dhal, Bengal gram, and Kabuli chana. The seeds are enclosed in a black, beige or brown skin that is brittle upon drying. The cotyledonory seeds inside are pale yellow in color. Seeds with or without skin are consumed as food after cooking. In many cases, the skin is removed and the seeds inside are split and used for preparing culinary items. Powdered seeds without skin are also used for making Hummus (Middle East) or many different food products in different parts of the globe. There are three main varieties of chickpeas namely: Desi with small dark brown seeds, Bombay chana with larger seeds and Kabuli with large seeds and lighter skin. A fourth variety with large black seed coats is grown in Italy. Seeds are generally cooked and used as food in salads, cooked foods and garbanzo flour known as besan in India is used to make various foods. In addition, the whole seed with skin are also fried and popped as a snack food. Chickpea leaves are also rich in protein and can be consumed as a leaf vegetable.

The plant grows to 20–50 cm (8–20 in) high and has small, feathery leaves on either side of the stem. Chickpeas are a type of pulse, with one seedpod containing two or three peas. It has white flowers with blue, violet, or pink veins. **Health:** Chickpeas have a high protein and carbohydrate content. Like all legumes, the seeds contain anti-nutrients that can impair absorption of minerals and digestibility but these are overcome by food processing.

Soybeans *(Glycine max)*: **Kingdom: Plantae; Division: Angiospermae, Class: Eudicots; Family: Fabaceae/**

Leguminosae; Genus and species: *Glycine max.* **Chromosome number: 2n = 40**

Soybean plants are erect annuals growing like bushes to a height

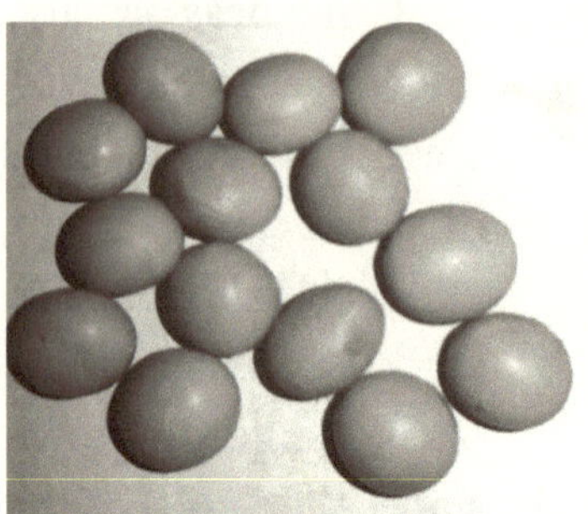

Soybeans

ranging from 0.6 – 7 ft. depending on the variety. The leaves are trifoliate and are typically palmate veined as in all dicots. The flowers that are small with colors ranging from white to pink and purple arise from the axils of the leaves. The flowers are self-pollinated and set fruits in the form of pods that contain 24 seeds per pod. The seeds are leguminous seeds. The cotyledons are rich in protein, carbohydrates, vitamins, minerals and fats. The oil has 16% saturated fat 23% monounsaturated fat and 58% polyunsaturated fat (Table). The leaves, stems and especially the pods are red-hairy. Pods are held close to the stems and are 2–3 in (5–7.5 cm) long with 2–4 black, yellow, white, or green seeds. There are three main types of soybeans: 1. Yellow seeded: These are used for making soybean flour, oil and fermented soybean cheese etc. 2. The black seeded types are usually fermented and made into sauces and fermented black beans. 3. The green and white seeded (or edamame) beans are the most tender and flavorful, and are often used as vegetables.

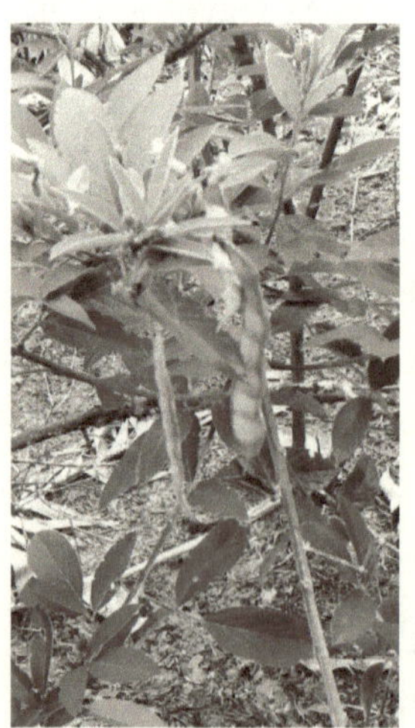

7. Other bean Types:

Wing bean/Goa bean/Manila bean/ (*Psophocarpus tetragonolobus*) Kingdom: Plantae, Division: Angiospermae, Class: Eudicots, Order: Fabales, Family: Fabaceae. Chromosome number: 2n = 18

The winged bean is a multi-use plant wherein the leaves, tubers, flowers and seeds are edible after processing. Plants grow in tropical and subtropical conditions mainly in

Southern India, Sri Lanka, and Malaysian archipelago, Indonesia, the Philippines, Thailand and Papua New Guinea. Plants are perennial herbs with twining stems, tuberous roots and seeds in pods with wings. Pods are waxy and semi-translucent. The beans inside the winged pods are a rich source of protein (~ 30%). Tuberous roots are also a good source of protein. Leaves and flowers are also edible. The pods have to be picked from plants at an early stage in development if it is being harvested as a vegetable source. Mature pods are inedible but the seeds are edible. Wing bean seed-flour can be used for culinary purposes. Winged bean flour can be used for making wing bean milk similar to soymilk.

Peas *(Pisum sativum)*: Garden peas *(Pisum sativum var sativum)*, Protein pea *(P. sativum var arvense)*, Kingdom: Plantae, Division: Angiospermae, Class: Eudicots, Order: Fabales, Family: Fabaceae, Chromosome number: 2n = 14.

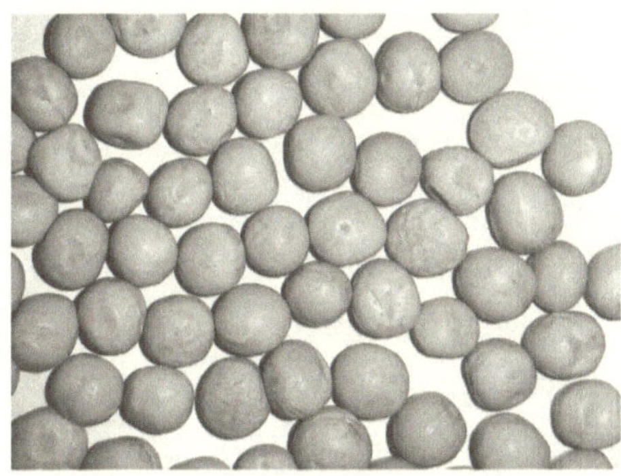

Dry Peas

There are many different varieties of garden peas. Most pea varieties require supports to grow. They are annual climbing herbs with tendrils. The field peas used as dry peas for soups, curries and broth belong to arvense variety. Snap peas are used mostly as vegetables.

Plants are rapid-growing, glabrous annual with angular or roundish hollow stems covered with a waxy bloom. Flowers are self-pollinated. In leafy types, leaves consist of one or more pairs of opposite leaflets borne on petioles together with several pairs of tendrils and a single or compound terminal tendril. Leaflets are broad and ovate with distinct ribs, and slightly toothed or entire. The plants are tap-rooted, 1 meter or more in depth, with numerous lateral roots. On each plant, inflorescences comprising one or two self-fertile flowers are borne on the end of axillary peduncles. Flower colour differs according to cultivar with white, pink, lavender, blue and purple represented. Pods containing several seeds, flattened when young but becoming roundish later are dehiscent along two sides. Seeds range in colour from green, yellow to brown and may be mottled.

Peanut *(Arachis)*: Peanut/groundnut *(Arachis hypogea):* **Kingdom: Plantae, Division: Angiospermae, Class: Eudicots, Order: Fabales, Family: Fabaceae Chromosome number: 2n = 40.** Peanuts are described under section on oil seeds.

Medicinal value and Toxicity

The seeds of all legumes are poor in the essential amino acid methionine and hence beans and other grain legumes should be enriched by adding other methionine containing grains, milk and milk products and or meat products.

Soybeans are rich in flavonoid compounds and plant estrogens. Soybeans are regarded as a natural remedy for menopause related problems. Soybeans contain natural estrogens geistein, daidzein and other phytoestrogens that help to control hot flashes, night sweats and vaginal drying inherent in menopause. Isoflavones in soy may also offer some relief for the pain, swelling, nausea and bleeding of endometriosis. Eating soybean products might also help in preventing hormone induced breast cancer.

Beans and lentils contain dietary fiber that in turn would help reduce or control gastrointestinal distress although the glycoprotein in legumes can also generate flatulence. Velvet beans (*Mucuna pruriens*) contain L-DOPA that is a precursor for dopamine and used in herbal medicine for treating Parkinson's disease.

Certain bean seeds like those of hyacinth beans contain cyanide and these have to be removed by boiling and cooking to destroy cyanoglucocides. Certain individuals with a mutation in the X-linked gene coding for the key enzyme glucose-6-phosphate dehydrogenase should not eat Fava beans since this bean triggers a reaction in this enzyme and causes a type of anemia called favism. Favism is endemic in the Mediterranean region and in particular in Egypt.

Most legume grains contain Phytohemagglutinin that causes diahorrea, bloating and nausea if consumed without processing by boiling in water for at least 10 minutes and in some cases 30 minutes. The legume Castor beans contains ricin that is a powerful cytotoxin and hence this bean is not edible. Caster bean oil is a powerful purgative.

Hemp/*Cannabis Sativa* as a Protein Food

Kingdom: Plantae, Division: Angiospermae, Class: Eudicots, Rosids, Order: Rosales, Family: Cannabaceae. Genus and Species: *Cannabis sativa*, Chromosome number: 2n = 16. Cannabis Sativa.

Modern plant taxonomists include *C. sativa*, *C. indica* and *C. ruderalis* as a single species namely C. sativa. The others are considered as sub species. The Cannabis known commonly as hemp is a variety that contains less than between 4–10 ppm of the psychoactive delta tetra hydro cannabinol (THC) and other cannabinoids. The plant is mainly used as a source of protein from seeds and as fiber from the stems. Hemp protein is made up of 35% albumin and 65% edestin, both being globulin types of protein. Seeds are small and contain Hemp oil which is a low smoking non-cooking oil rich in Omega 3 and omega 6 oils. The seeds are rich in hemp protein, which is consumed mainly as a protein supplement in drinks and used to enrich bakery products. Hemp should not be confused with other varieties of the same species that contain many cannabinoids especially THC and Cannabidiol (CBD).

Table 6 – Nutritional profile of important Phaseolus bean varieties per 100 g.

Nutrient	Black	Fava	French	Kidney	Lima	Navy	Northern	Pinto
Protein, G	21.25	26.12	18.81	23.58	21.46	22.33	21.86	21.42
Total lipid (fat), g	0.9	1.53	2.02	0.83	0.69	1.5	1.14	1.23
Carbohydrate, g	63.25	58.29	64.11	60.01	63.38	60.75	62.37	62.55
Fiber, total dietary, g	15.5	25	25.2	24.9	19	15.3	20.2	15.5
Sugars, total, G	2.12	5.7	NA	2.23	8.5	3.88	2.26	2.11
Calcium, Mg	160	103	186	143	81	147	175	113
Iron, Mg	8.7	6.7	3.4	8.2	7.51	5.49	5.47	5.07
Magnesium, Mg	160	192	188	140	224	175	189	176
Phosphorus, Mg	440	421	304	407	385	407	447	411
Potassium, Mg	1500	1062	1316	1406	1724	1185	1387	1393
Sodium, Mg	9	13	18	24	18	5	14	12
Zinc, Mg	2.2	3.14	1.9	2.79	2.83	3.65	2.31	2.28
Vitamin C, Mg	0	1.4	4.6	4.5	0	0	5.3	6.3
Thiamin, Mg	0.9	0.555	0.535	0.529	0.507	0.775	0.653	0.713
Riboflavin, Mg	0.193	0.333	0.221	0.219	0.202	0.164	0.237	0.212
Niacin, Mg	1.955	2.832	2.083	2.06	1.537	2.188	1.955	1.174
Vitamin B-6, Mg	0.286	0.366	0.401	0.397	0.512	0.428	0.447	0.474
Folates, DFE, µg	444	423	399	394	395	364	482	525
Vitamin B-12, µg	0	0	0	0	0	0	0	0
Vitamin A, µg	0	3	0	0	0	0	0	0
Vitamin A, IU	17	53	8	0	0	0	0	0
Vitamin E, mg	0.21	0.05	0	0.22	0.72	0.02	0.22	0.21
Vitamin D (D2 + D3)	0	0	0	0	0	0	0	0
Vitamin D µg	0	0	0	0	0	0	0	0
Vitamin K, µg	5.6	9	19	6	2.5	6	5.6	
Fatty acids, total, G	0.232	0.254	0.221	0.12	0.161	0.17	0.356	0.235
Fatty acids, mono, G	0.078	0.303	0.138	0.064	0.062	0.128	0.053	0.229
Fatty acids, polyun, G	0.387	0.627	1.207	0.457	0.309	0.873	0.477	0.407
Cholesterol, mg	0	0		0	0	0	0	0
Other	Lectins	Lectins	Lectins		Lectins		Lectins	

Table 7: Nutritional profile of Legume seed per 100 g

Nutrient	Adzuki	Black	Chick	Cow	Black	Lentils	Moth	Mung	Mungo	Peas	Pigeon	Soy
	Beans	Beans	peas	pea	Eye		Bean	Bean	Bean		Peas	beans
Protein	19.87	21.6	20.47	23.85	23.52	24.63	22.94	23.86	25.21	23.82	21.7	36.5
Total lipid (fat), G	0.53	1.42	6.04	2.07	1.26	1.06	1.61	1.15	1.64	1.16	1.49	19.9
Carbohydrate, g	62.9	62.36	62.95	59.64	60.03	63.35	61.52	62.62	58.99	63.74	62.78	30.2
Fiber, total dietary	12.7	15.5	12.2	10.7	10.6	10.7		16.3	18.3	25.5	15	9.3
Sugars, G		2.12	10.7		6.9	2.03		6.6		8		7.33
Calcium, Mg	66	123	57	85	110	35	150	132	138	37	130	277
Iron, Mg	4.98	5.02	4.31	9.95	8.27	6.51	10.85	6.74	7.57	4.82	5.23	15.7
Magnesium, Mg	127	171	79	333	184	47	381	189	267	49	183	280
Phosphorus, Mg	381	352	252	438	424	281	489	367	379	321	367	704
Potassium, Mg	1254	1483	718	1375	1112	677	1191	1246	983	823	1392	1797
Sodium, Mg	5	5	24	58	16	6	30	15	38	15	17	2
Zinc, Mg	5.04	3.65	2.76	6.11	3.37	3.27	1.92	2.68	3.35	3.55	2.76	4.89
Vitamin C, Mg	0	0	4	1.5	1.5	4.5	4	4.8	0	1.8	0	6
Thiamin, Mg	0.455	0.9	0.477	0.68	0.853	0.873	0.562	0.621	0.273	0.726	0.643	0.87
Riboflavin, Mg	0.22	0.193	0.212	0.17	0.226	0.211	0.091	0.233	0.254	0.215	0.187	0.87
Niacin, Mg	2.63	1.955	1.541	2.795	2.075	2.605	2.8	2.251	1.447	2.889	2.965	1.62
Vitamin B-6, mg	0.351	0.286	0.535	0.361	0.357	0.54	0.366	0.382	0.281	0.174	0.283	0.38
Folates, DFE, µg	622	444	557	639	633	479	649	625	216	274	456	375
Vitamin B-12, µg	0	0	0	0	0	0	0	0	0	0	0	0

Vitamin A, µg	1	0	3	2	3	2	2	6	1	7	1	1
Vitamin A, IU	17	17	67	33	50	39	32	114	23	149	28	22
Vitamin D (D2 + D3)	0	0	0.82	0	0.39	0.49	0	0.51	0	0.09	0	0.85
Vitamin E, µg		0.21	0		0	0		0		0	NA	0
Vitamin Klug		5.6	9		5	5		9		1.45	NA	47
Fatty acids, sat, g	0.191	0.366	0.603	0.542	0.331	0.154	0.364	0.348	0.114	0.161	0.33	2.88
Fatty acids, mooning	0.05	0.123	1.377	0.173	0.106	0.193	0.129	0.161	0.085	0.242	0.012	4.4
Fatty acids, polyun, g	113	0.61	2.731	0.889	0.542	0.526	0.75	0.384	1.071	0.495	0.814	11.3
Cholesterol		0	0		0	0		0		0	0	0
Other	Lectin	Lectin	Lectin	Lectin	Lectin	Lectin	Lectin	Lectin	Lectin	Lectin	Lectin	Lectin

References

Davis, D.W., Oelke, E.A., Oplinger, E.S., Doll, J.D., Hanson, C.V., and D.H. Putnam (1991): Cowpea. https://www.hort.purdue.edu/newcrop/cropmap/missouri/crop/pulse.html

Deshpande, U.S. and Deshpande, S.S. (1991) Legumes, In Foods of Plant origin; Production, Technology and Human Nutrition, Eds. Salunkhe, D.K.M and Deshpande, S.S. Pp137-300, Van Nostrand, Reinhold, New York, Pp 499.

Hardman, L.L., Oplinger, E.S. Schulte, E.E Doll, J.D., and G.L. Worf (1990): Fieldbean. https://hort.purdue.edu/newcrop/afcm/fieldbean.html.

http://www.oardc.ohio-state.edu/seedid/single.asp?strId = 159

http://www.uniprot.org/taxonomy/3916

https://www.hort.purdue.edu/newcrop/cropmap/missouri/crop/pulse.html

Hymowitz, T, Boyd, J. "Ethnobotany and Agriculture Potential of the Winged Bean," Economic Botany 31 (2): 180. Doi: 10.1007/bf02866589.

Kadam, S.S, Salunkhe DK (1985). Nutritional composition, processing, and utilization of horse gram and moth bean, Crit Rev Food Sci Nutr 22 (1): 1–26. Doi: 10.1080/10408398509527416, PMID 3899515.

Ladizinsky G. (1987). Pulse domestication: Fact & Fiction. Economic Botany, 43(1): 31-34 19

Muddy AN, Yu N, Arkoma HM (2014). Nutritional and health benefits of pulses, Appl Physiol Nutr Metab 39 (11): 1197–204. Doi: 10.1139/apnm-2013-0557, PMID 25061763.

National Research Council (U.S.), (1975): Underexploited Tropical Plants with Promising Economic Value, 2nd Edition, U.S. National Academies.

Oelke, E.A., Oplinger, E.S. Hanson, C.V. Davis, D.W. Putnam, D.H… Fuller, E.I and C.J. Rosen (1991): Dry pea. https://hort.purdue.edu/newcrop/afcm/drypea.html

Oplinger, E.S.. Hardman, L.L, Oelke, E.A. Kaminski, A.R. Schulte, E.E., and J.D. Doll (1990): Chickpea: https://hort.purdue.edu/newcrop/afcm/chickpea.html

Oplinger, E.S., Hardman, L.L. Kaminski, A.R. Combs, S.M., and J.D. Doll (1990): Moonbeam. https://hort.purdue.edu/newcrop/afcm/mungbean.html

Oplinger, E.S., Putnam, D.H., Doll, J.D., and S.M. Combs (1989): Fababean.https://hort.purdue.edu/newcrop/afcm.htm.

Yadav, S.S. et al. Lentil: An Ancient Crop for Modern Times, (2007): Springer Verlag, ISBN 97814020633121.

Tovar J (1996): "Bioavailability of carbohydrates in legumes: digestible and indigestible fractions." Arch Latinoam Nutr 44 (4 Suppl 1): 36S–40S, PMID 9137637.

USDA, NRCS. (2011): The PLANTS Database (http://plants.usda.gov, 19 April 2011). National Plant Data Center, Baton Rouge, LA 70874-4490 USA:

Vidal-Valverde C, Frias F, Estrella I, Gorospe MJ, Ruiz R, Bacon J (1994).:"Effect of processing on some antinutritional factors of lentils," J Agric Food Chem 42 (10): 2291–2295. Doi: 10.1021/jf00046a039.

Chapter 7

Oil Seeds

Oils extracted from various plant seeds are an essential part of human nutrition. These oils known as vegetable oils are used extensively in food preparations. These oils may be saturated, monounsaturated and polyunsaturated fatty acids. The major oil seed producing plants are Palm, Soybean, Rape seed, Canola, sunflower, peanut, and Cotton seeds, African Palm, Coconut, Olive, Corn, Sesame, Mustard and Safflower. Other oil seeds which have a minor role but which may have some cooking and medicinal value include Rice bran, walnut, almond, and flax seed oils. The relative content of Omega 3, Omega 6 or Omega 9 oils are considered important for cardio-protective effects such as reducing triglycerides, raising high density lipo-protein (HDL) and lowering Low density lipoprotein (LDL).

All fatty acids are composed of chains of carbon, hydrogen and oxygen atoms. The differences between fatty acids lie in the molecular configuration, producing differing health effects between fats. Saturated fats are defined as those where the c-c linkages are single bonds, whereas, mono unsaturated fats are those which have at least one double bond and rest are single bonds, polyunsaturated are those with more than 2 double bonds and trans fats are those unsaturated oils/fats that have been hydrogenated at their double bonds. Monounsaturated and polyunsaturated fats are known by another name: omega fatty acids. There are three types of omega fatty acids: omega-3, omega-6 and omega-9. Omega-3 and omega-6 fatty acids are essential polyunsaturated fats that cannot be made by the body. Therefore, Omega 3 and 6 fatty acids have to be obtained from food such as fish oil and certain plant seeds as Flax seeds (See Table). They are considered essential fatty acids because the body cannot manufacture them. Omega-9 fatty acids are from a family of monounsaturated fats that also are beneficial when obtained in food. Canola and Sunflower Oils are uniquely high in Omega-9 (monounsaturated) fatty acid.

Omega-3 fatty acid (Alpha-linolenic acid) is an essential fatty acid that plays an important role in brain function and may help fight against cardiovascular disease. The American Heart Association recommends a diet in which fatty fish, like salmon, herring, sardines and tuna are consumed at least twice a week. However, most plant oils do not provide Omega 3 but Flax seeds, walnut seeds and oil, brazil nuts seed and oil, canola oil, hemp oil, wheat germ oil, many grains and nuts supply moderate amounts. Oils like Hemp oil have a low smoking range and are not usable for frying. Within the body, omega-3 fatty acids are converted to DHA and EPA (docosahexaenoic acid and eicosapentaenoic acid, respectively). DHA and EPA are highly unsaturated fats that play very important roles in the vision development and brain function of infants. Lack of DHA has been associated with Alzheimer's disease that implies that a proper supply of Omega – 3 is needed to prevent occurrence or progression of this disease. Omega 3 oils are considered beneficial for controlling asthma, diabetes, arthritis, osteoporesis, skin conditions, cholestrol control, high blood pressure, attention deficit syndrome, depression, macular degeneration and digestive problems. Anecdotal and limited population studies indicate that foods rich in Omega-3 oils tend to reduce incidence and or progression of breast, colon and prostate cancers but these studies are inconclusive since some studies indicate that alpha linolenic acid from Omega – 3 is not converted in some patients to the metabolically active DHA and EPA and hence not effective.

Olive oil, wheat germ oil, grape seed oil, pistachios, sesame oil, sunflower oil, safflower oil, cottonseed oil, most nuts, pumpkin seeds and green vegetables contain Omega-6 oil.

Omega-9 fatty acids are mono unsaturated fatty acids that are produced by the body naturally provided there are sufficient omega 3 and 6 fatty acids that are obtained from food. Omega 9 is present in avacados, pecans, cashews, almonds, hazel-nuts, pistachio, macadamia, chia seeds, olives, and many nuts (Refer to table).This type of fatty acid is important for maintaining improved immune function and proper levels of cholesterol which is a part of cell membranes.

Although omega-3, omega-6 and omega-9 fatty acids all serve different functions within the body, the evidence points out that incorporating balanced proportions of both essential and non-essential fatty acids are necessary for maintaining overall heart health and general wellness. Omega-6 fatty acids are more inflammatory than those of omega-3 are. Balanced amounts of both Omega-6 and Omega-3 are considered essential for good health. While a ratio of 1:1 is good, many consider a ratio of Omega 6 to Omega-3 of 1:4 but some authors report that a ratio of 4:1 is a good balance. The ratios of omega-6 to omega-3 fatty acids in some common vegetable oils are: canola 1:2, hemp 3:1, soybean 7:1, olive 13:1, flax 1:3, cottonseed (almost no omega-3), peanut (no omega-3), grape seed oil (almost no omega-3) and corn oil 46:1 ratio of omega-6 to omega-3.

Caution: Omega-3 fatty acids may increase the effects of blood-thinning medications, including aspirin, warfarin (Coumadin), and clopedigrel (Plavix). Taking aspirin and omega-3 fatty acids may be helpful in some circumstances (such as in heart disease), but they should only be taken together under the supervision of a provider.Taking omega-3 fatty acid supplements may increase fasting blood sugar levels. Caution should be exercised while also taking medications to lower blood sugar, such as glipizide (Glucotrol and Glucotrol XL), glyburide (Micronase or Diabeta), glucophage (Metformin), or insulin since omega 3 fatty acids could offset the effects of anti-diabetic medications.

Coconuts *(Cocos nucifera):* Kingdom: Plantae, Division: Angiospermae, Class: Monocotyledonae, Order: Arecales, Family: Arecaceae, Genus: *Cocos nucifera.* Chromosome number: 2n = 32

Coconuts are large palm trees that can grow to a height of about 100 ft or more. There are shorter varieties that grow to about 10 ft. The plants are monocots. The tree trunk is woody and ribbed. The ribs indicate the position of older leaves that have fallen off when the tree grows. Ultimately, when the tree has fully matured, it will have a crown of pinnate compound leaves wherein, the leaflets are more than 2 ft long. Flowers and fruits are produced in bunches at the tree crown. The coconut is not a nut but a fruit called a drupe. It has an outer green or yellowish brown/ orange exocarp enclosing the fibrous mesocarp known as the coir and enclosing the "nut" with a hard shell. The shell encloses a liquid endosperm with many nuclei and the cellular endosperm that is the edible coconut meat. The coconut water that is the liquid endosperm is nutritious. It contains sugars, minerals and nutrients. It is considered good as an osmotically valuable drink to avoid dehydration. There is a tiny embryo that eventually grows on germination. The white colored edible cellular endosperm when dried is called as copra. The copra is extracted to produce coconut oil.

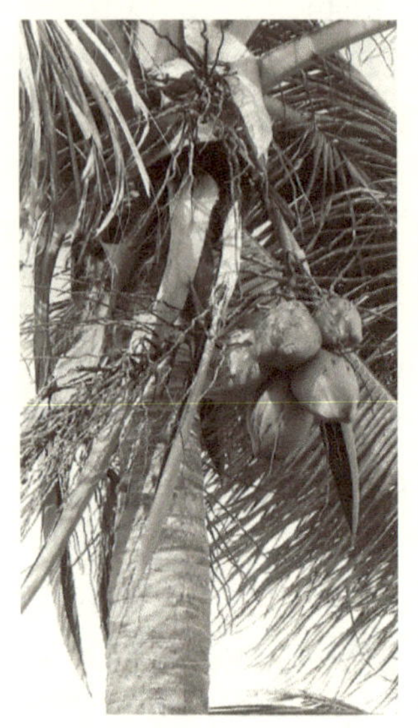

Coconut palm

Coconut oil is highly saturated medium chain triglycerides. Natural coconut oil contains 91 % saturated fats 6% monounsaturated fats and 3% polyunsaturated fats. Coconut oil freezes even at room temperatures. **Health:** Most health organizations like the World Health Organization, U.S. Food and Drugs Administration, American heart Association and several others warn against the use of coconut oil because of its high saturated fat level. However, some recent studies indicate that consumption of coconut oil is not as harmful as originally thought and that there are benefits for people suffering from Alzheimer's disease. Since a high percentage of the saturated fats in Coconut oil are made of lauric acid, which raises HDL levels, it is thought that coconut oil may actually be beneficial. The question of the interrelationships of consuming coconut oil and heart disease is now being debated. Many health food and mainstream grocery stores market Coconut oil. In traditional folk medicine, coconut oil is a base for many Ayurvedic preparations of India and in many cosmetic preparations worldwide since it is believed to control candidiasis and improve skin health.

Coconut oil is used for treating diabetes, heart disease, chronic fatigue, Crohn's disease, irritable bowel syndrome (IBS), Alzheimer's disease, thyroid conditions, raising energy levels and boosting the immune system. Ironically, despite coconut oil's high calorie and saturated fat content, some people use it to lose weight and lower cholesterol. However, the popular usage claims cited above have not been scientifically evaluated.

Corn *(Zea Mays):* Kingdom: Plantae, Division: Angiospermae, Class: Monocotyledonae, Order: Poales Family: Poaceae. Chromosome number: 2n = 20.

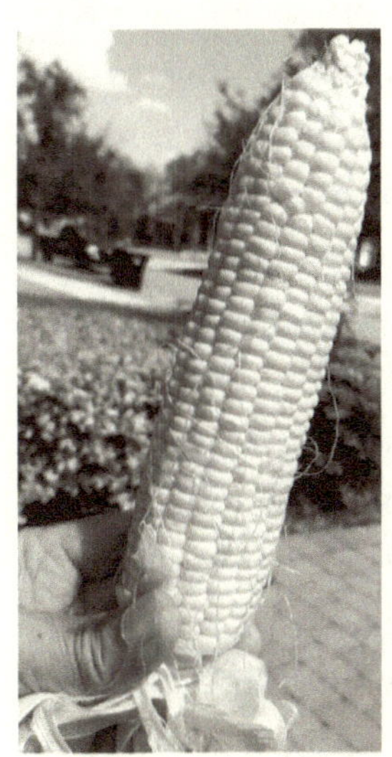

Corn on cob

The section on Cereals has already covered relevant details about corn (see cereals page). Here we will confine ourselves to corn oil. Corn oil contains about 13% saturated fats, 27 % monounsaturated fats and 57% polyunsaturated fats. The polyunsaturated fat contains high amounts of linoleic acid that is a dietary essential necessary for integrity of the skin, cell membranes, and the immune system and for synthesis of icosanoids. Icosanoids are necessary for reproductive, cardiovascular, renal and gastrointestinal functions and resistance to disease. Because of its low content of saturated fatty acids, which raises cholesterol, and its high content of polyunsaturated fatty acids, which lowers cholesterol, consumption of corn oil can be effective in lowering cholesterol. At the same time, it has a high amount of omega 6 fatty acids compared to omega 3 fatty acids and hence, consumption of large amounts of corn oil products may increase the chances of breast cancer in postmenopausal women and also prostate cancer in older patients. Corn oil contains vitamin E and phytosterols. Phytosterols are said to help lower cholesterol uptake from the intestine and also production of cholesterol in the liver.

Cotton (*Gossypium sp*): Kingdom: Plantae, Division: Angiospermae, Class: Eudicots, Order: Malvales, Family: Malvaceae. Chromosome number: 4n = 52. Wild cotton, 2n = 26

Cotton is basically divided into two major groups namely, Asiatic old world cotton *Gossypium arboretum* and *G. herbaceum* and new world or American cotton *Gossypium hirsutum* and *G. barbadense*. The plant is a shrub grown mostly for harvesting the fiber but the seeds are valuable sources of oil and of potentially valuable phytomedicine such as Gossypol. The dicotyledonous seeds germinate in five to ten days, producing palmate five lobed leaves. Branches arise from the nodes and produce flower buds that are called squares. The squares mature into bisexual flowers that after fertilization turn into fruits called bolls that contain the fiber and seeds. The cotton fiber is separated from the seeds by ginning. The seeds are dicotyledonous. The seeds contain about 26% saturated fats 18% monounsaturated and 52% polyunsaturated fats with hardly any omega-3 oil. **Health:** The highly saturated fat content is a cause for concern since saturated fats are linked to coronary diseases. The seeds contain gossypol that is a toxic polyphenol. Gossypol is a natural contraceptive and has been used particularly in China for this purpose. Gossypol also has antimalarial properties and is also under investigation as a potential anticancer compound. The crude oil is processed and refined to remove gossypol before it is marketed for edible commercial purposes.

Mustard (*Brassica nigra/B. juncea/Sinapis alba/B.alba*): Kingdom: Plantae; Division: Angiospermae, Class: Eudicots Order: Brassicales Family: Brassicaceae, Genus and species: *Brassica nigra* (Black); B.juncea (Brown), Sinapis *alba/B.alba* (White). Chromosome number: Amphi diploid = 18

Mustard is an annual herb related to rape, cauliflower, cabbage, turnip and horse radish. Oriental brown mustard (*B. juncea*), black mustard (*B. nigra*) and white mustard (*Sinapis Alba*) are three common types of mustard grown in different regions of the world. From very small seedlings, the plants grow rapidly and enter a phase of dense flowering. The blooms have an intense yellow color. The plants reach their full height of 1.5 to 2 m/5 to 61/2 feet after numerous green seedpods appear on their

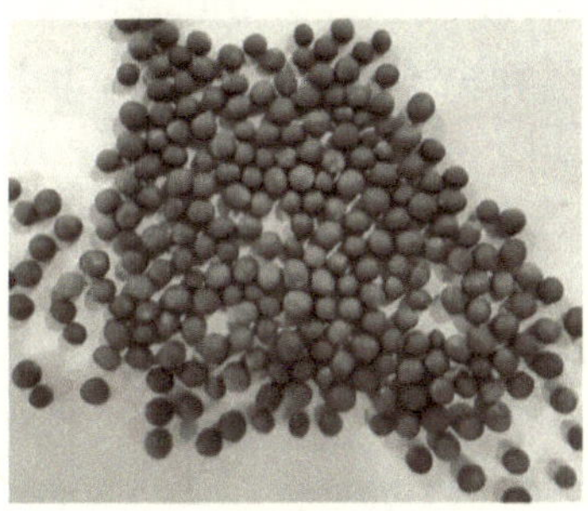

Mustard

branches. The pods of brown mustard contain up to 20 seeds each, those of white mustard contain up to 8 seeds. Mustard seeds are nearly globular in shape finely pitted, odorless when whole and pungent-tasting. White mustard seeds are light yellow in color and about 2.5 mm 1/10 inch in diameter; brown mustard seeds are about the same size but are a darker yellow in color. The seeds of both types contain similar constituents: about 30 to 40 percent vegetable oil, a slightly smaller proportion of protein and a strong enzyme called myrosin. When dry or when ground into flour, the seeds are odorless but when the seed is chewed or when the flour is mixed with water a chemical reaction occurs between two of the constituents within mustard. In brown mustard, this action yields the volatile oil of mustard that has a pungent irritating odor and an acrid taste. In white mustard, the result is sinalbin mustard oil that is odorless nonvolatile oil that produces a sensation of heat on the tongue. The stem and leaves are used as a green vegetable. The seeds are used as a condiment/spice and mustard paste is used as a flavoring agent for various dishes. The oil from mustard seeds is used for cooking although it has been largely replaced by canola oil in the North American continent. The oil is pungent due to the presence of allyl isothiocyanate. Mustard oil is 60% monounsaturated fatty acids, 21% polyunsaturated fats and 12 % saturated fats. The oil is rich in alpha lineolic acid and erucic acid. **Health:** Mustard oil contains over 45% erucic acid.

Erucic acid is considered toxic to heart and sale of mustard oil in the USA and European Union is allowed only for external use and not as cooking oil. However, data regarding the harmful effects of mustard oil on heart health is not conclusive and there are many reports questioning the rationale in banning the oil for cooking. The oil has been in use in sub continental India and in China for centuries. In the Indian subcontinent, Mustard oil is used for oil massages in order to strengthen muscles, improve peripheral circulation and development of bones

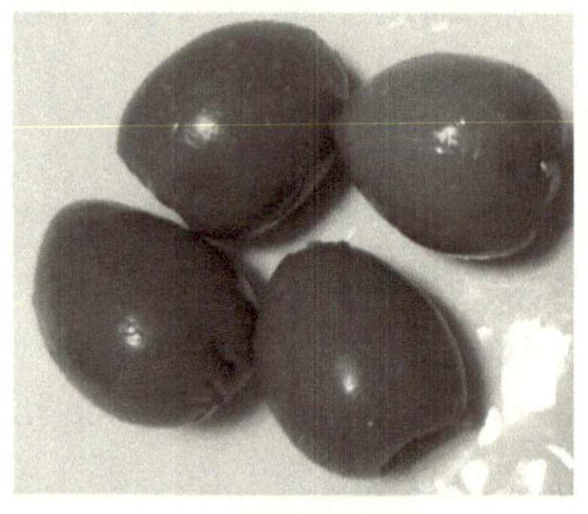

Olives

Olive *(Olea europeae):* **Kingdom: Plantae Division: Angiospermae, Class: Eudicots, Order: Lamiales Family:** *Oleaceae Genus* **and species:** Olea europeae. **Chromosome number, 2n = 46.**

The olive plant is one of the oldest cultivated plants originally grown in North Africa, and Mediterranean basin including Italy. Now, it is cultivated in many countries. The plant is an evergreen perennial tree growing to a height of about 25–50 ft depending on the variety. The leaves are green and oblong and flowers are found in inflorescences called racemes and are white in color. Fruits that develop after fertilization are green initially but become golden yellow to purple to black as they mature fully. The fruits enclose a typical dicotyledonous seed. The fruit contains oil glands from which oil is extracted. The olive fruit contains about 4% carbohydrates, 0.5% sugars, 1% protein, 34% dietary fibers and about 16 % fat and the rest of the fruit is made of cellulose, small amounts of vitamins and minerals and polyphenols. The oil contains 14% saturated fats, 73% monounsaturated fats, 13 % polyunsaturated fats. The actual amount of oil varies from variety to variety.

Green-yellow olives are those harvested after full development but just before they ripen, red-brown olives are harvested after full development of fruit but at mid ripening stage (not fully ripe) and black olives fully developed and ripened. At all stages, the fruits are bitter due to the presence of high quantities of polyphenols and other bitter chemicals that have to be removed before they can be consumed. The polyphenols are removed by one or more of several methods,. Generally by curing in lye and brine and fermenting followed by extensive washing to remove the lye, brine and fermentation by microbes. In some cases, instead of soaking in lye, the olives are allowed to shrink by soaking them in several layers of salt that draw out the water and phenolics from the olives and then they are soaked in water to rehydrate the olives. **Health relevance:** Since olive oil is relatively poor in saturated fats, it is considered as a heart –healthy oil. Virgin olive oil contains Oleocanthal which is an inhibitor of cyclooxygenase 1(COX-1), COX-2, 5-lipoxygenase and hence consumption of olive oil may be responsible for the lower incidence of heart disease in Mediterranean populations although, these populations also consume large quantities of red wine which is also implicated in reduction of heart disease. Olive oil is used for treating skin diseases and for good dermal health.

Palm/Oil palm *(Elaeis guineensis):* **Kingdom: Plantae; Division: Angiospermae, Class: Monocotyledonae, Order: Arecales; Family: Aricaceae, Tribe: Cocoseae Genus and species:** *Elaeis guineensis.* **Chromosome number 2n = 32.**

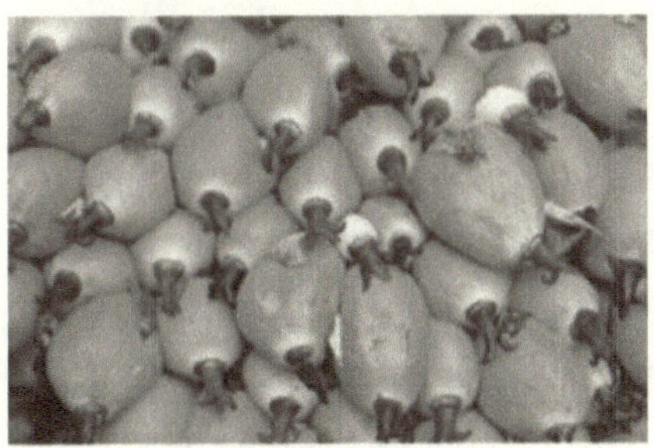
Oil palm fruit

The plant is a native of Africa and is grown extensively in Indonesia, Malaysia, Thailand, India, West Africa, Columbia and Brazil. The trees are single stemmed with a crown of compound leaves. Flowers are produced in clusters with three sepals and three petals in each flower. Fruits are reddish in color weighing about 100 pounds. The fruit encloses a single monocotyledonous seed. Both the fruit and the seed kernel are rich in oil. Oil from the fruit mesocarp is used for cooking wheras, the oil from the kernel is mostly used for manufacture of soaps and detergents. The palm oil from the fruit is rich in carotene and hence has a red color. Both the oil from the fruit as well as kernel is rich in saturated fats and hence they solidify at lower temperatures. Palm oil contains high amounts of Palmitic acid, which is linked to cardiovascular disease. **Health relevance**: Although palm oil is the leading cooking oil in Asia and Africa, it is very rich in saturated fats and thus many studies link the consumption of this oil in large amounts to the risk of cardiovascular disease. Unrefined oil from the fruit is rich in alpha and beta-carotene as well as lycopene.

Peanuts/Groundnuts *(Arachis hypogea):* **Kingdom: Plantae Group: Angiospermae, Class: Eudicots, Order: Fabales, Family, Fabaceae Genus and species:** *Arachis hypogeae.* **Chromosome number 2n = 40.**

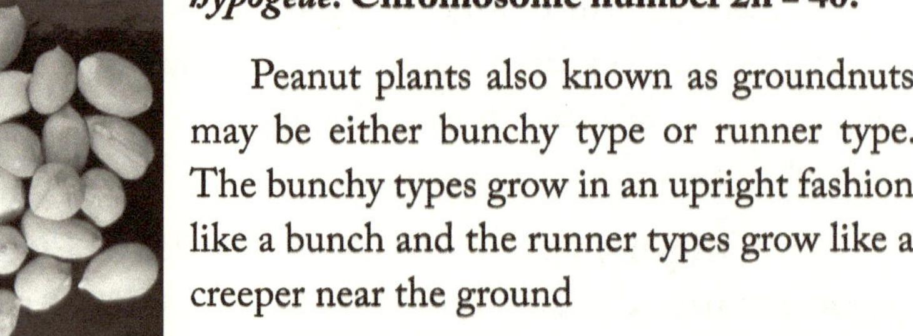

Peanuts

Peanut plants also known as groundnuts may be either bunchy type or runner type. The bunchy types grow in an upright fashion like a bunch and the runner types grow like a creeper near the ground

The various types are distinguished by branching habit and branch length. There are numerous varieties of each type of peanut. Both bunchy and creeper types produce compound leaves with each leaflet taking an oval penny sized shape. Flowers are pink or yellow in color. The bottom part of the flower known as the pedicel bends down after fertilization, and buries into the ground near the surface. The fruits that develop are pods that contain nuts. The nuts have a thin outer hull that is rich in antioxidants. The edible nuts are the cotyledons that are rich in oil and protein apart from carbohydrates, minerals and vitamins. The nuts are classified into Spanish runner, Virginia, Valencia, Tennessee red and white groups. The Spanish nuts are small. The Virginia types are even larger and Valencia types produce tightly clustered seeds in the pods. The Tennessee red and whites are Valencia types with red or white skins. Peanut oil contains about 18% saturated fat, 49% monounsaturated fat and 33% polyunsaturated fat. **Health relevance:** Peanut oil is used for cooking/ frying as also in various massage oils but the unrefined oil contains protein allergens. Even the smell of oil can initiate allergic responses in susceptible individuals. Those who are sensitive can have very severe and sometimes fatal reaction. Since the seeds can easily be infected by the fungus *Aspergillus* which produces a potent toxin – aflatoxin, moldy seeds should not be consumed.

Rapeseed/Canola *(Brassica napus):* **Kingdom: Plantae; Division: Angiospermae, Class: Eudicots; Order: Brassicales, Family: Brassicaceae, Genus and Species:** *Brassica Napus. Chromosome number 2n = 4x = 38 (Genome AA CC).*

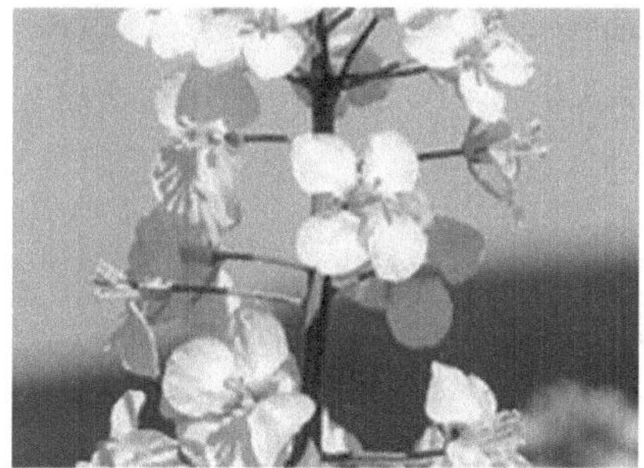

Canola

The plant is an herb related to mustard, cabbage and turnips. This species is a hybrid of B. campestris X B. oleracea. The natural rapeseeds are small and contain high concentrations of oil that is rich in erucic acid and glucoseinolates that are not considered good for cardiovascular health. However, new varieties that has been bred and marketed as canola oil are now available that has much lower concentrations of these two chemicals. The newly bred varieties are referred as Rapeseed 00 or Rapeseed double zero in order to indicate that they have very low levels of erucic acid and glucosinolates. Canola rapeseed oil contains 7.365% saturated fats 63.276 % Monounsaturated fats and 28.142% polyunsaturated fats. **Health relevance:** The naturally occurring B. *napus* seeds have oil that is high in erucic acid and glucoseinolates that are unhealthy for the heart muscle. But oil from the natural varieties that are rich in these two chemicals have been consumed by the people of India and China for thousands of years without any evidence of being harmful according to research conducted in India. Nevertheless, it must be noted that the life expectancy until recently in both these cultures were low and hence such arguments may not be relevant. However, new varieties originally bred at the University of Manitoba and since improved further are low in these two chemicals and hence consumption of canola oil derived from these new varieties is safe and approved for human consumption. Canola oil is low in saturated fats and contains both omega 3 fatty acids and omega 6 fatty acids with as ratio of Omega 6: Omega-3 of 2: 1. The United States Food and Drug Administration have given a qualified health claim of reducing coronary disease due to its cholesterol lowering abilities.

Safflower *(Carthamus tinctorius)*: Kingdom: Plantae, Division: Angiospermae, Class: Eudicots, Order: Asterales, Family: Asteraceae. Other names: American saffron Azafran, Bastard Saffron, False saffron. Chromosome number, 2n = 24

Safflower is an annual herb with many branches. Safflower is related to sunflower and has globular flower heads with many flowers in each head. The seeds are dicotyledonous and contain oil made of 6.2% saturated fats 14.3% monounsaturated fats and 74.6% polyunsaturated fats. There are two types of safflower varieties, the type that produces oil that is high in monounsaturated fatty acids oleic acid and those with high concentrations of polyunsaturated fatty acids linoleic acid. **Health relevance:** Safflower seed oil is used for preventing heart disease including hardening of the arteries (atherosclerosis) and stroke. It is also used to treat coughs, breathing problems, clotting conditions, pain, heart disease, chest pain and traumatic injuries. Some people use it for inducing sweating; and as a laxative stimulant, antiperspirant and expectorant to help loosen phlegm. Women sometimes use safflower oil for absent or painful menstrual periods. They use safflower flower to cause an abortion. However, data on use of safflower oil for cooking to improve cardiovascular health is inconclusive. Transgenic safflower plants expressing plant generated human insulin have been created by molecular techniques but these have proved to be of no commercial viability yet.

Sesame/Gingelly *(Sesamum indicum)*: Kingdom: Plantae, Division: Angiospermae, Class: Eudicots, Order: Lamiales Family: Pedaliaceae, Genus and species: *Sesamum indicum.* Chromosome number, 2n = 26

Sesame is a dicotyledonous annual herb plant grown in semiarid regions for its valuable oil and seed protein. The plants have soft stems from which non-serrated, lanceolate oblong leaves arise opposite to each other. The flowers are white, pink, purple blue or yellow. The seeds grow in capsule pods. The seeds are tiny and oval shaped and generally black or beige in color. The seeds contain 26% carbohydrate, 0.5% sugars, 17% protein, 48% fat and 17% dietary fiber. The oil is rich in antioxidants, lignans and vitamin E and has a high percentage of omega 6 fatty acids. **Health relevance:** When used as cooking oil, it is said to be beneficial in lowering cholesterol levels. The oil is used as carrier for various herbal preparations used in massage and other oil treatments in the Ayurvedic system. Ayurvedic physicians also recommend gargling of mouth with sesame oil for good dental hygiene. **Allergy:** The seeds and potentially the oil are potent allergens to people who are allergic to peanut, rye, poppy seeds, cashew, hazel, walnut, macadamia, pistachio and other tree nuts. There appears to be a correlation between sesame allergy and other allergic conditions such as asthma. Sesame allergy can manifest systemically including anaphylactic reactions as well as skin reactions, hives, itching, flushing etc. In Canada, food labels are required to mention presence of sesame if the preparation contains sesame.

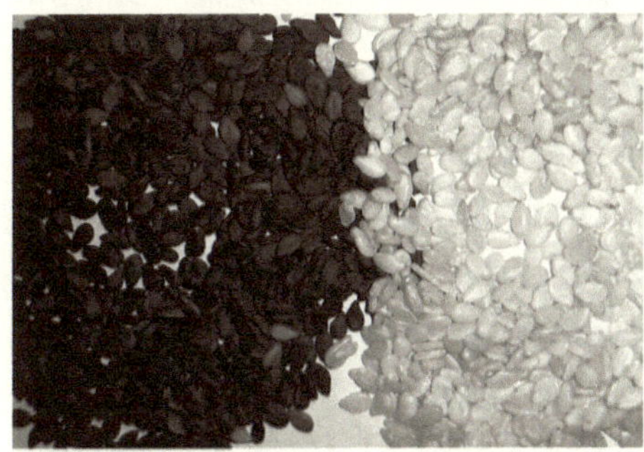

Sesame Black   **Sesame White**

Soybeans *(Glycine max)*: Kingdom: Plantae; Division: Angiospermae, Class: Eudicots; Family: Fabaceae/Leguminosae; *Genus and species: Glycine* max. Chromosome number, 2n = 40.

Soybeans are an important source of oil. The oil is rich in both mono and poly unsaturated fats as shown in the table below. Details about the plant are given in the section on legumes.

Sunflower *(Helianthus annua):* **Kingdom: Plantae, Division: Angiospermae, Class: Eudicots Order: Asterales, Family: Asteraceae Genus and Species:** *Helianthus annus.* **Chromosome number, 2n = 2x = 34.**

The plants are annuals growing in temperate countries. They have a long hairy stem from which serrated leaves arise in an alternate fashion. The terminal bud of the stem is modified into a floral meristem that generates the inflorescence or flower head that contains many individual florets. The outer rows of florets are called ray flowers and the inner smaller florets are called disk flowers. The center of the flower head contains disk flowers that are arranged in a specific spiral fashion and these set seeds. The seeds are small with a thick shell or hull that has to be removed for edible purposes. The dicotyledonous seeds are rich in oil. The oil is rich in both omega-6 and omega-9 oils. Sunflower oil degrades and becomes rancid when stored at higher temperatures and in light. **Health relevance:** The oil is rich in Vitamin E and omega – 6 and 0mega-9 fatty acids and low in saturated fats. Hence, sunflower oil is considered good for cardiovascular health. The oil is also used as a dental rinse. Sunflower oil is also used in many skin treatment preparations for good skin health.

Other Oils

a. **Rice Bran oil:** Rice bran oil is extracted from the outer layers of the seed after the hull is removed. This layer known as bran contains protein, vitamins and minerals besides oil. The oil derived from this bran contains 35% saturated fats, 38% monounsaturated and 37% polyunsaturated fats. The oil is rich in gamma orizanol, alpha tocopherols and other phytosterols that are considered useful for maintaining good health. Consumption of the oil has been shown to reduce serum triglycerides and total cholesterols while at the same time increasing HDL with a concurrent drop in LDL values. There are some reports suggesting that the oil when used as a supplement reduces troublesome hot flashes in menopausal women. Rice bran oil is used for cooking/frying in South East Asia but is not common oil for frying.

b. **Other edible Oils:** These are not significant oils for general edibility but are used in supplements, cosmetics and for other medicinal purposes. Examples are; Almond oil, Avocado oil, Grape seed oil, Hazelnut oil, flaxseed oil, Macadamia oil, Moringa oil; Pecan oil, Perilla oil, Pine nut oil, Pistachio oil, Poppyseed oil, Pumpkin seed oil, Walnut oil, Watermelon seed oil.

Table 8 – Fatty acid profile of different edible oils

OIL	Sat fat	Mono – unsat	Poly-Unsat	Trasnsfat	Omega-3	Omega-6	Omega-9	Vita-E	Vita-K
	g	g	g	g	g	g	g	mg	µg
Canola	7.365	63.276	28.142	0.4	11	21	NA	17.46	71.3
Coconut	86.5	5.8	1.8	0.028	NA	2	6	0.11	0.6
Corn	12.948	27.576	54.677	NA	1	58	28	14.3	1.9
Cotton	25.9	17.8	51.9	NA	1	54	19	35.3	24.7
Flax	3.663	7.527	28.73	0.094	64	15	11	0.47	9.3
Mustard	11.582	59.187	21.23	NA	6	15	NA	NA	NA
Olive	13.808	72.961	10.523	NA	1.5	15	0	14.35	60.2
Palm	49.3	37	9.3	NA	0	10	40	15.94	8
Peanut	16.9	46.2	32	NA	0	32	48	15.69	0.7
Rice bran	19.7	39.3	35	NA	2.2	34.4	38	32.3	24.3
Safflower	8	15	75	0.096	NA	NA	NA	34	7.1
Sesame	14.2	39.7	41.7	NA	NA	41	39	1.4	13.6
Soybean	15.34	21.701	58.208	NA	7	50	24	8.18	183.9
Sunflower 10.1	45.4	40.1	NA	0.2	39.8	45.3	41.08	5.4	

References

Balk E.M, Lichtenstein A.H, Chung, and M et al. (2006): Effects of omega-3 fatty acids on serum markers of cardiovascular disease risk: A systematic review, Atherosclerosis. 2006 Nov 189 (1): 19-30.

Belluzzi A, Boschi S, Brignola C, Munarini A, Cariani C, Miglio F. (2000): Polyunsaturated fatty acids and inflammatory bowel disease, Am J Clin Nutr. 2000; 71(suppl): 339S-342S.

Boskou, D. (2000): Olive oil, World Rev Nutr Diet. 2000; 87: 56-77

Chan E.J, Cho L. (2009): what can we expect from omega-3 fatty acids? Cleve Clin J Med. 2009 Apr; 76(4): 245-51.

Duke, J.A., (1983): Cocos nucifera –Nariel. https://www.hort.purdue.edu/newcrop/duke_energy/Cocos_nucifera.html

Freund-Levi Y, Hjorth E, Lindberg C, Cederholm T, Faxen-Irving G, Vedin I, Palmblad J, Wahlund LO, Schultzberg M, Basun H, Eriksdotter Jönhagen M. (2009).Effects of omega-3 fatty acids on inflammatory markers in cerebrospinal fluid and plasma in Alzheimer's disease: the OmegAD study. Dement Geriatr Cogn Disord. 2009, 27(5): 481-90.

Freund-Levi YF, Eriksdotter-Jonhagen M, and Cederholm T, et al. (2006): Omega-3 fatty acid treatment in 174 patients with mild to moderate Alzheimer disease: Omega AD Study, Arch Neurol. 2006; 63: 1402-8.

Geerling BJ, Badart-Smook A, van Deursen C, et al. (2000): Nutritional supplementation with N-3 fatty acids and antioxidants in patients with Crohn's disease in remission: effects on antioxidant status and fatty acid profile. Inflamm Bowel Dis. 2000, 6(2): 77-84.

Goldberg RJ, Katz J.A. (2007): Meta-analysis of the analgesic effects of omega-3 polyunsaturated fatty acid supplementation for inflammatory joint pain. Pain, 2007 Feb 28;

Hooper L, Thompson R, Harrison R et al. (2004): Omega 3 fatty acids for prevention and treatment of cardiovascular disease, (2004), Cochrane Database Syst Rev. 2004; CD003177.

Jing K, Wu T, Lim K. (2013): Omega-3 polyunsaturated fatty acids and cancer. Anticancer Agents Med Chem. 2013, 13(8): 1162-77.

McKinney JM, Sica D. (2006): Prescription omega-3 fatty acids for the treatment of hypertriglyceridemia, Review, Am J Health Syst Pharm. 2007 Mar 15, 64(6): 595-605.

Oplinger, E.S. Hardman, L.L. Gritton, E.T., Doll, J.D. and K.A. Kelling, (1989): Canola (Rapeseed): https://hort.purdue.edu/newcrop/afcm/canola.html

Oplinger, E.S. Putnam, D.H. Kaminski, A.R. Hanson, C.V., Oelke, E.A. Schulte, E.E., and J.D. Doll (1990): Sesame, https://hort.purdue.edu/newcrop/afcm/sesame.html

Oplinger, E.S., Oelke, E.A., Putnam, D.H., Kelling, K.A., Kaminsid, A.R., Teynor, T.M., Doll, J.D. and B.R. Durgan (1991): Mustard. https://hort.purdue.edu/newcrop/afcm/mustard.html.

Putnam, D.H., Oplinger, E.S., Hicks, D.R., Durgan, B.R. Noetzel, D.M., Meronuck, R.A. (1989): https://hort.purdue.edu/newcrop/afcm/sunflower.html.

Putnam, D.H. Oplinger, E.S. Teynor, T.M. Oelke, E.A. Kelling, K.A., and J.D. Doll (1991): Peanut. https://hort.purdue.edu/newcrop/afcm/peanut.html.

University of Maryland Medical Center, (2007): Omega-3 fatty acids, overview, The University of Maryland Medical System, https://www.umms.org/ummc/patients-visitors/health-library/medical-encyclopedia/images/omega3-fatty-acids

Chapter 8
Tuber Crops as Staple Food

Apart from cereals, legumes and oil crop plants, certain plants that produce underground storage tissues collectively called tubers contain substantial amounts of carbohydrates that are used as secondary or even primary sources of carbohydrates in all continents. Chief among these is potato that is the fourth largest source of food energy following Rice, Wheat and Corn in that order. In Africa, parts of South America and Asia another crop plant namely tapioca also known as Cassava/Yuca/Tapioca/Manihot root '(*Manihot utilissima*) plays major role as a food crop. A somewhat similar crop namely sweet potato is also a major food crop in South America, Asia, Africa and Polynesian islands. All three are also used as vegetables to complement other sources of food. All three are underground stems or roots wherein, carbohydrates mainly in the form of starch are stored. Certain other underground storage plants include various types of Yams, Taro and Arrowroot that provide energy in the form of stored starch and other carbohydrates. The tubers also contain smaller amounts of protein and are rich in minerals, some vitamins and phytochemicals. Since these are underground tubers, the plants have evolved a mechanism to protect themselves from attacks by soil borne fungi, bacteria, nematodes and other plant disease-causing agents by producing various phytochemicals including cyanide, alkaloids like solanine, toxic glycosides, oxalates and other chemicals. In order to prevent toxicity to humans, the outer skin from the tubers should be removed and the tubers should be processed further by dehydration through drying in the sun or by machinery or boiling in water, frying in oil and other processes.

Arrowroot/East Indian Arrowroot *(Curcuma angustifolia)*: Kingdom: Plantae; Division: Angiospermae, Monocotyledonae, Order: Zingiberales; Family: Zingiberaceae, Chromosome number, 2n = 42

This is not a staple food plant except among poorer populations and under conditions where other staple may not be available. This plant is a native of the Indian subcontinent and is related to ginger and turmeric. It is a perennial with leaves that are dark green on the upper surface and less green on lower surface. Leaves are long with parallel veins. Flowers grow on inflorescences containing 3-4 bisexual flowers with 3 white petals. Stamens have double anthers and style ends with a globular stigma. The underground stem called a rhizome grows to about 5 ft long and is the nutritive edible part of the plant. The rhizomes contain complex carbohydrates that are easily digestible, have a high binding capacity, and hence considered good for treating diahorrea. The dried powdered rhizome is used as a carbohydrate component of gruel and in baby foods. It is used as a source of starch among poorer populations. **Health**: The arrowroot starch is used in many baby foods and is a staple component of alternative medicinal preparations for controlling digestive ailments.

Bermuda arrowroot/Arrowroot/West-Indian Arrowroot/ *(Maranta arundanaceae)*: Kingdom: Plantae; Division: Angiospermae, Class: Monocotyledonae, Order: Zingiberales; Family: Zingiberaceae. Chromosome number: 2n = 18

This is a perennial rain forest plant grown in the West Indian (Carribean) islands and in other tropical and sub-tropical climes. It grows to a height of about 2 ft and is morphologically similar to East Indian arrowroot (*Curcuma angustifolia*). It produces white flowers with 3 sepals and petals. The rootstock containing starch grows to about a foot long and contains complex carbohydrates. It has no gluten. It is used for making biscuits, cakes and gruel. **Health**: Since the starch is not contaminated with gluten, it is a source of carbohydrate for those allergic to gluten.

Polynesian Arrowroot *(Tacca leontopetaloides)*: Kingdom: Plantae; Division: Angiospermae, Class: Monocotyledonae, Order: Dioscoriales; Family: Dioscoriaceae.

This plant is similar to many yams and is a food plant in the Polynesian islands (Fiji, Guam, Tonga, Hawaii, and Samoa, New Guinea). The tubers are hard and potato-like. The tuber flour is used to make puddings and other edible dishes. **Health:** The flour mixed with red clay is used to control diahorrea and dysentery.

Cassava/Tapioca/Manioc/Mogo/Yuca *(Manihot esculenta/ M. utilissima)*: Kingdom: Plantae Group: Angiospermae, Class: Eudicots, Order: Ephorbiales, Family: Euphorbiaceae Chromosome number, 2n = 36. This plant is a native of South America and is now grown extensively in the tropical and subtropical parts of the world particularly in Brazil, Nigeria, Kenya and many countries of Africa, India, Sri Lanka, Myanmar, Malaysia, Indonesia,

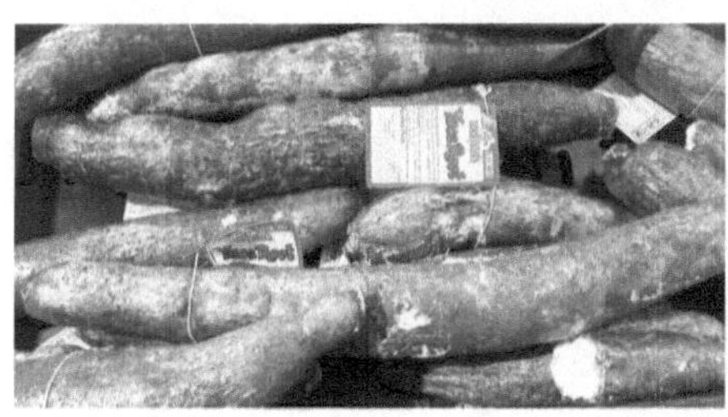

Cassava

Philippines, Thailand Viet Nam, Cambodia and China. The tuber from this plant is the third largest source of carbohydrates in the tropics after rice and corn. The plant is closely related to the rubber plant. It is a perennial shrub that grows to a height of about 10 ft with leaves that have 7-9 lobes on long petioles. Tuberous roots range from 6 inches to 30 inches in length and taper from top to bottom much like a cone. They grow in outward pointing clusters from the base of the stem just below the soil surface. There are essentially two varieties of Manihot and these are the bitter variety and the sweet variety. Both varieties contain glycosides that are converted into hydrogen cyanide when oxidized on exposure to air and hence are toxic unless the outer hard rind is removed and the white/yellow edible portion is then processed further by soaking in water, boiling, frying and or drying. The tubers are rich in carbohydrates amylopectin and amylose but very poor in protein. The tubers after mashing can be fermented to produce various alcoholic beverages. **Health:** Apart from its nutritional value, there are no medicinal uses although there are some unverified reports that the tuber contains anticancer compounds. Consumption of poorly processed cassava causes acute toxicity including vomiting, nausea, goiter, ataxia and other neuro muscular conditions. Cassava roots, peels and leaves should not be consumed raw because they contain two cyanogenic glucosides linamarin and lotaustralin. These are decomposed by linamarase, a naturally occurring enzyme in cassava liberating hydrogen cyanide (HCN). The amount of cyanide released can be as high as 2 mg/100 g of tuber. Chronic low-level cyanide exposure results in development of goiter and tropical ataxic neuropathy, a disorder that renders a person unsteady and uncoordinated. Severe cyanide poisoning particularly during famines is associated with outbreaks of a debilitating irreversible paralytic disorder called konzo and in some cases death. The incidence of konzo and tropical ataxic neuropathy can be as high as 3% in some areas. However, boiling and cooking can remove most of the cyanides. Drying, fermenting and frying to prepare tapioca chips can eliminate the toxicity.

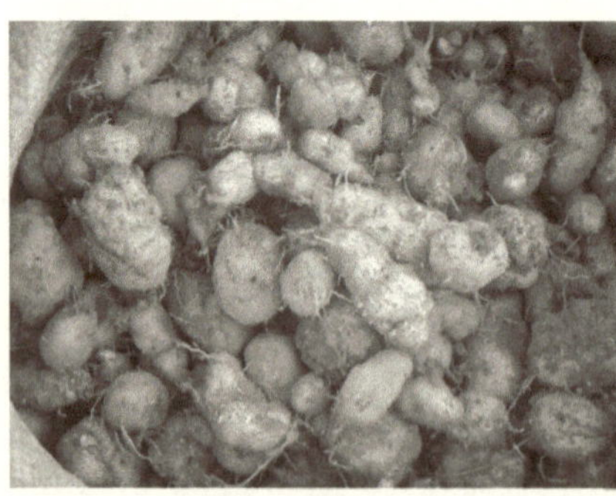

Hausa potato

Country Potato/Hausa potato/Chinese potato/Koorka/ *(Plectranthus rotundifolius/ Solenostemon rotundifolius):* **Kingdom: Plantae, Division: Angiospermae, Class: Eudicots, Order: Lamiales, Family: Lamiaceae. Chromosome number, 2n = 64.**

The small rounded or slightly elongated aromatic tubers of this plant are edible and used as a stir-fry vegetable in Southern India (Koorka (Malayalam), Siru Kizhangu (Tamil), and sambrali (Karnataka)), Sri Lanka (Innala), and Indonesia (Kentang), Malaysia (ubi keling) and in Africa (Zulu Potato, ngaboyo). The name Chinese potato is more aptly applied to Taro roots but in India, it is used for *Plectranthes* also. It is also a subsistence crop and the tubers are consumed as a famine-food after boiling or toasting the tubers. The tubers have an aromatic medicine flavor. The plants are herbaceous perennials with a mint-like appearance. **Health:** The tubers and leaves of the closely related *P. barbatus* contains the di-terpene Forskolin used to treat allergies, psoriasis, obesity, bladder infections, irritable bowel syndrome.

Elephant yam *(Amorphophallus paeoniifolius):* Kingdom: Plantae; Group: Angiospermae; Class: Monocotyledonae; Order: Alismatales; Family: Araceae. Genus and Species: Amorphophallus paeoniifolius, **Synonyms:** A. campanulatus, A. bangkokensis, A. chatty, and A. decurrens. **Chromosome number 2n = 28.** This is a tropical plant grown in Africa, India, Sri Lanka, Indonesia, and Malaysia, Philippines and other South Asian countries, Pacific and Carribean islands. The plants are grown in order to harvest their very large corm/tubers which are used mainly as a vegetable although it can be processed (baked, fried) as a source of food. However, the tubers contain substantial amounts of oxalic acid crystals that have to be leached by cooking

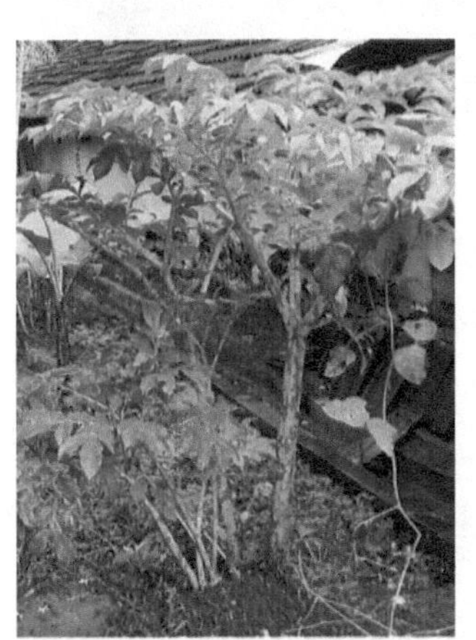

Yam plant

before usage. The plants have a large underground stem called as corm from which a fleshy stem arises with a crown of large leaves. The flower is huge and smells of rotting flesh. **Health:** Toxic oxalates have to be removed by various cooking processes before consumption. Cooked elephant yams are used by Ayurvedic, Unani and Siddha medicine practioners for treating prostate hyperplasia.

Jicama/Yard bean *(Pachyrhizus tuberosus):* **kingdom: Plantae; Division: Angiospermae, Class: Eudicots, Order: Fabales, Family: Fabaceae. Chromosome number, 2n = 22**

This is a legume plant grown mainly in the carribean islands and in Florida, USA. It is a vine producing large spherical or elongated taproot, which can weigh as much as 40 Lb. (20 Kg). The tuber has brown skin, which has to be removed for cooking. The edible root after removing skin is white in color. It is a rich source of carbohydrates. The seeds are poisonous since they contain rotenone, which is a rodenticide.

Potato *(Solanum tuberosum):* **Kingdom: Plantae, Group; Angiospermae, Class: Eudicots Order: Solanales Family: Solanacease Genus and species:** *Solanum tuberosum.* **Chromosome number: 2n = 48**

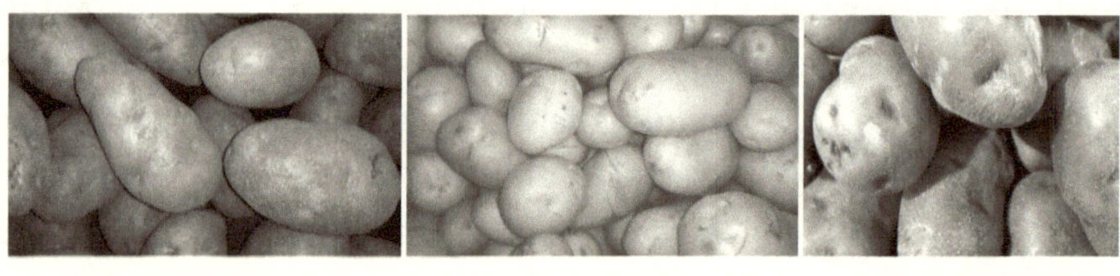

Russet	**White Potato**	**Red Potato**

The potato is the fourth most important food crop after Rice, wheat and corn and is used as a staple food in many parts of South America and Europe and as vegetable in many other parts of the world. There are over 5000 varieties of potato of which only a few are cultivated extensively for food consumption. Besides *S. tuberosum,* there are other species of potato namely, *S. stenotomum, S. phureja,* S. *goniocalyx* and *S.ajanhuiri* which are diploids. Two triploid species with 36 chromosomes: *S. chaucha* and *S. juzepczukii* and one pentaploid cultivated species with 60 chromosomes: S. *curtilobum* are also cultivated. The plants are natives of the Andes region of South America and have been introduced to all other parts of the world. The plants are annuals that produce elongated oblong or round tubers under the ground. The tubers contain essentially two major types of starches namely amylopectin and amylose.

Those varieties with high amylopectin are sticky and good for making potato starch, potato soup etc. Since the tubers are rich in starch, they are rated as having high glycemic index and hence diabetic patients should avoid consuming large quantities of potato products. If the tubers are exposed to light while still on the plant, the tuber skin turns green and the level of the toxic glycol alkaloid solanine goes up. Certain varieties of potato are red, some purple and even blue due to presence of various pigments. Deep-frying and sautéing potato result in the formation of acrylamides that are potential carcinogens/neurotoxins when consumed in large amounts. The leaves and stems and greening sprouts contain large amounts of the toxic glycoalkaloids and hence not suitable as sources of food. Dicotyledonous seeds are produced in small round fruits that are not edible. New plants are grown from seeds although they may also be grown from the "eyes" of the tubers themselves. **Health relevance:** The potato skin is used in India to prevent burn injuries. When stir-fried or fried in oil at a temperature above 120 C, a potent neurotoxin and carcinogen acrylamide is produced in small quantities. Boiled or cooked potatoes at temperatures below 120 C do not generate this toxin. Some new varieties that do not produce acrylamide have been developed by a commercial organization (Simplot) in the USA.

Sweet Potato *(Ipoemea batatas)*: Kingdom: Plantae, Division: Angiospermae, Class: Eudicots, Order: Solanales Family: Comvolvulaceae, Genus: *Ipoemoea batatas*. Chromosome number, 2n = 90

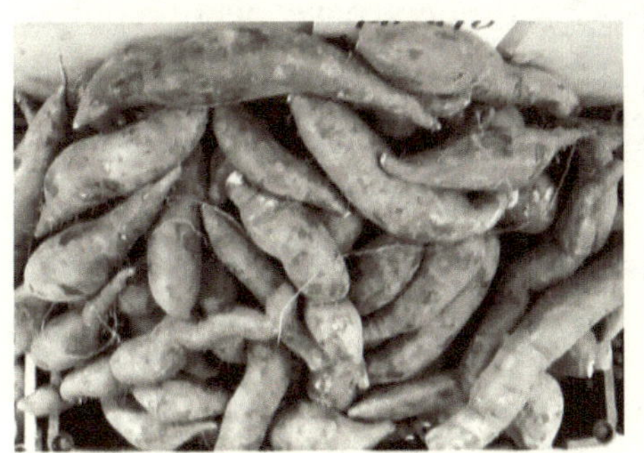

Red Sweet potato tuber

Sweet potato plants are dicotyledonous members of the morning glory family. The plants are natives of South America and are grown extensively for harvesting the tubers in South America, Africa the carribean islands, Polynesia and Asia. It is a perennial vine with heart shaped alternate leaves. The related morning glory often grown in gardens is considered to have anti-cancerous properties. The tuberous roots may be pink, yellow or purple in color. The edible portion of the tuber after removal of the outer skin may also be white, yellow or pink-purple and the latter in particular contains antioxidents chemicals such as anthocyanin and carotene. The tubers are sweet and rich in carbohydrates. The tubers are eaten raw, cooked in fire or in boiling water or deep-fried. The tubers apart from being staple foods in some cultures such as Maori, Papua New Guinea, Solomon Islands and Uganda in Africa are generally consumed as vegetables in many other countries. The plants do not tolerate drought or frost. Plants produce edible harvestable tubers in about 9 months after planting. The tubers are rich in Carbohydrates, soluble fiber, vitamin A from carotene and important minerals. Apart from the tubers, the young leaves are consumed as leaf-vegetables after cooking. **Health relevance:** Mainly nutritional value. The antioxidants in the colored varieties may have some protective value in preventing tumors in the GI tract.

Taro *(Colocasia esculenta):* Kingdom: Plantae; Division: Angiospermae, Class: Monocotyledonae; Order: Arales; Family: Araceae; Genus and Species; *Colocassia esculente.*

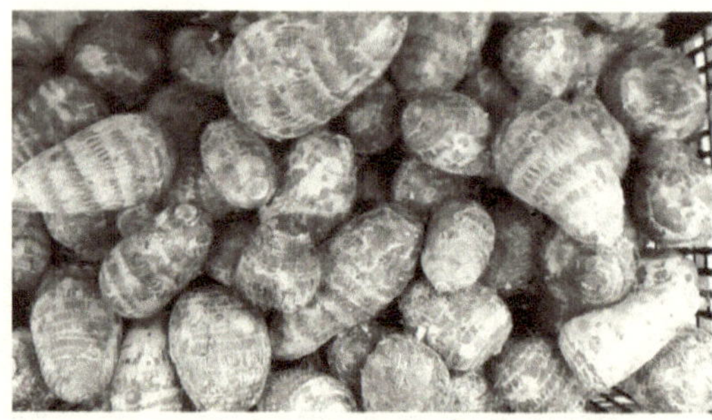

Taro corm

Chromosome number: 2n = 28, 42. Different numbers have been reported based on collection. Pacific including Japan, Thailand are 2n = 28 whereas accessions from Australia, New Zealand, India, Nepal are 2n = 42.

This plant is a native of Sothern India and South East Asia and is grown now in many parts of Africa, Oceana, Caribbean islands and Mediterranean countries for harvesting their starchy corms, which are bulbous underground stems as well as their leaves and stems for use as vegetables and as a staple food. The plants are perennials with an underground fleshy corm, fleshy stem with very large heart-shaped leaves. The corm and the petiolate leaves contain large quantities of calcium oxalate and hence they can be very irritating to touch. The skin of the corm, which irritates the human skin, has to be peeled off before processing for edibility. Leaves and petioles are cooked and cannot be eaten as raw vegetable. **Health:** The starchy corms are a good source of complex carbohydrates. Leaves and stem provide roughage and small quantities of vitamins and minerals.

Yam *(Dioscorea sp):* Kingdom: Plantae; Division: Angiospermae; Class: Monocotyledonae, Order: Dioscoriales, Family: Dioscoriaceae. Genus and Species: *D. rotundata,* (white yam), *D. cayenensis,* (yellow yam), *D. alata* (Winged yam), *D.opposita* (Chinese yam), *D. bulbifera* (Air potato), *D.esculenta* (lesser yam), D. dumetorum (bitter yam), *D.trifuda* (Cush Cush yam). Chromosome number: 2n = 40, 3n = 60, 4n = 80, different ploidy levels.

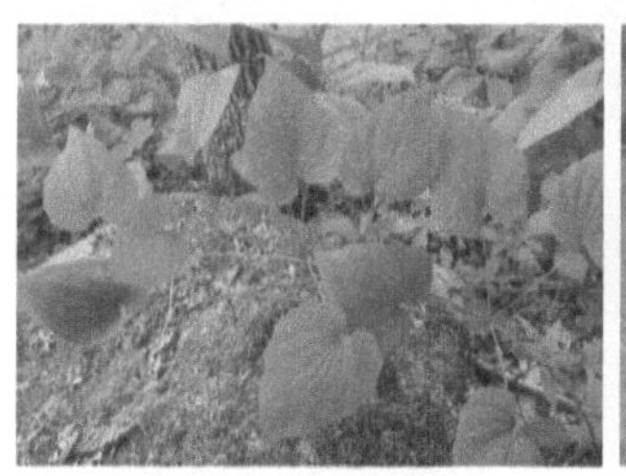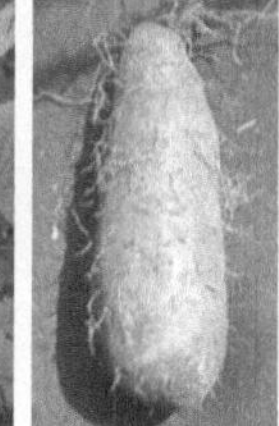

Dioscorea vine   D. alata

As noted above, there are several species of yam, all belonging to the same family and possessing many similar qualities. All are vines which produce underground tubers which are rich in carbohydrates (about 30%) serving both as a significant source of food and used also as a vegetable. The bulk of yams is produced in Africa but is also grown in Asia, South America, carribean and pacific islands.

The white and yellow yams (*D.rotunda, D.cayenensis*) are the most important cultivated yams. Both are large vines reaching a length of 40 ft and produce tubers that are 5.5–11.0 lbs.

The winged yam or purple yam or ratalu (*D. alata*) is grown mostly in South Asia and pacific countries. Chinese yam (*D. opposita*) is grown mostly in china and has smaller vines with smaller tubers. Air potato (*D. bulbifera*) plants are vines about 20 ft long producing smaller tubers about 1–4 lbs. The lower leaves have bulbils which are edible after cooking. The lesser yams (*D.esculenta*) are vines about 10 ft long with small tubers grown mostly in Southeast Asia. The bitter yam (*D.dumitorum*) is used mainly as a vegetable in West Africa after boiling to remove toxic principles. The Cush Cush yam (*D.trifida*) is grown mostly in the Central and South Americas under rain forest conditions.

Yams are among the most important sources of nutrition in Africa. Yams contain about 2% protein but the protein lacks essential amino acids like cysteine, methionine and tryptophan. It has a low glycemic index. **Health:** Yams contain allergens, certain varieties have toxic chemicals like thiocyanates, and hence the tubers have to be processed by boiling, frying or soaking in salt water to remove harmful chemicals. At the same time, they contain Diosegnin that is the starting point for synthesis of various steroids

Table 9: Nutritional value of Tuber crops

Metabolite	Arrowroot Rhizome	Cassava tuber	Dioscorea yam	Elephant yam	Potato tuber	Sweet Potato	Taro corm
Water, g	80.75	59.68	81.44	69.6	79.34	77.28	70.64
Protein-g	4.24	1.36	1.34	1.53	2.02	1.57	1.5
Total lipid (fat), g	0.2	0.28	0.1	0.17	0.09	0.05	0.2
Carbohydrate, g	13.39	38.06	16.3	27.88	17.47	20.12	26.46
Fiber, g	1.3	1.8	2.5	4.1	2.2	3	4.1
Sugar, g	NA	1.7	0.31	0.5	0.78	4.18	0.4
Calcium, mg	6	16	26	17	12	30	43
Iron, mg	2.22	0.27	0.44	0.54	0.78	0.61	0.55
Magnesium, mg	25	21	12	21	23	25	33
Phosphorus, mg	98	27	34	55	57	47	84
Potassium, mg	454	271	418	816	421	337	591
Sodium, mg	26	14	13	9	6	55	11
Zinc, mg	0.63	0.34	0.27	0.24	0.29	0.3	0.23
Vitamin C, mg	1.9	20.6	2.6	17.1	19.7	2.4	4.5
Thiamin, mg	0.143	0.087	0.102	0.112	0.08	0.078	0.095
Riboflavin, mg	0.059	0.048	0.019	0.032	0.032	0.061	0.025
Niacin, mg	1.693	0.854	0.481	0.552	1.054	0.557	0.6
Vitamin B-6, mg	0.266	0.088	0.179	0.293	0.295	0.209	0.283
Folate, DFE, µg	338	27	14	23	16	11	22
Vitamin B-12, µg	0	0	0	0	0	0	0
Vitamin A, µg	1	1	0	7	0	709	4
Vitamin A, IU	19	13	138	2	14187	76	
Vitamin E, mg	0	0.19	0.21	0.35	0.01	0.26	2.38
Vitamin D, ug	0	0	0	0	0	0	0
Vitamin D, IU	0	0	0	0	0	0	0
Vitamin K, µg	0	1.9	1.4	2.3	1.9	1.8	1
Fatty acids, g	0.039	0.074	0.022	0.037	0.026	0.018	0.041
Fats, monoun, g	0.004	0.075	0.004	0.006	0.002	0.001	0.016
Fats, polyun, g	0.092	0.048	0.045	0.076	0.043	0.014	0.083
Cholesterol, mg	0	0	0	0	0	0	0

References

Arnau, G., Nemorin, A., Maledon, E., Abraham, K. (2009): Revision of ploidy status of Dioscorea alata L. (Dioscoreaceae) by cytogenetic and microsatellite segregation analysis. Theor Appl Genet. 118 (7): 1239-49. Doi: 10.1007/s00122-009-0977-6. Epub 2009 Mar 1.

Coates, D.J., Yen, D.E., and P.M. Gaffe (1988): Chromosome Variation in Taro, Colocasia esculenta: Implications for origin in the Pacific. Cytologia 53: 551-560,

Coursey, D.G. (1967): Yams, London: Longmans, Green and Co. Ltd, 230 pp

http://aggie-horticulture.tamu.edu/vegetable/guides/the-crops-of-texas/root-and-tuber-crops/

http://www.celkau.in/Crops/Tuber%20Crops/TuberCrops.aspx

http://www.fao.org/docrep/s8620e/S8620E09.htm

http://www.gcp21.org/wcrtc/

Martin, F.W. and Sadik, S. (1977): Tropical yams and their potential, Part 4 Dioscorea rotundata and Dioscorea cayenensis. United States Department of agriculture, Agriculture Handbook, No. 502, Washington, DC: USDA Agricultural Research Service, 36 pp

National Research Council (2006): Lost crops of Africa, Volume II: Vegetables Washington, D.C., National Academies Press, pp. 269–285, ISBN 0-309-66582-5

Ravi V.J., Balagopalan, C. (1996): Review on tropical root and tuber crops. I. Storage methods and quality changes Crit. Rev. Food Sci. Nutr. 1996, 36 (7): 661-709.

Sanginga, N., Mbabu, and A., (2015): *In* Feeding Africa, United Nations Commission for Africa, (http://www.afdb.org/fileadmin/uploads/afdb/Documents/Events/DakAgri2015/Root and Tuber Crops Cassava Yam Potato and Sweet Potato.pdf)

Chapter 9

Vegetables for Good Health

The term vegetable as used here refers to any plant part including roots, stems, leaves, flowers, botanical fruits and certain seeds used to supplement a diet when eaten raw as salads or cooked as part of a meal or alone as snacks or desserts. Herein, we include eggplant, tomatoes, various chilli and bell peppers, cucumber, bitter melon, pumpkin and various other gourds as vegetables although, in reality they are fruits in the botanical nomenclature. Vegetables also include many cereal plant parts (eg. Corn), legumes (eg. Peas, various bean types) and oil seeds (coconuts meat), Some of the vegetable plants have already been described in the sections on cereals, legumes, oil and tuber plants. The list of such plants is very long and hence, we will confine ourselves to descriptions of a selected number of the major vegetable plants and a general description of this group.

Some Vegetables contain large amounts of carbohydrates as in the case of banana/plantain, potatoes, sweet potatoes, yams, taro roots, beetroots and other underground stems and roots. Others, particularly in the legume family, contain substantial amounts of protein as in the case of peas *(Pisum sativum)*, lentils *(Lens culinaris)*, soybeans *(Glycine max)*, field beans *(Phaselus sp)* and other bean species. Yet others are high in fats exemplified by coconuts *(Cocos nucifera)*, soybeans *(Glycine max)* etc. Some vegetables may also be main sources of food. However, when consumed as a vegetable the nutrient content would not be the same as the mature seed/grain.

In general, vegetables contain various vitamins, minerals and soluble fiber that help to supplement the body's requirements for these essential vitamins and minerals. In addition, many vegetables contain antioxidants, antimicrobial chemicals, various other phytochemicals, which may have a role in preventing cancers, cardiovascular disease, and gastrointestinal disease and improve neurological functions etc. Thus, inclusion of various vegetables in the diet helps to improve the general well-being and health of individuals. At the same time, some vegetables contain toxic principles such as cyanides (yucca roots), oxalic acid (various yams, celery) and other potentially toxic chemicals that can be removed through processing by soaking and boiling before consumption.

Vegetables used for culinary purposes may be derived from underground parts of plants including underground stems and roots exemplified by potato, carrots radish, beet, sweet potato, yams, taro roots, lotus roots, turnips, onions and garlic. Vegetables consumed from stems and leaves include Asparagus, cabbage, Brussels sprouts, celery, bamboo shoots, spinach, amaranth leaves, rhubarb, collard greens, mustard greens, lettuce, taro leaves, beet, chard and lotus stem. Floral parts used as vegetables include banana florets, broccoli and cauliflower. Botanically defined fruit vegetables are cucumbers, squashes, chayote squash, pumpkin, tomatoes, eggplant/Brinjal, chilli peppers, okra, bitter melon, ash gourd, snake gourd, drum stick, variety of bean pods, soybean pods and seeds, pea pods, cowpea, garbanzo, guar, Dolichos. Seed vegetables are fresh peas, soybeans, various bean seeds, mung bean, lentils, mustard, sesame etc.

Most alternative medicine systems as well as modern allopathic systems of medicine recommend the inclusion of vegetables in the daily diet in order to help improve and maintain good health. The nutrient value of major vegetables is given in Tables 10 to 13. Descriptions of some of these vegetable plants are given in the sections on cereals, legumes oilseeds, tubers and other chapters.

Leaf Vegetables

Leaves of many plants are consumed as salads or after cooking. This group includes various Amaranthus species, Brussels sprouts, Cabbage, Collard green, Kale, Lettuce, Moringa (Drumstick), Mustard green, and Spinach. The leaves in all cases are nutritious and generally are rich in minerals, fiber and useful phytochemicals. The leaves also contain about 20% protein but they are not significant contributors of protein or carbohydrates since vegetables are only supplements in the meal eaten. Nevertheless, under famine conditions, leaf vegetables can be of substantial nutritive value as a source of protein apart from vitamins, minerals, fiber and antioxidants. Humans are not equipped to digest the high cellulose content of these leaves but the undigested cellulose gives bulk by absorbing water from the gut and enabling relief from constipation.

Agathi/Vegetable hummingbird *(Sesbania grandiflora)***: Kingdom: Plantae, Division: Angiospermae, Class: Eudicots, Order: Fabales, Family: Fabaceae, Genus: and species:** *Sesbania grandiflora.*

Agathi is a small tree growing in South East Asia, Southern India and Sri Lanka. It has been introduced in Mexico, Southern USA, Central and South America as well as the Carribean islands. Both the leaves and flowers are cooked and consumed as a vegetable. **Health:** The leaves are rich in some essential amino acids and contain about 20% protein. It is considered a diuretic, emetic, emmenagogue, febrifuge, laxative, and tonic. Agathi is a folk remedy for bruises, catarrh, dysentery, fevers, headaches, sores, sore throat, and stomatitis. Bark, leaves, gums, and flowers are considered medicinal. Cooked leaves in particular are consumed after a fast in order to provide bulk.

Amaranths *(Amaranthus sp)***: Amaranth: Kingdom: Plantae, Division: Angiospermae, Class: Eudicots, Order: Caryophyllales, Family: Amaranthaceae Genus: and species:** *Amaranthus caudatus (2n = 32), A.cruentes (2n = 34), A.hypochondriacus (2n = 32).* **Chromosome numbers for the three species is given in parenthesis.**

Amaranthus grain is a pseudo cereal and details of the plant have been described earlier. The leaves of grain Amaranth and other species of

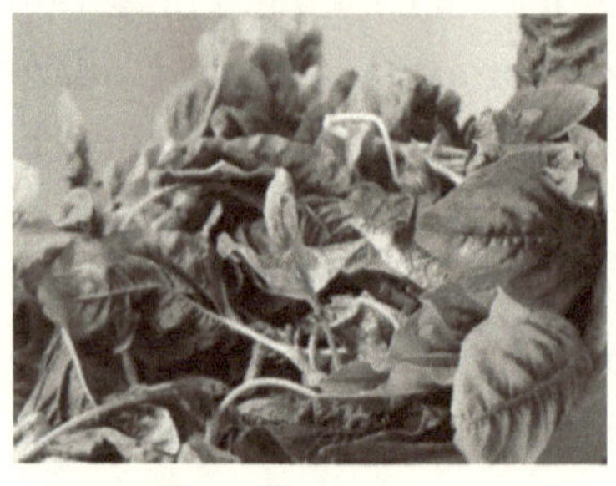

Amaranth leaves

Amaranthus are also edible as leafy greens and are cooked and consumed as part of a meal in different parts of the world. These are: *Amaranthus Cruentes* (Purple amaranth-Vietnamese); *Amaranthus retroflexus* (Common amaranth – Thailand); *Amaranthus spinosus* (Prickly amaranth – Thailand); *Amaranthus tricolor* (Amaranth – China, Asia); *Amaranthus viridis* (Slender amaranth-South India); They are rich in antioxidants, saponins, triterpinoids and ecdysteroids. All have similar botanical features with some morphological variations. **Health:** High fiber and antioxidants.

Green Amaranth/Slender Amaranth *(Amaranthus viridis):* Amaranth: Kingdom: Plantae, Division: Angiospermae, Class: Eudicots, Order: Caryophyllales, Family: Amaranthaceae Genus: and species: *A. viridis*. Chromosome number, 2n = 34

This tropical spinach-like green leaf plant has some medicinal properties. The plant bears all the characteristics of the family Amaranthaceae. The leaves are cooked and eaten as a vegetable in North Eastern China (Cheng-Kruk, Shak) and Southern India (Kuppa Cheera), Africa, by Australian natives, Carribean Islands (Callaloo) and in Greece (Vlita). The hard nutty black seeds borne on catkins are edible. **Health:** Leaves have antioxidants and leaf extracts are being recommended as green medicine.

The family Brassicaceae contains the largest number of leaf vegetables and hence all members of this family are grouped together below.

Brussel sprouts *(Brassica oleraceae*-Gemmifera group): Kingdom: Plantae; Division: Angiospermae; Class: Eudicots; Order: Brassicales;

Family: Brassicaceae; Genus and Species: Brassica oleracea **Gemmifera group. Chromosome number: 2n = 18.** The plants are biennials growing

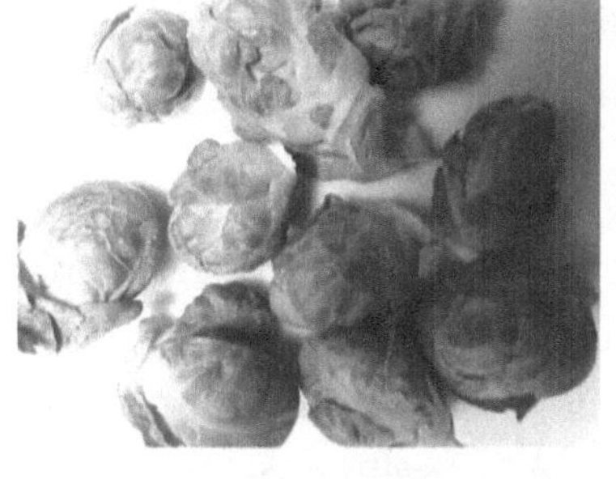

Brussels sprouts

to an average height Of 2 Ft with thick cabbage-like leaves. The stem produces a number of leafy buds that are the edible Brussels sprouts. The name is derived from the fact that the sprouts were a common source of vegetable in the Brussels region of Belgium since ancient times. The sprouts are rich in Vitamins C, K, B6 and minerals. The rich vitamin K levels in the sprouts indicate that the sprouts are contra-indicated in patients on blood thinning agents.

Cabbage *(Brassica oleraceae)*: Kingdom: Plantae; Division: Angiospermae, Class: Eudicots Order: Brassicales Family: Brassicaceae Capitata group; Genus and species: Green cabbage (B. oleracea L. var. capitata, **L.f. Alba DC) Red cabbage: *(B. oleracea L. var. capitata L.f. rubra L. Thell)*; Savoy cabbage: *(B. oleracea L. var. sabauda L.)*. Chromosome number: 2n = 18.**

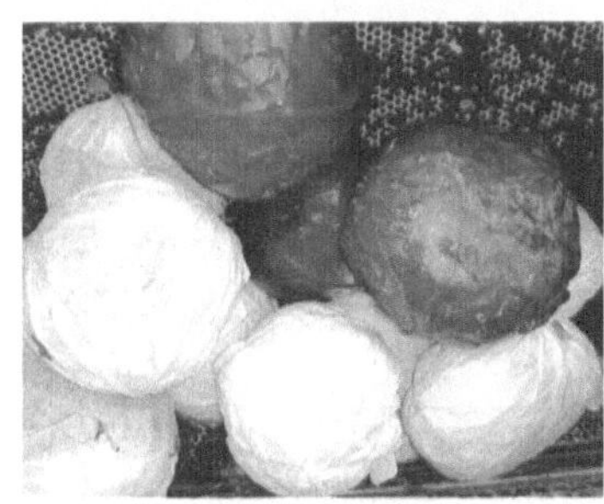

Cabbage

Cabbage is a leafy green biennial plant with leaves that bunch into a tight globular head, which is the leafy vegetable. These cabbage heads range in weight from 1–9 lbs. The heads can be beige green or purple. It is a good source for vitamins and minerals plus many phytochemicals. This vegetable like others in the cabbage family have anticancer properties. **Health relevance:** The purple cabbage contains anthocyanin that is an antioxidant. They have a low glycemic index and have high fiber content. Cabbage juice is recommended by traditional medical practitioners for treating ulcers. Folk medicinal practioners recommend the use of leaves to treat sore feet and as a poultice for treating boils and warts.

Chard *(Beta vulgaris subsp. vulgaris*, Cicla-Group and Flavescens-Group): Kingdom: Plantae; Division: Angiospermae, Class: Eudicots; Order: Caryophyllales; Family: Amaranthaceae, Genus and species: *Beta vulgaris subsp. Vulgaris.* Chromosome number: 2n = 18.

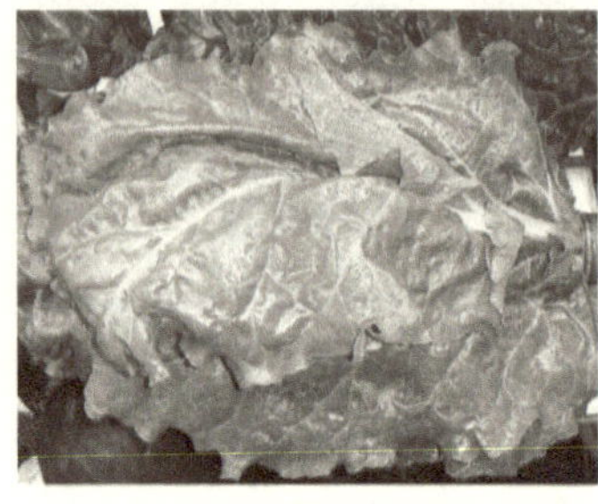

Chard

Chard s a leafy green vegetable often used in Mediterranean cooking. The plants are biennials. The leaf blade can be green or reddish in color; the leaf stalks also vary in color, usually white, yellow, or red. Swiss chard is high in vitamins A, K, and C; it is also rich in minerals, dietary fiber, and protein. The leaves contain oxalic acid and hence the leaves are preferably cooked to remove the oxalates. Since the leaves contain approximately 300% of the daily requirement of Vitamin K, caution should be exercised by people on blood thinning agents like warfarin in eating this leaf vegetable.

Chinese cabbage *(Brassica Rapa sub sp.pekinensis):* Kingdom: Plantae; Division: Angiospermae, Class: Eudicots Order: Brassicales Family: Brassicaceae. Chromosome number, 2n = 20

Chinese cabbage is a leafy vegetable that is very popular in Chinese, Japanese and Korean cuisine. The plants are very similar to cabbage. The oblong heads are nutritious.

Collard Green: Collard greens *(Brassica oleracea):* Kingdom: Plantae; Division: angiospermae, Class: Eudicots, Order: Brassicales, Family: Brassicaceae; Binomial name: *Brassica oleracea.* Chromosome number, 2n = 18

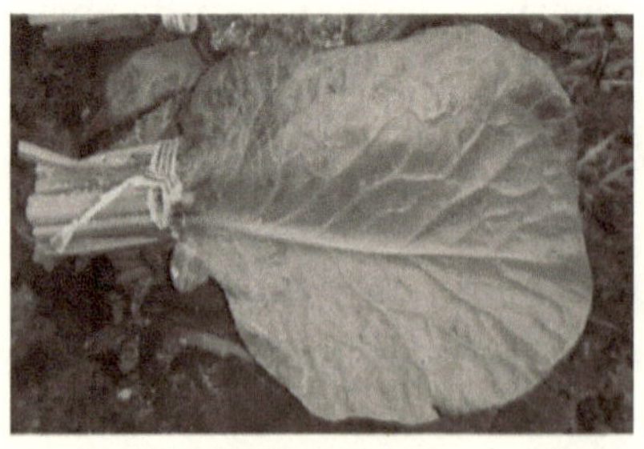

Collard Greens

Collard greens are close relatives of Cabbage, Broccoli, and Kale etc. The plants have dark brown or purple-tinged leaves. Collards that do not produce a head as in cabbage and are referred to as Acephala. Plants may be biennial or perennial. Leaves are slightly bitter and after cooking, are a good source for minerals, soluble fiber, vitamins and antioxidants. **Health:** The leaves contain Sulforaphene and diindolylmethane that have anti-microbial properties.

Kale: *(Brassica oleracea):* **Kingdom: Plantae; Division: Angiospermae; Class: Eudicots; Order: Brassicales; Family: Brassicaceae; Genus and Species:** Brassica oleracea **Acephala group. Chromosome number, 2n = 18**

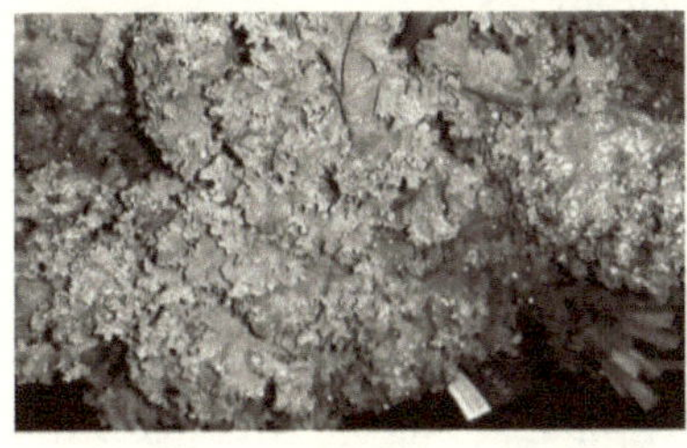

Kale

It is a leafy vegetable related to mustard, cabbage and cauliflower where in the central leaves do not form a head. There are at least five varieties of Kale namely, Scots Kale that is curly leaved; plain leaved, Rape Kale, leaf Cavalo Nero or Tuscan Kale and spear Kale. Kale is a fast growing leafy vegetable. Kale contains many phytonutrients and anti-oxidants. **Health relevance:** Kale leaves are rich in carotenoids and Sulforaphene. Sulforaphene is an anticancer agent. Kale leaves also contain indole-3-carbinol that helps to repair DNA damage in cells. Kale juice is a popular health food drink. Kale has been found to contain a group of resins known as bile acid sequestrants that have been shown to lower cholesterol and decrease absorption of dietary fat. Steaming significantly increases these bile acid binding properties.

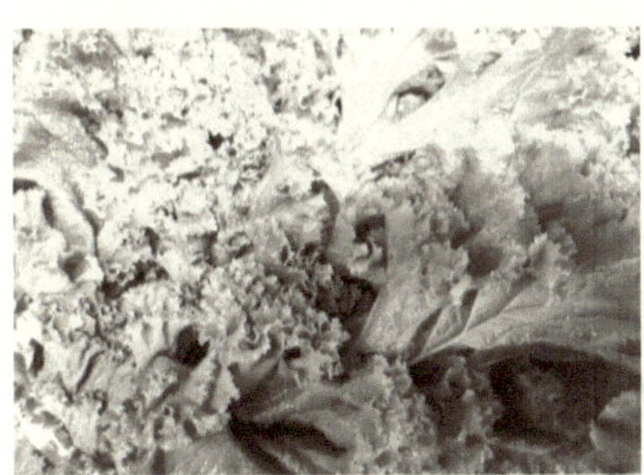

Mustard Green

Mustard greens *(Brassica juncea):* Kingdom: Plantae, Division: Angiosperms, Class Eudicots, and Rosids Order: Brassicales, Family: Brassicaceae, Binomial name: *Brassica juncea.* **Chromosome number, 2n = 4x = 36**

Mustard greens have a botanical profile similar to that of *B. napa* described earlier under oil seeds. The leaves and stem are used as a green vegeatable. In Russia, this variety is grown as the main source of mustard oil. The plant accumulates cadmium from soils and hence a good crop for phytoremediation of soils.

Other Brassica/Cabbage family: Leaves of several other plants of Brassicaceae named below are consumed either in salads or after cooking as part of specific ethnic cultures. These may serve as alternate sources of leaf-food under famine conditions. Apart from leaves, other parts of these plants such as radish are edible roots or stems.

Brassica napus (Rutabaga – India, Nepal); *Brassica nigra* (Black Mustard); *Brassica oleracea* var. alboglabra (Chinese kale); *Brassica rapa* subsp. Chinensis (Bok Choi); *Brassica rapa* subsp. Narinosa (Chinese Savoy); *Brassica rapa* subsp. Nipposinica (Mizuna, Japan, China); *Brassica rapa* subsp. Pekinensis (Chinese/Napa Cabbage); *Brassica rapa* subsp. Rapa (Rapini).

Other Major Green leafy vegetables

Dandelion (Taraxacum officianale): Kingdom: Plantae; Division: angiospermae, Class: Eudicots, Order: Asterales, Family: Asteraceae; Binomial name: Taraxacum officianale. Chromosome number, 2n = 24

Dandelion is a European native perennial plant whose low spreading, deeply notched leaves form a rosette pattern as they emerge from a weak central taproot. The plants are often found as weeds in lawns. It closely resembles endive in form and in cultural requirements. The hollow flower stalks form a single compound flower of many golden colored florets. Like chicory, varieties differ in leaf shape, ranging from very curly leaved to broad-leaved.

Endive: Two species of Endive are edible. These are Belgian endive and Endiva that contains two varieties namely curly endive and Escarole respectively.

1. Belgian Endive/Chicory *(Cichorium intybus)*: Kingdom: Plantae; Division: Angiospermae, Eudicots, Order: Asterales, Family: Asteraceae; Binomial Name: Cichorium intybus. Chromosome number, 2n = 18

This type of Chicory is more known for the powdered dry Chicory roots that are added to some types of coffee powders. However, the leaves that have a somewhat bitter taste are also edible after cooking in boiling water. **Health:** Chicory has anti-hepatotoxic properties as shown by animal studies. In alternative medicine, chicory is listed under Bach flower remedies for cancer treatment without scientific basis.

2. Endiva *(Cichorium endiva)*: Kingdom: Plantae; Division: angiospermae, Class: Eudicots, Order: Asterales, Family: Asteraceae; Binomial Name: Cichorium endiva. Chromosome number, 2n = 18.

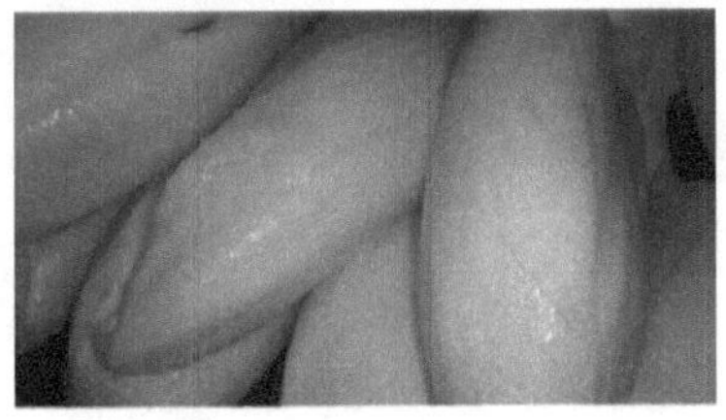

Endiva

Tender Endive leaves are used in salads and in soup preparations. There are two types of endive: 1. Curly endive *(C.endiva var crispum)* with curly leaves and 2. Escarole/Broad leaved Endive *(C. endiva var latifolia)* with broad pale yellow leaves. Both types of endive are used as green vegetables in salads and in soups.

Fenugreek *(Trigonella foenum-graecum)*: Kingdom: Plantae; Division: Angiospermae; Class: Eudicots, Order: Fabales, Family: Fabaceae. Chromosome number, 2n = 16

The plants are annual herbs with trifoliate leaves. The leaves of Fenugreek are used as a cooked leaf vegetable in various soups, stew independently or as a mix with other greens. Details of this plant are given under the section on spices. **Health:** Fenugreek leaves and seeds are considered effective in controlling diabetes and are recommended as lactating agents to induce milk production for breast-feeding.

Garden Cress *(Lepidium sativum);* Kingdom: Plantae; Division: Angiospermae, Class: Eudicots, Order: Brassicales; Family: Brassicaceae. Binomial name: Lepidium sativum, **Chromosome number: 2n = 16. However, there are 7X, 9X, 11X and 14 X ploids depending on variety and accession.**

These annual herbs can be grown hydroponically and known variously as garden cress, mustard cress, garden peppercress and poor man's pepper because of the tangy peppery taste of the leaves. Leaves and sprouts are harvested for use in salads, soups and as a flavor condiment. **Health:** Seed powders/extracts are reported to be useful for treating Asthma by improving lung functions and possibly have hypoglycemic properties.

Gonkura/Roselle/*(Hibiscus subdariffa):* Kingdom: Plantae; Division: Angiospermae, Class: Eudicots; Order: Malvales; Family: Malvaceae.

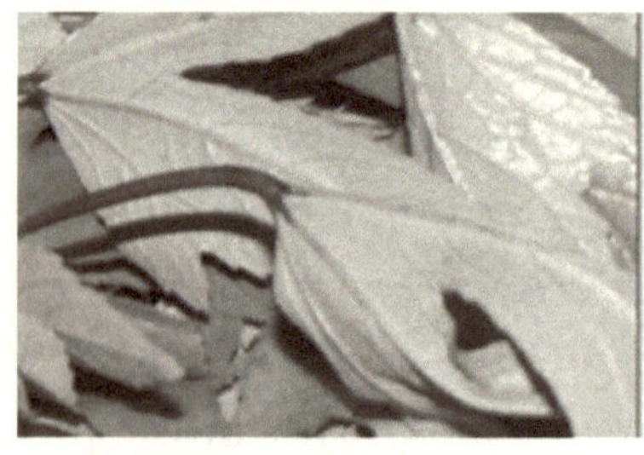

Gonkura

The plant is known variously as; Sour leaf and Red Sorrel (English), Gonkura, Pulicha Keerai, Pundi, Ambadi, Mathipuli, Lalchatni (India) Chin Baung (Myanmar), T Flor de Jamaica (Mexico), Karkade (Arabic); Sorrel (Caribbean islands). This plant is closely related to the taller, green stemmed Gongura/Kenaf/hemp *(Hibiscus cannabinus).* The leaves are a very important herb or vegetable in a good part of India (Andhra, Kerala, Karnataka, Assam and others), and valued for their iron content. They are used in a wide variety of pickles, dals and curries. The flowers are red in color and contain high levels of phytochemicals. **Health:** Leaf and flower broth contain phytochemicals and are recommended in native medicine of India for treating high blood pressure, liver disease and atherosclerosis.

Lettuce *(Lactuca sativa):* Kingdom: Plantae; Division: Angiospermae; Eudicots; Class: Order: astrales Family: asteraceae; Genus and species: *Lactuca sativa.* Chromosome number, 2n = 18

It is an annual plant grown in temperate countries. It is a leaf vegetable used mainly in salads but also in stir-fries and steamed food.

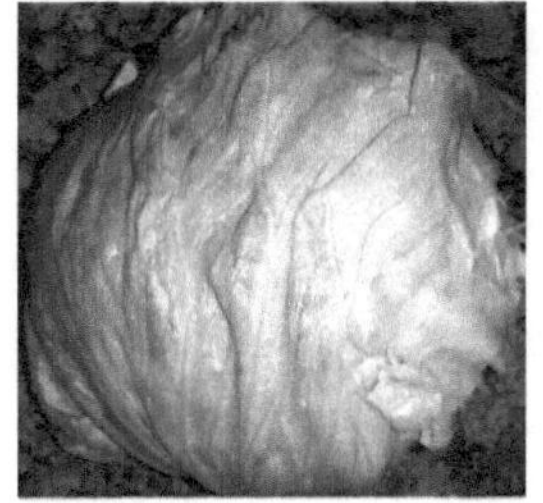

There are several varieties: Romaine, Iceberg or crisphead, Butterhead, Woju and French crisp. Plants grow to a height of 6–12 inches. Leaves are crisp in the salad and sandwich varieties. **Health relevance:** Lettuce leaves are high in fiber and have vitamins and minerals especially lithium.

Lettuce

Moringa *(Moringa Oleifera):* **Kingdom: Plantae; Division: Angiospermae, Class: Eudicots, Order: Brassicales, Family: Moringaceae; Genus and species:** *Moringa Oleifera.* **Others:** *Moringa ovalifolia,* **((South-west Africa, Namibia and southwestern Angola);** *Moringa stenopetala,* **(Ethiopian Moringa-Ethiopia/Africa) Chromosome number, 2n = 28.**

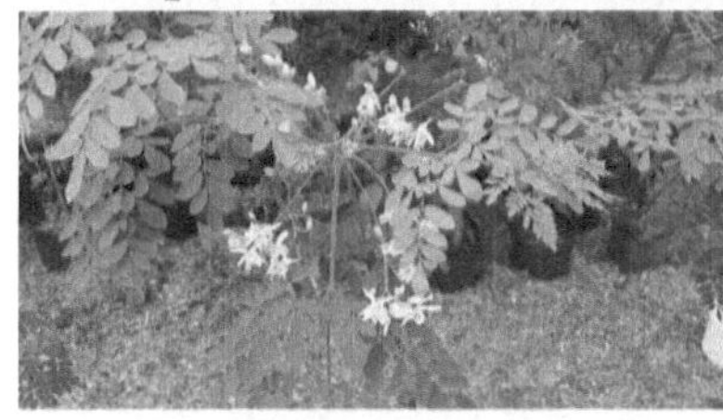

Moringa plants are tall, drought resistant, fast growing deciduous trees, growing in tropical/sub-tropical countries where the fruits, seeds and leaves are used as vegetables, salads and oil. The trees are also known as drumstick

Moringa

trees since they produce long stick like fruit-pods. Trees reach a height of 30 ft-40 ft. Trees produce fragile drooping branches with tri-pinnate small leaves. Flowers are yellowish-white and bisexual. Fruits are long about 8"-14" and are tri-capsulate. Seeds have three whitish wings that help dispersal when the capsule breaks open. However, the capsulate fruits are harvested for use as vegetables long before they break open naturally. Moringa is a sun and heat-loving plant and does not tolerate freezing or frost. Moringa is particularly suitable for dry regions as it can be grown using rainwater without expensive irrigation techniques. Plants can be generated from cuttings and seeds. Moringa is cultivated for its leaves, kernels and oil. The oil is used mainly for cosmetic purposes. The leaves are the most nutrient-containing part of the plant. The tree is recommended by the Food and agriculture organization of the

United Nations as a great source of nutrition to combat malnutrition. **Health:** Apart from its nutritional value, Moringa leaves and fruit are used for treating anemia, arthritis, diabetes, stomach ulcers and as an aphrodisiac. The leaves are also being promoted as anti-cancer green extract.

Spinach (Spinacea oleracea): Kingdom: Plantae; Division: Angiospermae Class: Eudicots; Order: Caryophyllales Family: Amaranthaceae formerly Chenapodiaceae; Genus and species: Spinacia oleraceae. Chromosome number, 2n = 10.

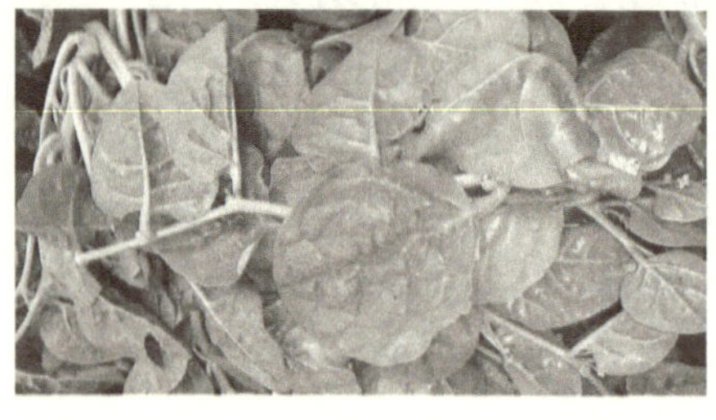

Spinach

It is an annual herb whose leaves are used as green vegetable. The plants grow to a height of about 1–2 ft. with soft stems from which long leaves with soft petioles arise in an alternate fashion. The leaves are generally green but Chinese spinach has purple stems and leaf veins containing anthocyanin. The leaves are a rich source of folates. **Health:** The leaves contain Oxalic acid that chelates the iron and calcium present in the leaves and make them poorly available. However, boiling the spinach can remove the oxalates but this also removes the nutrients. Spinach is one of the plants that receive heavy doses of pesticides and hence the leaves have to be washed well before use.

Wild Lettuce, spinach and radish types of leaf vegeatable:

The leaves of the following plants are consumed in salads or after cooking. They are, *Chenopodium album* (Lamb's Quarters), *Chenopodium giganteum* (Tree Spinach), *Basella alba* (Indian spinach/Malabar Spinach-India South Asia), *Cnidoscolus aconitifolius* (Chaya), *Ipomoea aquatica* (Water Spinach), *Gynura crepioides* (Okinawan Spinach), *Raphanus sativus* (Radish), *Raphanus sativus var. longipinnatus,* (Chinese radish), *Mycelis muralis,* (Wall lettuce), *Campanula rapunculus*

(Rampion), *Campanula versicolor* (Harebell), *Capparis spinosa* (Caper), *Centella asiatica* (Asian pennywort, Gotukola, Bai bua bok, Gotukola Sambola).

Table 11: Nutritional data of Leaf Vegetables

Used in salads and or cooking (continued). Data from National Nutrient Database for Standard Reference Release 28 Software v.2.3.5, The National Agricultural Library, United States Department of Agriculture Agricultural Research Service

Metabolite	Cabbage	Chard	Chicory	Cress	Dandelion	Endive	Roselle
	Chinese	Swiss					Gonkura
Water, g	95.32	92.66	92	89.4	85.6	93.79	86.58
Protein-g	1.5	1.8	1.7	2.6	2.7	1.25	0.96
Total lipid (fat), g	0.2	0.2	0.3	0.7	0.7	0.2	0.64
Carbohydrate, g	2.18	3.74	4.7	5.5	9.2	3.35	11.31
Fiber	1	1.6	4	1.1	3.5	3.1	NA
Sugar	1.18	1.1	0.7	4.4	0.71	0.25	NA
Calcium, mg	105	51	100	81	187	52	215
Iron, mg	0.8	1.8	0.9	1.3	3.1	0.83	1.48
Magnesium, mg	19	81	30	38	36	15	51
Phosphorus, mg	37	46	47	76	66	28	37
Potassium, mg	252	379	420	606	397	314	208
Sodium, mg	65	213	45	14	76	22	6
Zinc	0.19	0.36	0.42	0.23	0.41	0.79	NA
Vitamin C, mg	45	30	24	69	35	6.5	12
Thiamin, mg	0.04	0.04	0.06	0.08	0.19	0.08	0.011
Riboflavin, mg	0.07	0.09	0.1	0.26	0.26	0.075	0.028
Niacin, mg	0.5	0.4	0.5	1	0.806	0.4	0.31
Vitamin B-6, mg	0.194	0.099	0.105	0.247	0.251	0.02	0
Folate, DFE,	66	14	110	80	27	142	NA
Vitamin B-12, µg	0	0	0	0	0	0	NA
Vitamin A, µg	223	306	286	346	508	108	14
Vitamin A, IU	4468	6116	5717	6917	10161	2167	287
Vitamin E, mg	0.09	1.89	2.26	0.7	3.44	0.44	NA
Vitamin D, µg	0	0	0	0	0	0	NA
Vitamin D, IU	0	0	0	0	0	0	NA
Vitamin K	45.5	830	297.6	541.9	778.4	231	NA

Metabolite	Cabbage	Chard	Chicory	Cress	Dandelion	Endive	Roselle
Fatty acids, g	0.027	0.03	0.073	0.023	0.17	0.048	0
Monounsaturated, g	0.015	0.04	0.006	0.239	0.014	0.004	NA
Polyunsaturated, g	0.096	0.07	0.131	0.228	0.306	0.087	NA
Cholesterol, mg	0	0	0	0	0	0	NA
Caffeine	0	0	0	0	0	0	NA

Root, Stem and Bulb Vegetables

The plants described below are those vegetables used in salads or cooking derived from roots, stem or bulbs of various plants. Tubers like potato, sweet potato; taro, dioscorea and yams are also used as vegetables and have been described under staple foods since they provide significant calories as staples.

Asparagus: *(Asparagus officianalis):* Kingdom: Plantae Division: Angiospermae, Class: Monocotyledonae Order: Asperagales; Family: Asparagaceae; Genus and species: Asparagus officianalis. Chromosome number, 2n = 30.

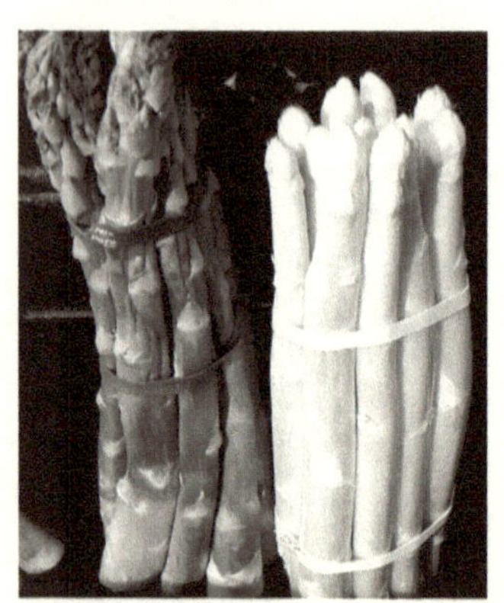

Asparagus

Asparagus is a perennial herbaceous monocot plant wherein, the tender shoots that are the stems with scaly leaves are the edible vegetable. The plants tolerate salinity and grow best in saline conditions. Male and female flowers grow on separate plants generally. Although the natural shoots are green in color, white or pale white shoots are artificially produced by a blanching process wherein the shoots are covered to prevent photosynthesis and the shoots become bleached.

Health relevance: The asparagus shoots are rich in vitamins and minerals. The shoots are also recommended as a medicinal herb known as shatavaari in the Ayurvedic system. The seeds of Asparagus are toxic.

Beets *(Beta vulgaris):* **Kingdom: Plantae, Division: Angiospermae, Class: Eudicots, Family: Chenopodiaceae/Amaranthaceae, Chromosome number, 2n = 18**

There are many varieties of this plant but chiefly, the purple colored roots of garden beet variety of this species is used as a vegetable whereas, the white colored root variety is mainly used to extract beet sugar and a third variety known as leaf chard is used as a leafy vegetable. All varieties of beet are herbaceous biennials with leafy stems with heart shaped leaves. The garden beet has roots that enlarge into bulbous deep purple heart-shaped structures containing valuable antioxidants, minerals, vitamins and sugar. Both the bulbous roots and leaves are used as vegetables. The red pigment in beets is due to presence of betalain pigments. The roots also contain indicaxanthin and vulgaxanthin that seem to have a protective effect in thalassemia patients by preventive oxidative damage to red blood cells. The roots and leaves also contain oxalic acid which are causative agents for developing kidney stones and hence eating cooked beet from which most of the oxalates are removed is better than eating raw beets in salads. Some people pass out red colored urine (beet urea) after consuming beets and this is because such individuals are unable to break down betacyanin present in beetroots.

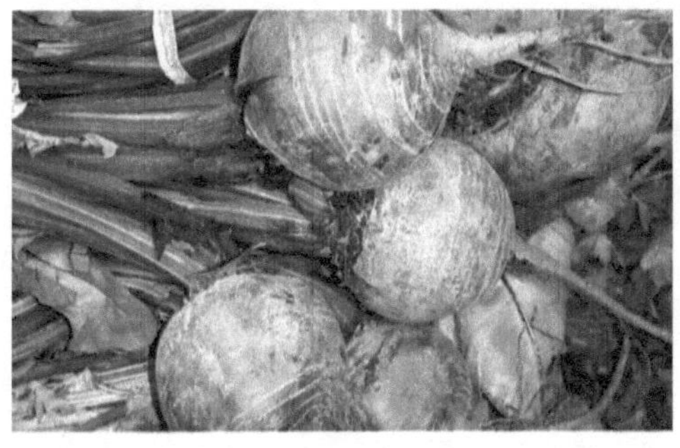

Beets

The sugarbeet variety contains large amounts of sugar, mainly used for extracting sugar, and has very little use as a vegetable. **Health relevance:** Rich source of antioxidants. It is reported to help protect red blood cells from oxidative damage. It contains oxalic acid that can lead to developing kidney stones if eaten as raw vegetable in salads.

Carrots *(Daucus carota)*: Kindgdom: Plantae Division: Angiospermae, Class: Eudicots Order: Apiales Family: Apiaceae; Genus and species: *Daucus carota*. 2n = 18

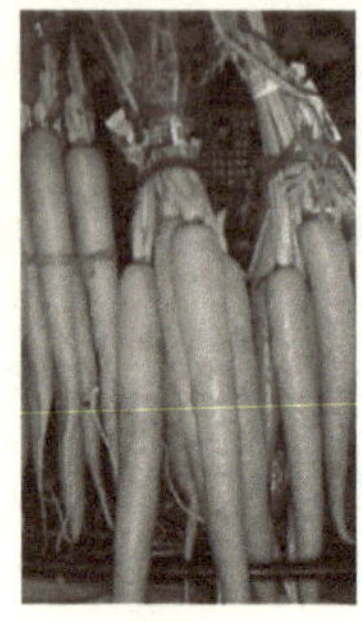

Carrots

The carrot plants are biennials growing to about 3 ft. tall producing small white or pink flowers arranged in an umbel. Stems have fine hairs and leaves are bi or tri pinnate. The taproots become enlarged like an inverted pyramid ranging in size from about 3–4 inches in the case of baby carrots to about 9 inches long in the longer variety. The roots range in color from pale yellow to orange-red and are the edible vegetable.

Health relevance: The edible roots contain fiber, cellulose, sugar, soluble amino acids and carotene. Carotene is a precursor for vitamin A. Besides carotene, it contains caffeic acid and polyacetylenes that have antifungal activities. Over consumption of carrots results in a condition known as Carotenemia. Carotenaemia (xanthaemia) wherein, the skin turns yellow-orange. This is reversible but the condition can be mistaken for jaundice.

Celery *(Apium graveolens)*: Kingdom: Plantae; Division: Angiospermae, Class: Eudicots; Order: Apiales; Family: Apiaceae; Genus and species: *Apium graveolens*. Chromosome number, 2n = 22.

The plants are herbaceous growing to a height of about 3 ft. The plants have fleshy greenish white stems that are edible. Celery is consumed as a raw vegetable salad. Leaves and flowers are similar to those of carrots. The plant has high fiber. **Health relevance:** Many people are allergic to celery and the celery allergens can cause severe anaphylactic shock. It is a uterine stimulant and so pregnant women should avoid celery. Celery also contains oxalates that cause formation of kidney stones.

Garlic *(Allium sativum):* Kingdom: Plantae; Division: Angiospermae, Class: Monocotyledonae; Order: Aliases; Family: Amaryllidaceae. Botanical name: *Allium sativum.* Chromosome number, 2n = 16

Garlic plants produce underground bulbs in clusters known as cloves. Garlic plants are herbaceous perennials but are treated as annuals for harvesting. Garlic cloves are used for cooking, medicine and as pest repellants. There are three morpho-types of garlic namely, A, U, H morpho-types with certain specific identifying morphological features. **Health:** Some studies indicate that garlic may reduce cholesterol and triglycerides. Garlic reduces platelet aggregation. Garlic has anti-bacterial and possibly anti-viral properties. Garlic causes bad breath and even body odor. Consuming milk simultaneously while consuming garlic products will reduce this odor. Other side effects include gastrointestinal discomfort, sweating, dizziness, allergic reactions, bleeding, and menstrual irregularities.

Jerusalem artichoke *(Helianthus tuberosus):* Kindgdom: Plantae; Division: Angiospermae; Class: Eudicots Order: Asterales, Family: Asteraceae. Chromosome number, 2n = 6x = 102

Helianthus tuberosus belongs to the same genus as the Sunflower. The tubers of the plant are edible. The tubers appear similar to ginger. Plants are perennial herbs. The root system survives year to year underground and above ground, they produce opposite leaves on top and alternate leaves in the lower part of stem. The tubers contain about 10% protein and 76% inulin that is a polymer of fructose. **Health:** Since the tubers have no sugar but only inulin that is converted to fructose, the tubers are recommended as a source of food for diabetics (type-2). Fructose is not directly used as a sugar by the body and yet is a carbohydrate source.

Kohlrabi/Knolkhol (*Brassica oleraceae,* Gongylodes): Kindgdom: Plantae; Division: Angiospermae; Class: Eudicots Order: Brassicale, Family: Brassicaceae. Chromosome number, 2n = 18.

This is a stem and leaf vegetable plant. The stems are pale green and swollen. The edible stem upon harvest contains many brownish scars 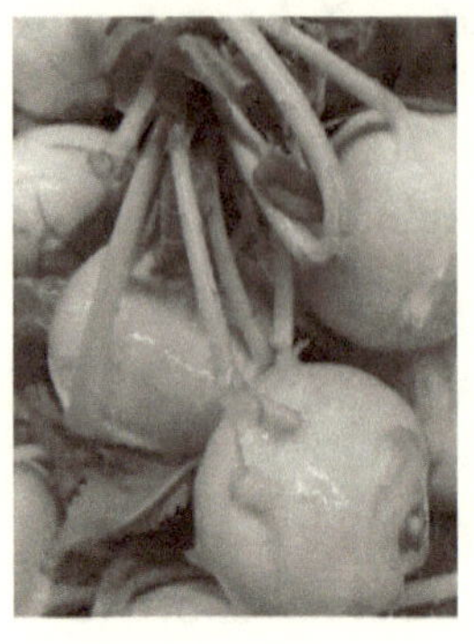 representing the position of previous leaves which had dropped during growth. The skin is tough and has to be peeled for cooking. The leaves arise in a bunch just above the swollen stem. Kohlrabi stems are surrounded by two distinct fibrous layers that do not soften appreciably when cooked. These layers are generally peeled away prior to cooking or serving raw. The long leaves are also consumable in salads or after cooking. **Health:** Source of minerals and soluble fiber.

Kohlrabi

Onion (*Allium* sp): Kingdom: Plantae; Division: Angiospermae, Class: Monocotyledonae, Order: Asperagales Family, Amaryllidaceae. Botanical names: *Allium Cepa* (Bulb Onion, 2n = 16), *A. ampeloprasum* var. sectivum (Pearl onion); *Allium cepa var. aggregatum* (Shallots, 2n = 16); *A. fistulosum* (Japanese bunching onion, welsh onion); *A. ampeloprasum var. sectivum* or *A. ampeloprasum* 'Pearl-Onion Group (Pearl onion); *A. ampeloprasum var. porrum* (Leek); *A.cepa – var-aggregatum* (Potato onion). Chromosome number: n = 8 in all species but since there are many hybrids the 2n or ploidy number are multiples of 8.

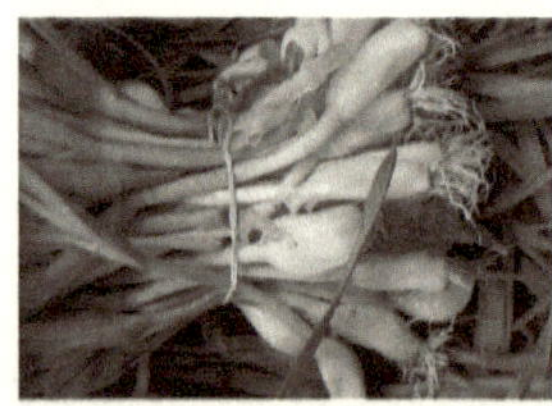

Green Onions

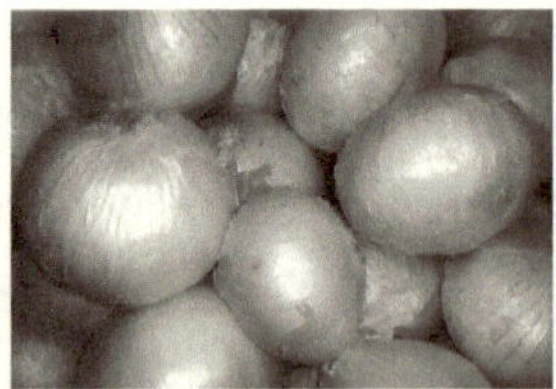

Yellow/White Onion

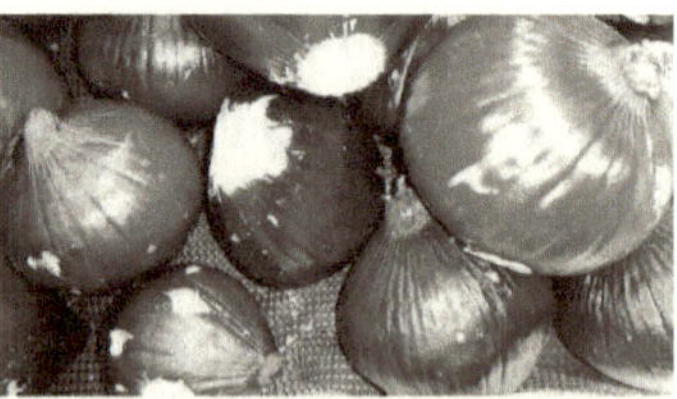

Red onion

Onions belong to the genus Allium. There are many types of onions as noted above but the most common onion in use is the bulb onion (*A.cepa*). Onion plants are perennial when grown in tropical/sub-tropical climates or generally annual in temperate regions. In either case, the bulbs are harvested in the very first year of growth.

Onion bulbs are bulbous stems from which hollow cylindrical leaves arise. Bulb Onions can be yellow, red or white. Plants are usually developed from seeds, sets or transplants. The plants generate hollow cylindrical, monocotyledonous leaves at the bottom of which the stem becomes bulbous with fleshy scaly leaves surrounding the bulb. There are two main groups of Onions namely the Common Bulb onion group (*A.cepa var.cepa*) and the aggregatum group (*A.cepa var.aggregatum*).

The Common bulb onion upon completion of the growth cycle produces a single bulb that may be yellow, red or white, of different shapes, and sizes depending on specific sub verities or hybrids. The aggregatum group contains potato onions, welsh onions and shallots wherein the plant produces clusters of smaller onion bulbs. Many hybrids are also known. Shallots are formed in clusters of offsets with a head composed of multiple cloves. The skin colour of shallots can vary from golden brown to gray to rose red, and their off-white flesh is usually tinged with green or magenta. Shallots are used mainly for cooking. Potato onions produce larger bulbs in clusters compared to shallots. These are also used for cooking purposes. Spring onions also known as scallions or green onions are used as vegetables and consist of many different *Allium* species or may refer to bulb onions harvested before full bulb formation. **Health**: Onions are rich in phytochemicals including Flavanoids, anthocyanin and polyphenols. They are considered good as cardio protective agents as well as diuretics. However, many people are allergic to onions and exhibit contact dermatitis, asthma, sweating, severe lacrimation and even anaphylaxis. However, cooking removes many allergens due to denaturation of allergic proteins. Onions can be quite lethal to animals including pets.

Parsnip *(Pastinaca sativa)*: Kindgdom: Plantae; Division: Angiospermae; Class: Eudicots Order: Apiales, Family: Apiaceae. Chromosome number, 2n = 22.

Parsnips are biennial herbs that had its origin in the Eurasian region. It is a root vegetable wherein the edible part is the swollen taproot.

The plant grows vegetatively during the first year and then produces flowers in umbels similar to those of carrots in the second year. Generally, the taproots are harvested after the winter before the second year growth. Parsnips can be eaten raw but most commonly they are cooked by baking or broiling. **Health:** Parsnip roots contain antioxidants such as falcarinol, falcarindiol, panaxydiol and methyl-falcarindiol that have anti-cancer, anti-inflammatory and anti-fungal properties. They have high fiber content.

Radish: *(Raphanus sativus):* **Kindgdom: Plantae; Division: Angiospermae; Class: Eudicots Order: Brassicales Family: Brassicaceae. 2n = 18**

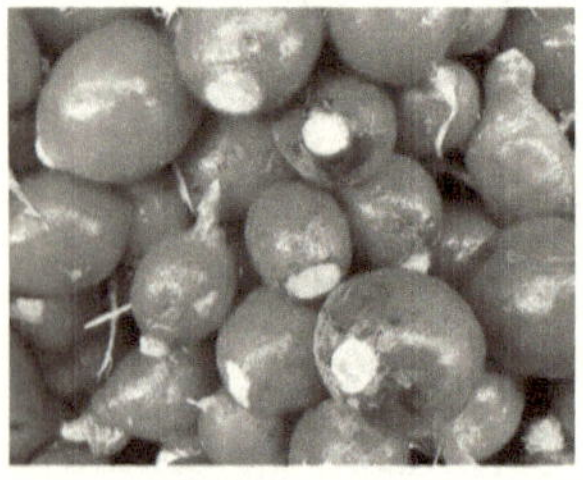

Red Radish

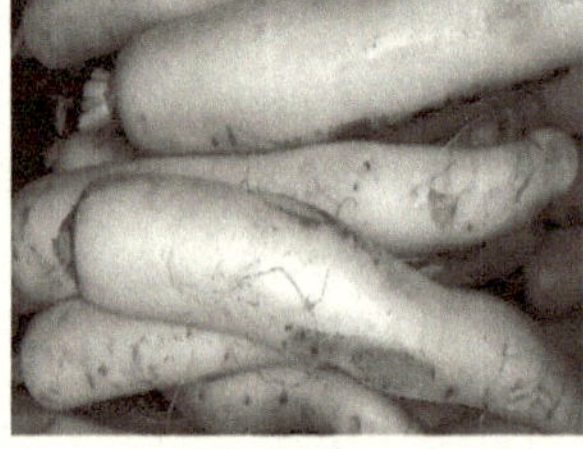

White Radish

Radishes are edible root vegetables that were domesticated in Europe in pre-Roman times. There are different varieties ranging from those with small bulbous red-pink roots to those that are elongate –white and very long white colored. Radishes are grown and consumed throughout the world both as a raw vegetable in salads and after cooking. Some radishes such as Daikon are grown both for their roots as well as for their oil-bearing seeds. They are biennial plants with globular or cylindro-conical fleshy roots. The Daikon variety has much longer fleshy roots. Leaves are arranged in a rosette form similar to turnips and beets. The white flowers are borne on a racemose inflorescence. The fruits are small pods that can be eaten when young. **Health:** Good source of minerals and fiber.

Rutabaga/Swedish turnip (Brassica napus var. napobrassica): Kindgdom: Plantae; Division: Angiospermae; Class: Eudicots Order: Brassicales, Family: Brassicaceae. Chromosome number, 2n = 38. The plants are a natural cross hybrid of turnips and cabbage. The roots as well as leaves are edible but are essentially considered as a food of last resort. The roots are cooked for edibility. **Health:** Roots and leaves contain cyanoglucosides and hence there is a possibility of developing goiter since cyanates released could make iodine unavailable for thyroid development.

Turnip: *(Brassica Rapa subsp. Rapa):* **Kindgdom: Plantae; Division: Angiospermae; Eudicots Order: Brassicales, Family: Brassicaceae. Chromosome number,** 2n = 38.

Turnip is a biennial root vegetable plant commonly grown in temperate climates worldwide for its white bulbous taproot. The taproot is globular about 3 inches to 10 inches in diameter with a thin skin and white flesh. About 1–2 inches of the root projects above ground and is pink or red in color. Leaves are thin and similar to mustard greens and consumed as a leaf vegetable after cooking. **Health:** Good source of minerals and fiber but also has cyanoglucosides that can be toxic. In view of this, turnip roots and leaves should be heat treated (stir-fry, boiling) before consumption so that the cyanoglucosides are destroyed.

Table10 – Nutritional data of Leaf

Vegetables used in salads and or cooking: Data from National Nutrient Database for Standard Reference Release 28 Software v.2.3.5. The National Agricultural Library, United States Department of Agriculture, Agricultural Research Service

Metabolite	Amaranth	Brussels sprouts	Cabbage	Collard	Kale	Lettuce Ice	Moringa	Mustard	Spinach	Sweet Potato	Turnip
Water g	91.69	86	92.18	89.62	84	95.64	78.66	90.7	91.4	86.81	89.67
Protein-g	2.11	3.38	1.28	3.02	4.28	0.9	9.4	2.86	2.86	2.49	1.5
Total lipid g	0.18	0.3	0.1	0.61	0.93	0.14	1.4	0.42	0.39	0.51	0.3
Carbohydrate, g	4.11	8.95	5.8	5.42	8.75	2.97	8.28	4.67	3.63	8.82	7.13
Fiber	NA	3.8	2.5	4	3.6	1.2	2	3.2	2.2	5.3	3.2
Sugar	NA	2.2	3.2	0.46	2.26	1.97	NA	1.32	0.42	0.81	
Calcium, mg	209	42	40	232	150	18	185	115	99	78	190
Iron, mg	2.26	1.4	0.47	0.47	1.47	0.41	4	1.64	2.71	0.97	1.1
Magnesium, mg	55	23	12	27	47	7	147	32	79	70	31
Phosphorus, mg	72	69	26	25	92	20	112	58	49	81	42
Potassium, mg	641	389	170	213	491	141	337	384	558	508	296
Sodium, mg	21	25	18	17	38	10	9	20	79	6	40
Zinc, mg	0.88	0.42	0.18	0.21	0.56	0.15	0.6	0.25	0.53	0.19	
Vitamin C, mg	41.1	85	36.6	35.3	120	2.8	51.7	70	28.1	11	60
Thiamin, mg	0.02	0.139	0.061	0.054	0.11	0.041	0.257	0.08	0.078	0.156	0.07
Riboflavin, mg	0.134	0.09	0.04	0.13	0.13	0.025	0.66	0.11	0.189	0.345	0.1

Metabolite	Amaranth	Brussels sprouts	Cabbage	Collard	Kale	Lettuce Ice	Moringa	Mustard	Spinach	Sweet Potato	Turnip
Niacin, mg	0.559	0.745	0.234	0.742	1	0.123	2.22	0.8	0.724	1.13	0.6
Vitamin B-6, mg	0.177	0.219	0.124	0.165	0.27	0.042	1.2	0.18	0.195	0.19	0.263
Folate, DFE,	57	61	43	129	141	29	40	12	194	1	194
Vitamin B-12, μg	0	0	0	0	0	0	0	0	0	0	0
Vitamin A, μg	139	38	5	251	500	25	378	151	469	189	579
Vitamin A, IU	2770	754	98	5019	9990	502	7564	3024	9377	3778	11587
Vitamin E, mg	0	0.88	0.15	2.26	1.54	0.18	0	2.01	2.03	0	2.86
Vitamin D, μg	0	0	0	0	0	0	0	0	NA	0	0
Vitamin D, IU	0	0	0	0	0	0	0	0	NA	0	0
Vitamin K	NA	177	76	437.1	705	24.1	NA	257.5	482.9	302.2	251
Fatty acids, g	0.05	0.062	0.034	0.055	0.09	0.018	0	0.01	0.063	0.111	0.07
Monounsat, g	0.041	0.023	0.017	0.03	0.05	0.006	0	0.092	0.01	0.02	0.02
Polyunsat, g	0.08	0.153	0.017	0.201	0.34	0.074	0	0.038	0.165	0.228	0.12
Cholesterol, mg	0	0	0	0	0	0	0	0	0	0	0

Fruit-Vegetables

The following are botanically called as fruits but are popularly known as vegetables. Here, the edible part is the fruit of the plant that develops after pollination. The completely un-ripened mature fruit along with the outer skin and tender seeds are consumed as vegetable. In some instances as in Avacados, certain cucurbits, the outer skin is removed before consumption.

Avocado/Vennai Pazham in Tamil *(Persea americana)*: Kingdom: Plantae; Division: Angiospermae, Class: Magnoliids; Order: Laurales; Family: Lauraceae. Chromosome number, 2n = 2 × = 24

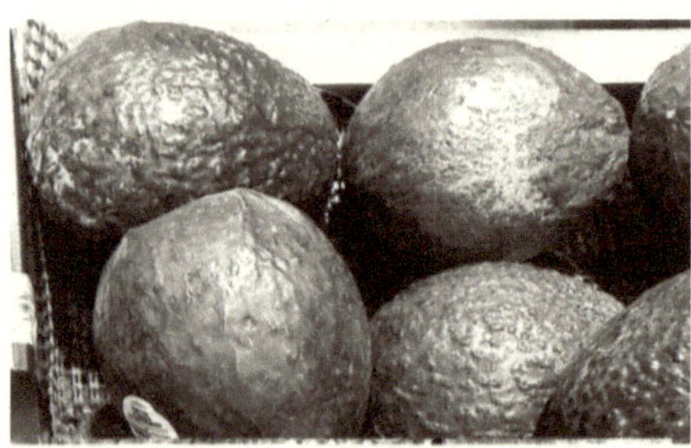

Avacados

The Avocado is a large tall tree growing to a height of about 70 ft. They grow in subtropical climates in areas which are not windy since high winds cause dehydration and early fall of the small greenish yellow flowers. The avocado plants exhibit a phenomenon called dichogamy wherein the flowers change from female-protogyny to male-protandry or male-protandry to female – protogyny. There are two main flowering types among avocados. In Cultivar A flowers open as female in the morning and close in the afternoon or evening of the first flowering day. On the second day of flowering, the same cultivar opens in the afternoon as male flowers. In cultivar B on the first day flowers open in the afternoon as female then close in the evening and open as male flowers on the second day. Leaves are arranged in an alternate fashion on stem. Fruits are fleshy, pear shaped with a central seed. The fruit does not ripen on the tree but ripens after harvesting or falling down naturally. The fruits are served raw since cooking can change the fruits to become bitter. The fruits are rich in monounsaturated oleic acid plus lesser amounts of palmitic acid and linoleic acids. Fruits are rich in Vitamins C, E and some of the B vitamins. Avocados also contain phytosterols and carotenoids such as lutein and zeaxanthin. **Health:** Several reports show that intake of avocado can reduce serum cholesterol levels with decrease in LDL cholesterol and increase in HDL cholesterol.

Banana/Plantain (Musa sp) Kingdom: Plantae Division: Angiospermae, Class: Monocotyledonae Order: Family: Musae, Genus and species: Cultivated bananas are *Musa acuminata Colla and Musa balbisiana Colla, Musa acuminata (Blood banana), M. paradisiaca syn. M. Sapientum (Plantain, Nendiran), M. balbisiana (wild banana),* are different species of cultivated banana. Most of the current edible bananas are hybrids.

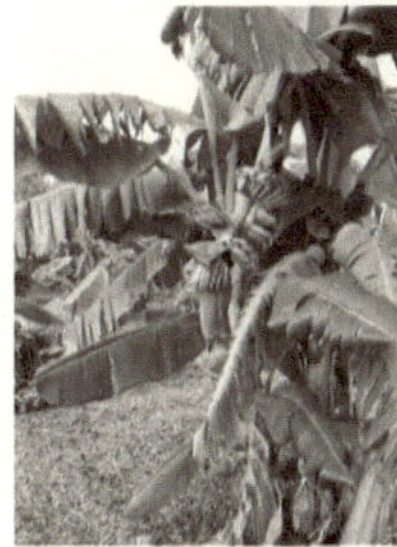

Banana bunch

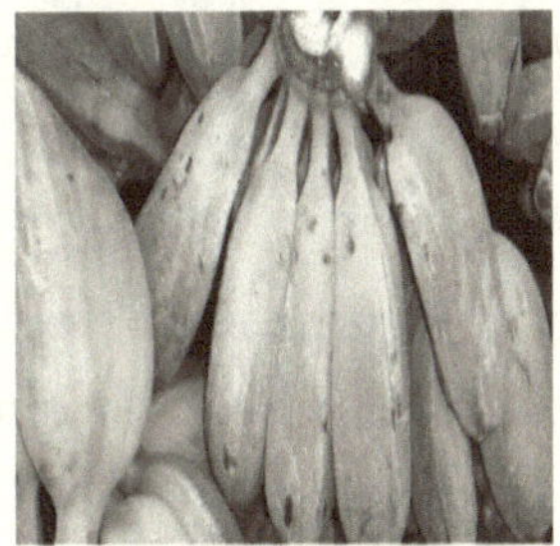

Raw banana

The banana fruits grow in a bunch of about 80–100 fruits. The unripe banana fruit is used as a culinary vegetable and as a source of carbohydrate. The unripe pulp is dried, powdered and consumed in baby foods and as a staple food in many Asian, African and South American cultures. The powdered fruit is also used for fermentation to prepare alcoholic beverages. Detailed description of Banana is given in the section on culinary fruits. The finely cut pieces of the skin of the plantain variety is cooked and or stir-fried as a vegetable side dish. The skin is rich in fiber and minerals. The aerial banana stem is a pseudo stem and can be seen when the outer layers are peeled off. This pseudo stem is white in color and is very shiny. The pseudo-stem is fibrous and is very juicy. This pseudo stem is edible after cooking. **Health:** The juice of the banana pseudo stem contains many chemicals, which can dissolve stones. It is prescribed as a remedy for dissolving kidney stones. The fruit vegetables are rich in carbohydrates and minerals. The skin of the fruit vegetable is a good source of dietary fiber.

Legume vegetables: All bean species, cluster beans, soybeans, cowpea, Crowder peas, lentils, peas, Dolichos beans and other legumes are also consumed as vegetables. These have been described elsewhere in this book. Usually, the pods along with the unripe seeds are the edible vegetables.

Common/Field beans: (Phaseolus vulgaris): Kingdom: Plantae Division: Angiospermae, Class: Eudicots, Order: Fabales, Family: Fabaceae, Chromosome number, 2n = 22

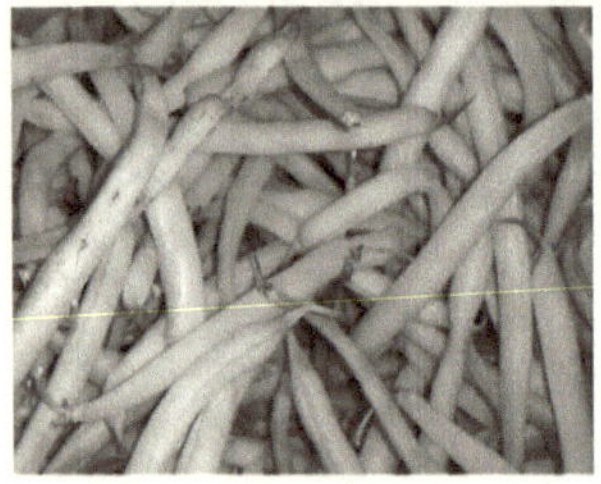

Wax

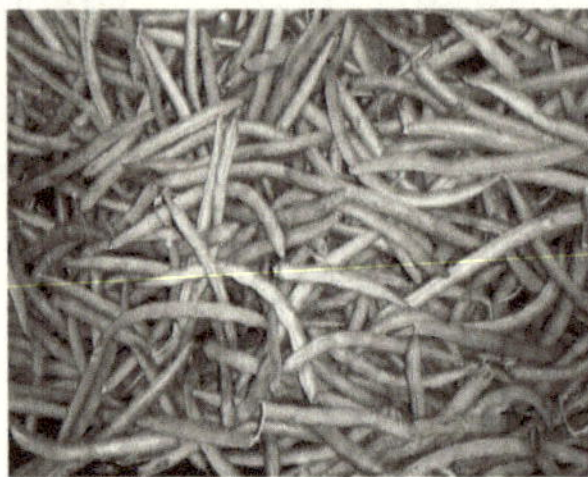

Field Beans

These are the most common type of beans used as vegetables when they are harvested before full maturity. If they are harvested after full maturity then, the seeds are used as legume seed staples. The common bean is also known as string bean, Snap beans, French bean, garden bean, green bean, haricot bean, pop bean, or snap bean. The plants are herbaceous annual plants grown worldwide. While the common field beans have a climbing habit, many cultivars are grouped as "bush beans" or "pole beans," depending on their style of growth. Bush beans are short bushes that grow without support. Pole beans are climbers needing poles for support. They twist around their supports that may be poles, trellis, cages or even other plants (trees/shrubs). The pod color can be green (most common), purple, and pink-red or striped.

Cowpea/black eyed pea/Crowder pea/Southern Pea *(Vigna unguiculata)*: **Kingdom: Plantae Division: Angiospermae, Class: Eudicots, Order: Fabales, Family: Fabaceae, Chromosome number, 2n = 22**

The tender green pods with immature seeds are consumed as cooked vegetable. Details of the plants are given in the Chapter on legumes.

Yard long bean/Asparagus bean/Chinese bean *(Vigna sesquipedalis)*: **Kingdom: Plantae Division: Angiospermae,**

Class: Eudicots, Order: Fabales, Family: Fabaceae, Chromosome number 2n = 22.

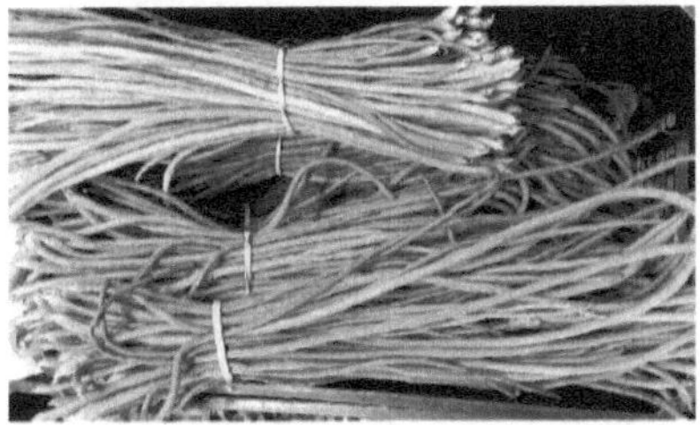

Pods

This is also a popular vegetable. Here, the tender pods that are about half a yard long are cut and cooked as vegetable. Botanical details and nutrition are given elsewhere in this book.

Dolichos/Hyacinth bean/Avara (Dolichos lab lab/lablab purpureus): Kingdom: Plantae Division: Angiospermae, Class: Eudicots, Order: Fabales, Family: Fabaceae Chromosome number, 2n = 22.

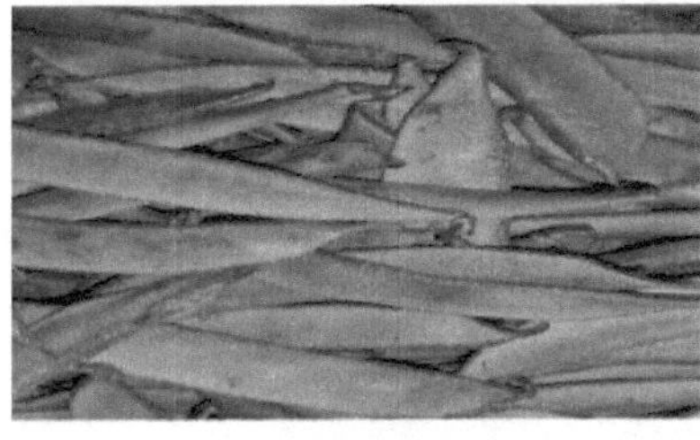

Lablab

Dolichos lablab bean is a popular bean grown mostly as a vegetable. However, the seeds are valuable sources of protein. They are twining herbs with broad leaflets in threes. The leaves are dark green with a tingle of purple. The flowers are pea-like rich, brilliant purple and arranged in loose clusters on long stems that extend above the foliage. The seedpods are green or purple, flat and slightly curved with a purple margin in some cases. The beans inside are dark colored with a conspicuous white hilum.

Garden peas *(Pisum sativum)*: Kingdom: Plantae Division: Angiospermae, Class: Eudicots, Order: Fabales, Family: Fabaceae, Chromosome number, 2n = 14.

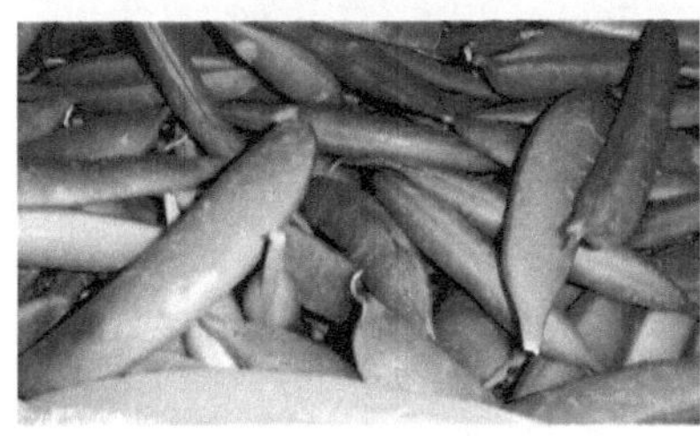

Garden Peas

The tender green pods before maturation of seeds are edible as vegetable. The green pods are cooked as is or sliced and cooked. They are a good source of fiber as well as vitamins and minerals. Botanical details are given elsewhere.

Guar *(Cyamopsis tetragonoloba)*: Kingdom: Plantae Division: Angiospermae, Class: Eudicots, Order: Fabales, Family: Fabaceae Chromosome number, 2n = 14.

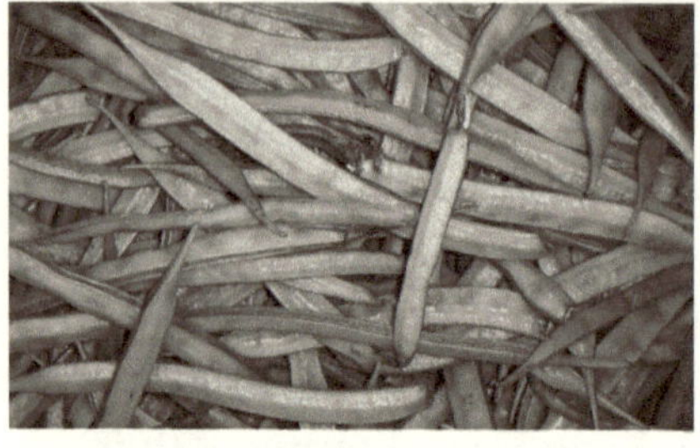

Guar

Cyamopsis tetragonoloba is an upright bush with branches along the tender fibrous stem. The plant grows upright; reaching a maximum height of up to 2–3 m.; Flowers grow in clusters in the axils. The green pods are flat and slender with 5–12 cm small brown seeds. Seeds are rich in guar gum that is used as a thickening agent in ice creams, coffee creams and other foods and is now increasingly used in the oil fracking industry. The slender pods are rich in fiber and are an edible vegetable.

Bitter Melon *(Momordica charantia)*: Kingdom: Plantae Division: Angiospermae, Class: Eudicots Family: Cucurbitaceae Genus and species: Other names are Goya – Japanese; Kho Kua – Viet nam; Pare – Indonesia; Karela/Karola/Pavakkai/Kaippakka etc India; Sopropo – Dominican Republic. Chromosome number, 2n = 22.

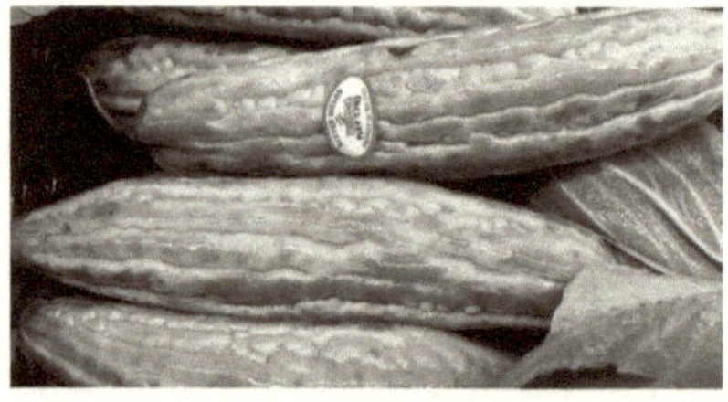

Bitter Melon

The plants are vines with palmate leaves. The flowers are small and yellow in color. Fruits vary in size depending on the variety. All have a serrated soft spinous exterior. The fruits are hollow and spongy inside with many seeds. The edible part is the fruit that has a bitter taste. The fruit vegetable is extensively used to prepare various food dishes in Asia, Africa in particular and in the Caribbean islands and South America. **Health relevance:** The green fruit juice as well as fruit powders have hypoglycemic properties. The plant has been used around the world from native healers in the Amazon to Ayurvedic doctors in India to treat diabetes, as it is a natural hypoglycemic. In India, the plant is also used for treating hemorrhoids, abdominal discomfort, fever, worm infections and skin diseases. Consumption of this fruit by pregnant women is contra-indicated, as it is known to cause bleeding and abortion.

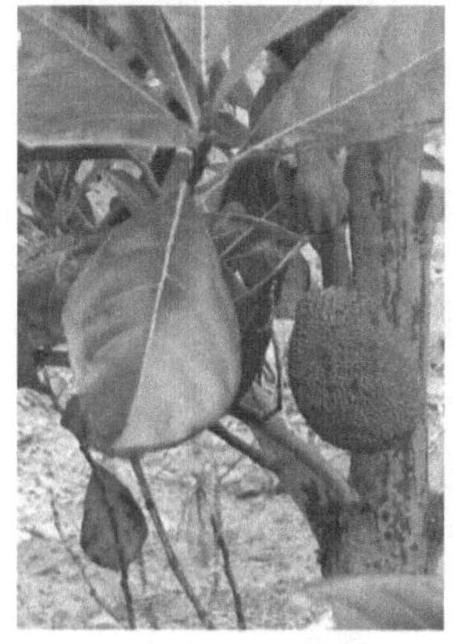

Bread Fruit

Breadfruit, *(Artocarpus altilis)*: Kingdom: Plantae, Division: Angiospermae, Class: Eudicots, Order: Rosales, Family: Moraceae. Chromosome number, n = 14, 4x = 56.

The breadfruit tree is related to Jack Fruit tree producing smaller globular fruits, which have a nutty bread-like taste when baked. The trees are natives of Polynesian and Carribean islands and grow in other sub-tropical climates including South India, Sri Lanka, Indonesia, Cambodia and other countries of South East Asia and in Central America. The fruits are known as Kada chakka or Seema Chakka or Jee Kujje or Jeev Khadgi in India. Unripe or slightly ripe fruits are sliced and baked or sautéed or pureed after removing skin. In many impoverished regions, the breadfruit is also a staple food. Normally, the breadfruit after cooking is consumed as a vegetable dish.

The plants are large trees producing unisexual flowers in the same tree (monoecious). After pollination, the compound false fruit emerges from the swollen perianth containing large numbers of flowers, which set seeds. Many cultivars are seedless. **Health:** It serves the carbohydrate needs in many island cultures. The fruit are rich in fiber.

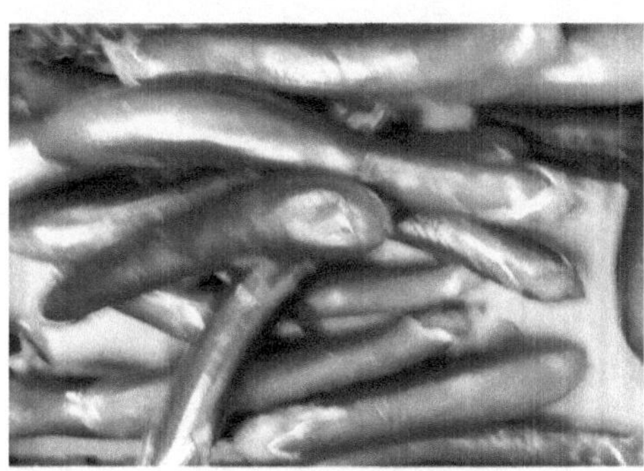

Japanese Long Egg Plant

B r i n j a l / E g g p l a n t / Aubergine/Guinea squash *(Solanum melongina)*: Kingdom: Plantae; Division: Angiospermae, Class: Eudicots, Order: Solanales, Family: Solanaceae. Other names:

melongene, garden egg, guinea squash, melanzana. Chromosome number, 2 n = 24. Many are hybrids with different ploidy numbers.

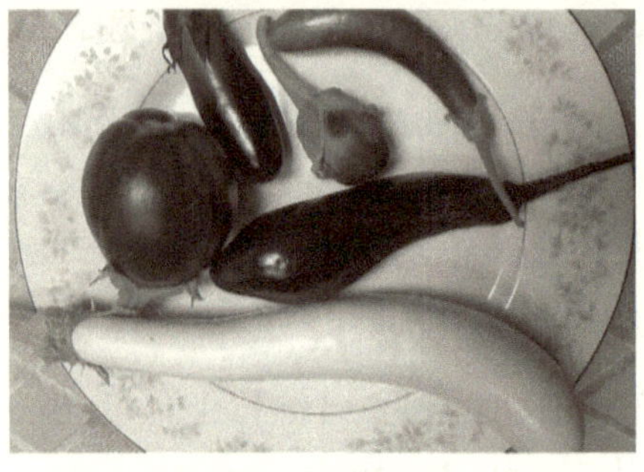

Egg plant Varieties

The plants belong to the same family as tomato, tomatillo, tobacco and various chili peppers. It is a plant native to the Indian subcontinent growing in tropical countries as a perennial and as an annual in colder temperate countries. It is a bushy plant growing to a height of 1–3 ft. tall with spiny or smooth stems bearing many wavy leaves. The plant bears white, pink or purple five petal flowers. The fruits may be white, beige, green or purple sometimes with stripes. Depending on the variety, they may be egg shaped, globular or elongated. There are no special health benefits known. The fruits are low in protein, vitamin and mineral content but are popular components of vegetable foods in Asia, Africa and Middle Eastern cuisine and in Italy, France, Greece and South America.

The wild eggplant/pea eggplant *(Solanum torvum)* also known as Turkey berry, Pea Aubergine, Chundakkai (Tamil), Susumber (Jamaica) is a close relative and is used as a minor component in the cuisine of many Asian, Indian and Pacific island cultures. The plants are herbs producing small globular marble-sized green fruits. The fruits soaked in buttermilk and dried are said to have unconfirmed medical benefits. **Health relevance:** The colored varieties contain antioxidants and phytonutrients. The skin contains the anthocyanin Nasunin that in animal studies has been shown to protect cell membranes from oxidative damage. The skin also contains high levels of the phenolic compound chlorogenic acid that is also an antioxidant.

Chili pepper (*Capsicum annum* and many other species): Kingdom: Plantae; Division: Angiospermae Class: Eudicots; Order: Solanales; Family: Solanaceae; Tribe: Capsiceae; Genus and species:

Capsicum annum; C.frutescens C.chinense; C.pubescens; C.baccatum. **Chromosome number is Variable, many. Haploid number can be 12, 24, 25, 26 and 27.**

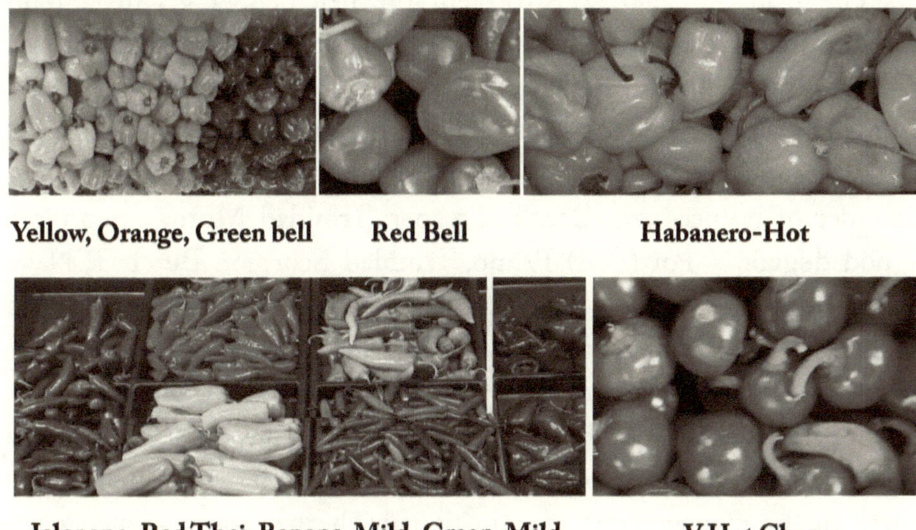

Yellow, Orange, Green bell   Red Bell   Habanero-Hot

Jalapeno, Red Thai, Banana-Mild, Green-Mild,   V.Hot Cherry
Cubanellee, Green Thai, Pablano

The *Capsicum* plant is an annual herb growing to a height of about 1 ft-4 ft. depending on species. The plant has glabrous leaves that may be small in some species or large in the bell pepper group. The flowers are bisexual and are white in color. Fruits vary in size from the size of an apple or only about the size of a newborn baby's finger. Chili peppers include five domesticated species namely: 1. *C. annum* that includes green, yellow and red bell peppers, wax, jalapeno, cayenne and chiltepen that are often referred to as capsicum peppers. 2. C. *frutescens* that include Thai malagueta, tabasco, piri piri and Kambuzi peppers. 3. *C. chinense* that include naga habanero, datil and scotch bonnet peppers. 4. *C. pubescens* that include the South American rocoto peppers and 5. *C. baccatum* that include the S. American Aji peppers.

Chili pepper commonly referred to simply as Chillies in India is actually a native of South America. It was introduced to India through Portugese traders and from there to other countries. Thus, until the introduction of these plants from S. America, the cuisines of the old world of Asia and Europe did not include chillies but depended on black pepper or peppercorn for generating the "Heat" in culinary practice.

The fruit of *Capsicum* sp except the bell pepper group contain variable quantities of the alkaloid Capsaicin and related phytochemicals known as capsaicinoids that give the pungent burning sensation to foods. Capsaicin is concentrated in the white pith tissue holding the seeds and in the fleshy parts of the fruit but not in the seeds. The hottest chillies in order of hotness are: Carolina reaper; Trinidad Moruga Scorpion, 7 pod duglah, 7 Pot (Pod) Primo, Trinidad Scorpion Butch T, Naga Viper, Bhut Jalokia, 7 Pot Barrackpore, 7 Pod red, Infinity chili and Red Habanero, Orange habenaro, Datil, Thai, Cayenne, Manzano, Serreno, Jalapeno, Pablano, Anaheim, Pepperoncini, Banana, Bell Pepper. The bell pepper group is the least "hot" and contains hardly any capsaicin. **Health relevance**: Capsaicin is considered a safe and effective topical analgesic agent in the management of arthritis pain, herpes zoster related pain, diabetic neuropathy, mastectomy pain and headaches. Some studies link consumption of highly spiced food with chillies to stomach cancer.

Cucurbits (Pumpkin, Cucumber, Gourds, Squashes and many others) Kingdom: Plantae; Division: Angiospermae Class: Eudicots; Order: Cucurbitales; Family: Cucurbitaceae; Genera and species: (*Benincasa hispida Ash gourd/Winter melon*); *Cucurbita pepo* (*Pumpkin and Zucchini*), *Cucumis sp* (*Cucumber*); *Lagenaria siceraria* (*Bottle gourd*), *Luffa acutanguila* (*Luffa*) *Momordica charantia* (*Bitter melon*) *Praecitrullus fistulosus*, *Sechium edule* (*Chayote squash*), *Trichosanthes* sp. (Snake gourd),

All the members of this family are herbaceous annual vines producing unisexual flowers either in the same plant or on separate plants. All have palmate leaves with hairy stems and tendrils. The fruits may be very large ovate-globular as in many Pumpkin varieties or cylindrical-elongated as in Zuchini and Cucumbers or very long and snake like as in the Snake gourds. The pumpkin vegetable is orange in color and has high quantities of carotene a precursor for vitamin

A. Pumpkin seeds are edible and contain pumpkin seed oil. **Health relevance:** All edible vegetable members are rich in minerals. Pumpkins contain trigonelline and nicotinic acid that can cause reductions in blood sugar. Winter melon juice is used in Ayurveda and other eastern forms of alternative medicine for control of peptic ulcers. It has diuretic properties and helps in dissolving kidney stones. Chayote squash is useful for diuretic, cardiovascular and anti-inflammatory properties. Snake gourds contain Trichosanthin that is an abortifacient and hence eating snake gourd dishes is not recommended for pregnant women. Many of the gourds and pumpkins contain a bitter principle called Cucurbitacin, which may be toxic.

The following is a brief description of some members of this family. These are grouped according to the genera.

Cucurbita Pepo Varieties: Chromosome Number, 2n = 20

1. Common pumpkin *(C. pepo):* **Chromosome number, 2n = 20.** The fruits are yellow/orange in color, weigh between 6–18 lbs. with some cultivars being able to grow to more than 75 lbs. The outer skin of the fruit-vegetable is smooth and ribbed. Certain varieties are white or green. The orange-yellow pumpkin contains lutein and beta-carotene that are converted to vitamin A upon ingestion. Some large cultivars of

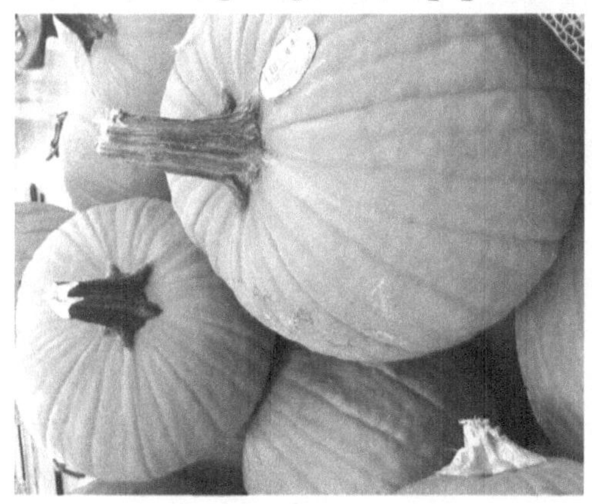

Pumpkin

squash with similar appearance have also been derived from *Cucurbita maxima*. Specific cultivars of winter squash derived from other species, including *C. argyrosperma*, and *C. moschata*, are also sometimes called "pumpkin." The seeds of pumpkin known, as Pepitas are rich in protein and the oil from seeds are used along with other oils for adding flavor. **Health:** Pumpkin is used for treating bladder irritation, kidney infections, intestinal worms, and trouble urinating due to benign prostatic hyperplasia (BPH). Pumpkin is sometimes used in combination with herbs to treat symptoms of BPH. The roasted pumpkin seeds are considered a snack food. The chemicals in the pumpkin seed cause an increase in urination (diuretic effect), which helps relieve bladder discomfort. Pumpkin seed also contains a chemical that might kill intestinal worms.

2. Acorn squash *(Cucurbita pepo var. turbinata)*: Chromosome number, 2n = 20

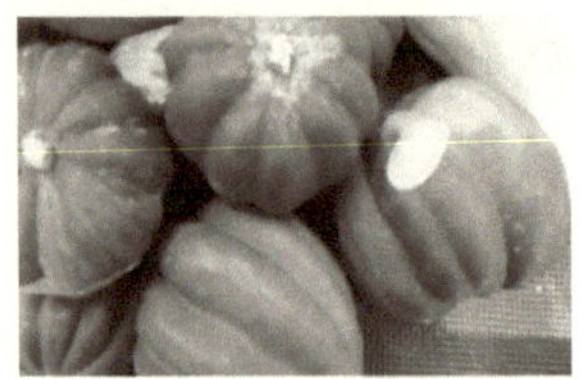

Acorn Squash

This is a winter squash with fruits with ridges. The fruits are green in color with tinges of yellow or orange. The skin is very thick and somewhat difficult to cut and peel. The flesh is yellow–orange in color and is rich in carotenoids. The flesh is cooked, baked or sautéed. **Health:** Source of good fiber, potassium, vitamin C.

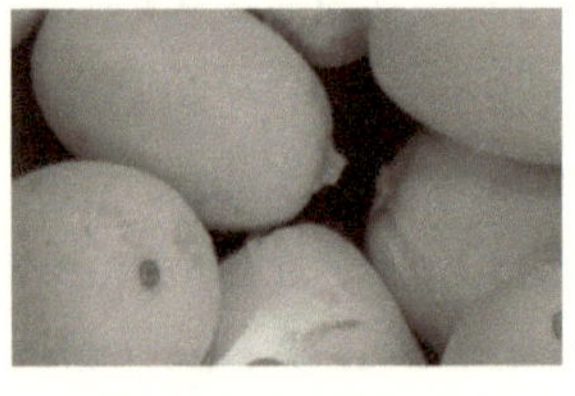

Spaghetti Squash

3. Spaghetti Squash/pumpkin *(C. pepo L. 'Spaghetti')*: Chromosome number, 2n = 20. This is a yellow skin fibrous squash variety with pale yellow flesh. The fruits are rich in carotenoids and fiber.

4. Zuchini *(C. pepo var Zuchini)*: Chromosome number, 2n = 20. Zuchini squash plants produce fruits that can be a meter long but are usually harvested when they are about 9 inches long. Fruits are pale green or dark green. Certain varieties are golden yellow in color. Both the green and yellow varieties have white or beige colored flesh. They are used in soups, salads or cooked. Some fruits

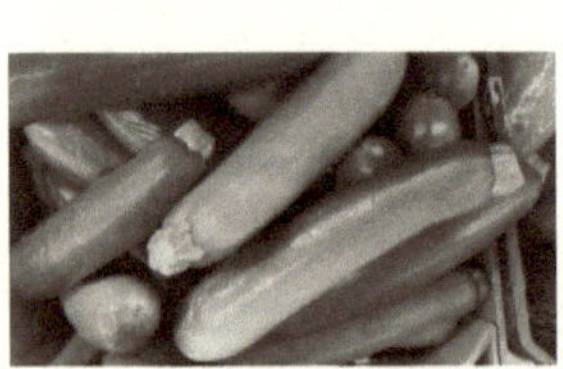

Zuchini

are bitter due to higher than normal content of toxic Cucurbitacin. Cucurbitacins are destroyed by heat.

Squash *(Cucurbita maxima)*: There are several subspecies of *C. maxima* namely: Buttercup squash *(C. maxima subsp. Andreana)*,

Hubbard Squash *(C. maxima Duchesne ssp. maxima convar. hubardiana Grebensc)*, **Banana squash** *(Maxima Duchesne ssp. maxima convar. Bananina)*; **Hokkaido squash** *(C. maxima Duchesne ssp. maxima cv. maxima 'Hokkaido')*; **Red Hokkaido** *(Maxima Duchesne ssp. maxima cv. maxima 'Red Hokkaido')*; **Red Kuri** *(Maxima Duchesne ssp. maxima cv. maxima 'Red Kuri')*, **Atlantic-Giant** *(C. maxima Duchesne 'Atlantic Giant')*, **Patty pan squash** *(Maxima var patty pan)*. **Cucurbita maxima varieties: Chromosome number, 2n = 40**

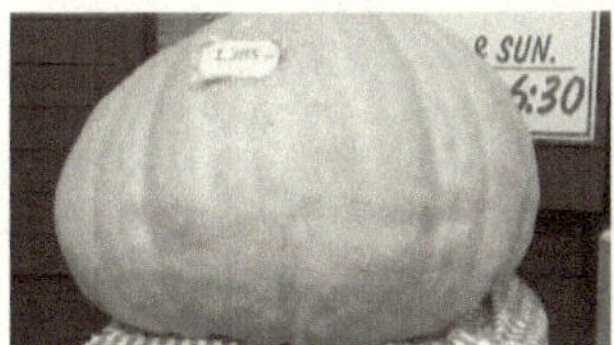 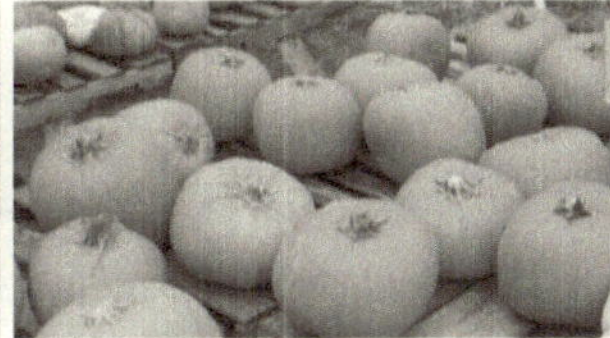 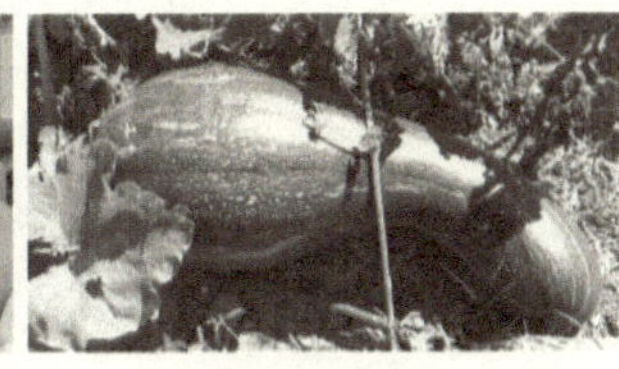

| **Giant pumpkin** | **Halloween red-orange** | **Buttercup** |

This species of Cucurbita probably originated in South America and spread to various parts of the world. All the giant "pumpkins" are really squashes belonging to *C. maxima*. This includes the giant documented pumpkin of about 2000 Lbs. The Halloween red-orange squashes are all *C. maxima* whereas the Jack-O-lanterns are the true pumpkins *C. pepo*.

There are many different cultivars of *C. maxima* as noted above. The buttercup squashes are smaller with a turban shape weighing 3–5 lbs. and used as vegetable, and in soups. The Banana squash has an elongated shape, with light blue, pink or orange skin and bright orange flesh. The Hubbard squash has a teardrop shape. All varieties are vines with typical cucurbit genus characters.

Cucumis Species (Cucumbers): Chromosome Number, 2N = 14

Cucumber *(Cucumis sativus)*: Cucumbers are among the most widely cultivated plants among the Cucurbitaceae. There are three main groups of cucumbers namely slicing cucumbers, pickling cucumbers and burp-less cucumbers. A fourth group known as Dosa kai is specific to

South Asian and Indian sub continental cooking. The fruits are elongated and vary in size and are used as vegetable in salads and after cooking. Water constitutes more than 90% of the fruits and hence very useful in controlling dehydration. Some cultivars of Cucumber are parthenocarpic producing seedless fruits without pollination wheras the majority require pollination by bees and are self-incompatible. Several varieties of cucumber have evolved to become the local favorite cucumbers.

Slicing Cucumber *(C. Sativus)* Chromosome Number, 2n = 14

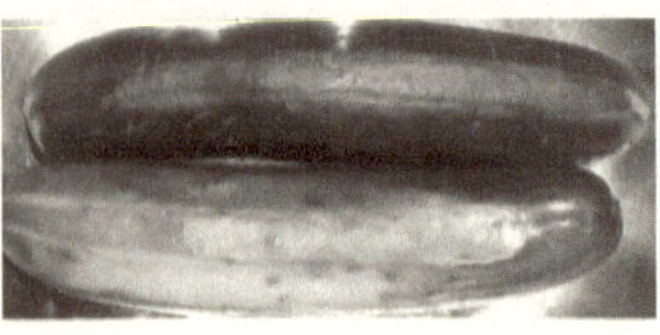

Slicing

These cucumbers are about 9 inches long and have a thin skin. They are green or pale green in color and are nearly cylindrical in shape. These are generally sliced and used in salads but they can also be cooked and or stir-fried. **Health:** Cucumber juice and fruit are used by dermatologists to improve skin health, puffed eyes and for control of heartburn.

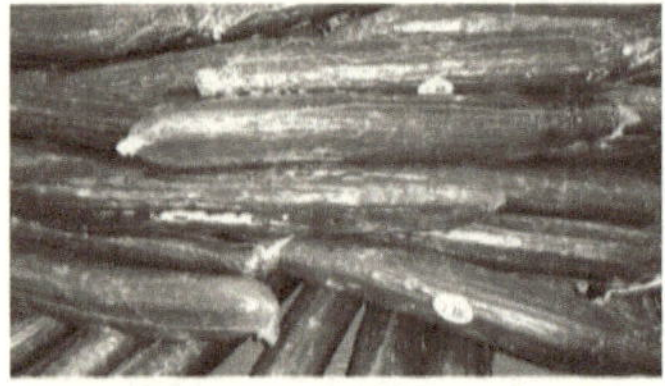

Burp less Cucumber

Burp less/English Cucumber *(C. sativus)*; Chromosome number, 2n = 14

These fruits are very long and the fruits are set without pollination and hence grown in bee-proof glass houses or areas. These are used in Salad preparations or cooked as per local customs.

Pickling Cucumber/Gherkin/Dill (C. sanguria) Chromosome number, 2n = 14.

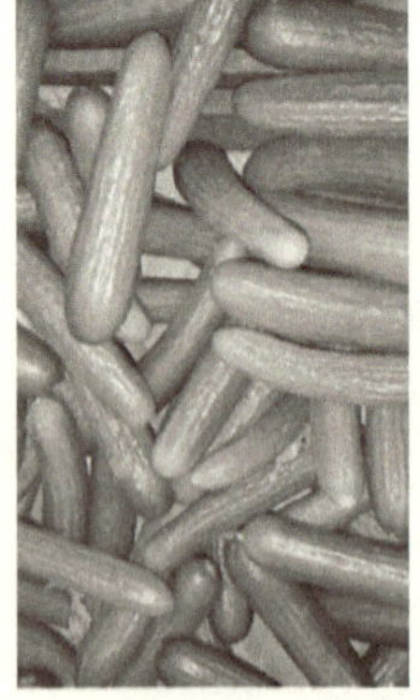

Pickle

This is a small cucumber known as pickling cucumber. The fruits are a miniature version of the garden cucumber *(C. sativus)*. The fruits are used to make pickles by a lacto-fermentation process, adding Dill, Allspice and soaking in brine and vinegar. There are many variations such as Kosher, Kool Aid, Hungarian, Polish and West Indian (Carribean) cucumber pickles.

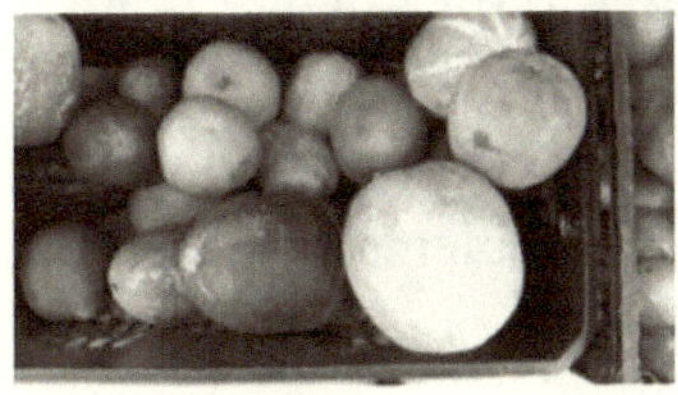

Dosa

Dosa kai; Chromosome number, 2n = 24. This is a popular green-yellow cucumber which is really a melon but called cucumber available in parts of India as well as many other regions including Mexico, California and Florida in the USA. These are cucumbers used to make various curries in India. The pulp is white.

Other cucurbit varieties, They are: 1. Lebanese cucumbers: These are small seedless cumbers popular in the middle east.2. East Asian cucumbers: These are burp less slender green cucumbers with a ridged skin used to make pickles as well as salads. 3. Persian cucumber: These are mini, seedless, sweet, cucumbers eaten with yogurt or salt and lime juice.4. Beit Alpha cucumbers: These are small, sweet parthenocarpic cucumbers found in the Middle east.5. Apple cucumbers: These are short, round cucumbers grown in Europe and New Zealand. 6. *Schälgurken*: These are German Cucumbers. 7. *Kakiri*: This is a smooth skinned cucumber, found in Southern India and Sri Lanka used in Salads or eaten raw in summer after smothering the cut slices with chili powder, salt and lemon juice.

Other Cucurbitaceae Vegetable Species

Ash gourd/Winter melon *(Benincasa hispida/B.cerifera)*: Chromosome number, 2n = 24.

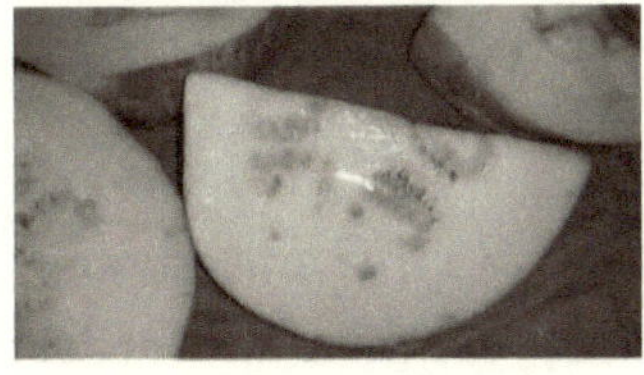

Ash Gourd

This plant variously called Ash gourd, Winter Gourd, Winter melon and white gourd is a vine exhibiting all general characters of Cucurbits. The fruit is not a true melon since it is not sweet when fully mature.

The fruits have a thick waxy coating with a white fleshy marrow. It has long shelf life of nearly a year. Ash gourds grown in India have a white waxy coating on the thick skin wheras, the variety grown in other South Asian countries like Thailand, Vietnam, China have a smooth waxy texture without the white coating. The shoot, tendril, leaves and flowers are edible. **Health:** The fruit is prescribed as a medicine in Ayurveda (Kushmanda rasayana) for treating urinary problems, emaciation, improve digestion and help to increase body weight.

Bottle gourd/Calabash/Dudhi/Sorakkai (*Lagenaria siceraria*): Chromosome number, 2n = 22.

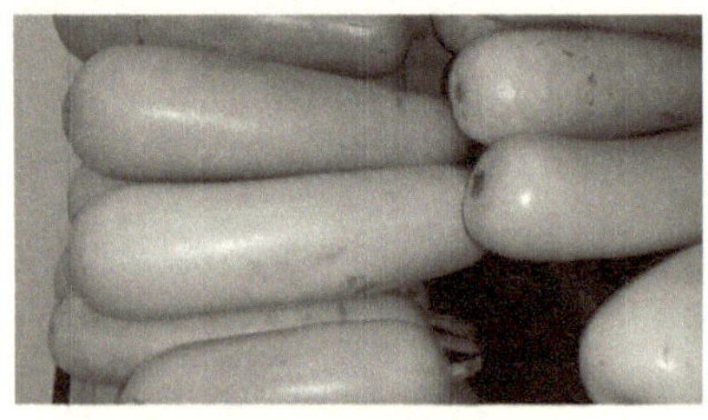

Bottle Gourd

L.ciceraria is the most common of six different species. The gourds of the various species may be harvested young and used as a vegetable. The plants are grown in Africa, Indian subcontinent and in many tropical, sub-tropical, and semi-arid regions. The mature fruit is dried and used as a container for storing water and for making certain musical instruments.

Health: The Indian sub-continental traditional medicine recommends use of bottle gourds for treating jaundice, diabetes, ulcer, piles, colitis, insanity, hypertension, congestive cardiac failure, and skin diseases. The fruit pulp is used as an emetic, sedative, purgative, and diuretic, anti – bilious, and pectoral agents. The flowers are an antidote to poison. The stem, bark and rind of the fruit are diuretic. The seeds are vermifuges. Extracts of the plant have shown antibiotic activity. Leaf juice is widely used for treating pre-mature baldness.

Loofah/vegetable gourd/Dish cloth gourd *(Luffa acutangula)*: Kingdom: Plantae; Division: Angiospermae, Eudicots; Order: Cucurbitales; Family: Cucurbitaceae: Chromosome number, 2n = 26

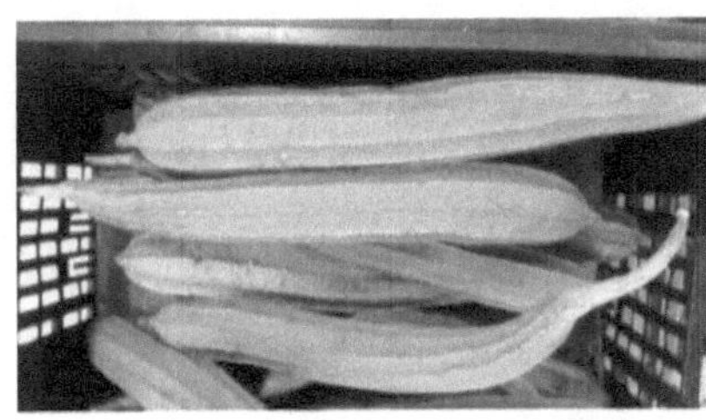

Loofah

This is a vine like other cucurbits and is a warm season cold sensitive plant. The vines produce separate male and female yellow colored flowers. The young fruit is edible as a vegetable. When the fruit gets old, it becomes very fibrous and is not useful as a vegetable but is processed into a scrubbing sponge. This plant-based scrubbing sponge is a good substitute for fabricated sponges especially for those with dermal problems. There is also a non-ridged smooth skin variety (*L. aegyptica*).

Snake Gourd/Padwal/Patole, *(Trichosanthes cucumeriana):* **Kingdom: Plantae; Division: Angiospermae, Eudicots; Order: Cucurbitales; Family: Cucurbitaceae. Chromosome number, 2n = 22.**

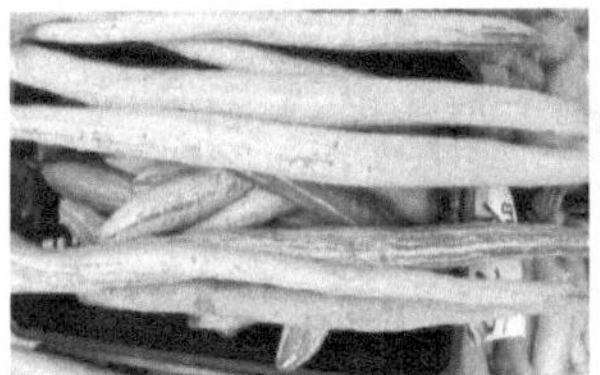

White Snake Gourd

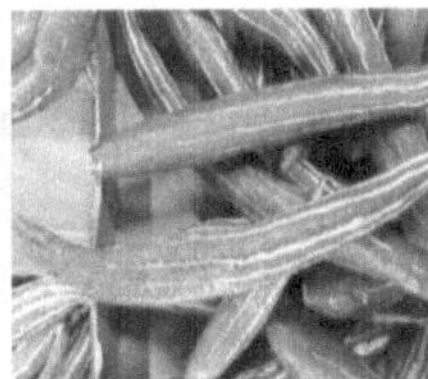

Snake Gourd

This is an annual climber grown in trellises in most countries of Asia and introduced as a vegetable crop in Europe and in Florida, USA during summer months Plants are monoecious and the white colored flowers are insect pollinated. The long snake-like fruits are edible as are the soft seeds. **Health:** Fruits have anti-helminthic properties. It may have anti-inflammatory properties as well. The fruits and leaves are abortifacient and pregnant women should not eat large amounts of this vegetable.

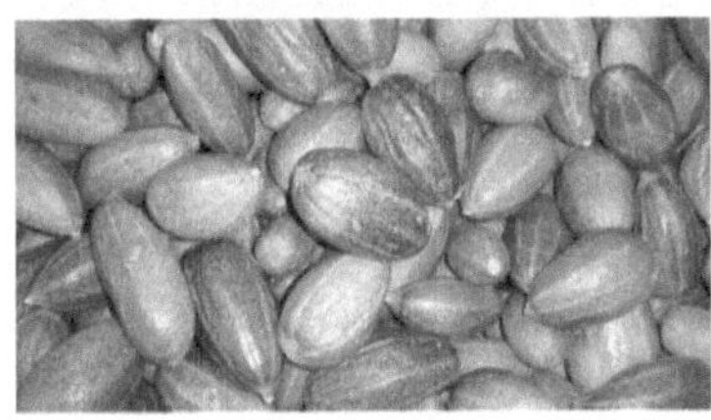

Tinda

Tinda/Indian baby pumpkin *(Praecitrullus citrullus):* **Kingdom: Plantae; Division: Angiosperms; Eudicots; Order: Cucurbitales; Family: Cucurbitaceae; Chromosome number, 2n = 24**

Plants are annual vines with palmate leaves. Tinda, also called Indian round gourd or apple gourd or Indian Baby Pumpkin, is a squash-like cucurbit grown for its immature fruit, a vegetable especially popular in South Asia. The fruit is approximately spherical, and 5–8 cm in diameter. Tinda are used as a vegetable in the Indian subcontinent

Tindora/Tendli/Ivy gourd/Kovakka *(Coccinia grandis):* **Kingdom: Plantae; Division: Angiosperms; Dicotyledonae, Eudicots; Order: Cucurbitales; Family: Cucurbitaceae. The plant is also referred to as C. India. Chromosome number, 2n = 20, 22, 24+ XX/Xy, heteromorphic sex chromosomes.**

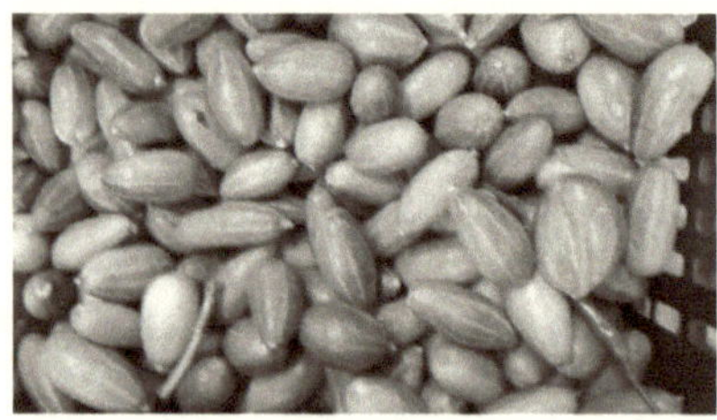
Tindora

The plant is a vine growing at a rapid rate of about 4 inches per day. The vine plant is grown India, the Philippines, Cambodia, China, Indonesia, Malaysia, Myanmar, Thailand, Vietnam, eastern Papua New Guinea, and the Northern Territories of Australia, Fiji islands, Samoa and Hawaii. Both the young shoots as well as fruits are edible. The fruits are rich in beta-carotene. The fruits in particular are cooked, stir-fried and added to soups. **Health:** Alternative medicine recommendations include use for treating leprosy, fever, asthma, bronchitis, and jaundice. It is also considered to have anti-histaminic properties.

Other fruit vegetables:

Black nightshade/Manathakkali *(Solanum nigrum):* **Kingdom: Plantae; Division: Angiospermae, Class: Eudicots, Order: Solanales; Family: Solanaceae. Chromosome number, 2n = 4x 48.**

Solanum nigrum commonly known as black nightshade, garden huckleberry or Manathakkali in Tamil, is considered as a medicinal fruit and the leaves and fruits are used to prepare various culinary dishes. The plants are herbs often growing as a weed in N. America but are cultivated in India, Indonesia and Africa. Although the leaves and berries contain toxic solanine alkaloids, the leaves and fruits are a common ingredient of traditional Indian medicines. Infusions are used in dysentery, stomach complaints, and fever. The juice of the plant is used on ulcers and other skin diseases. The fruits are used as a tonic, laxative, appetite stimulant, and for treating asthma and "excessive thirst." It is used as a cooked leaf vegetable. In North India, the boiled extracts of leaves and berries are also used to alleviate liver-related ailments, including jaundice. In Assam, the juice from its roots is used against asthma and whooping cough. So long as the leaves and fruits are used as medicinal plant through cuisines, the toxicity is not an issue but large quantities can cause abdominal distress and other toxicities because of the solanine content.

Chundakkai/Pea eggplant/Pea aubergine/Susumber/ Turkey berry, (Solanum torvum**): Kingdom: Plantae; Division: Angiospermae, Class: Eudicots, Order: Solanales; Family: Solanaceae. Chromosome number, 2n = 4x = 48.**

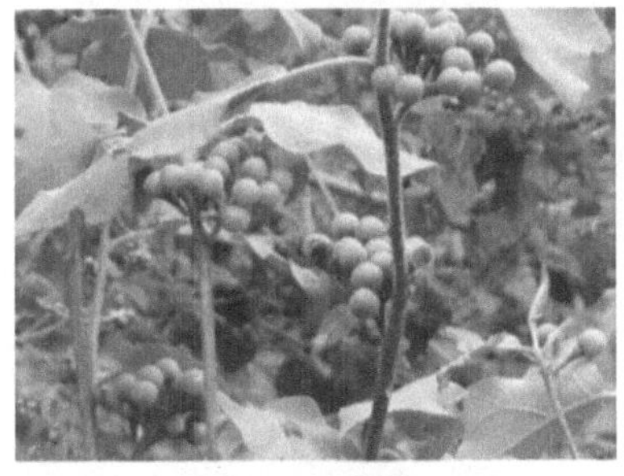

Chundakkai

This is a common fruit vegetable of Southern India as well as Thai, Laos and Jamaican cuisine. The plants produce small marble-sized (1–2 cm diameter) green fruits on slender shrubby bushes. Leaves are toxic due to high solanine alkaloid content. Both green fruits and dried fruits are sautéed or fried in culinary preparations. They are used more like a spice than a vegetable dish *per se*. **Health:** The leaf and seed extracts are prescribed as digestive aids in Siddha medicine practice. However, there are experimental reports to the effect that aqueous extracts of the berries are toxic to mice.

Moringa *(Moringa Oleifera)*: Kingdom: Plantae, Division: Angiospermae, Class: Edudicots, Order: Brassicales, Family: Moringaceae. Chromosome number, 2n = 28.

The fruits of Moringa known as drumsticks are edible. These long pod fruits have winged seeds. The outer pod of the fruit is very fibrous

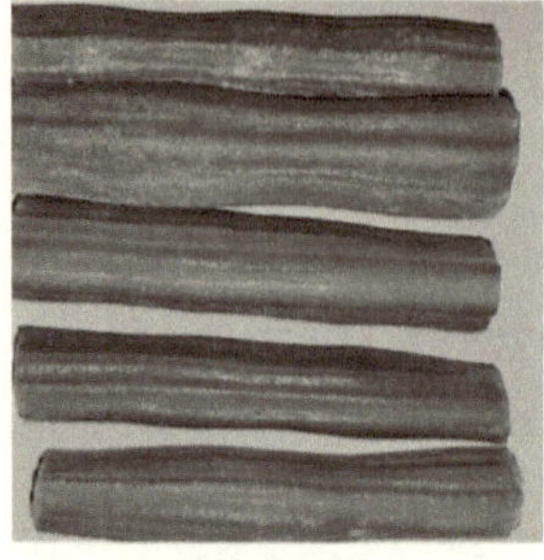

and non-edible but the juicy-slushy-fleshy mesocarp inside and seeds are edible. The botany of the plant is described under leafy vegetables.

Health: The flesh and seeds of the drumstick are said to have medicinal value. The seeds contain Moringa oil that is prescribed as a hair tonic and as an anti-ageing skin treatment.

Moringa Cut fruit

There are also claims that the oil helps to induce good sleep when massaged into scalp.

Okra/Ladies finger *(Abelmoscus esculentes/Hibiscus esculentes)*: Kingdom: Plantae; Division: Angiospermae, Class: Eudicots; Order: Malvales; Family: Malvaceae; Genus and Species: *Abelmoscus esculentes.* Chromosome number, 2n = 72–132, Amphi diploids with variable chromosome numbers.

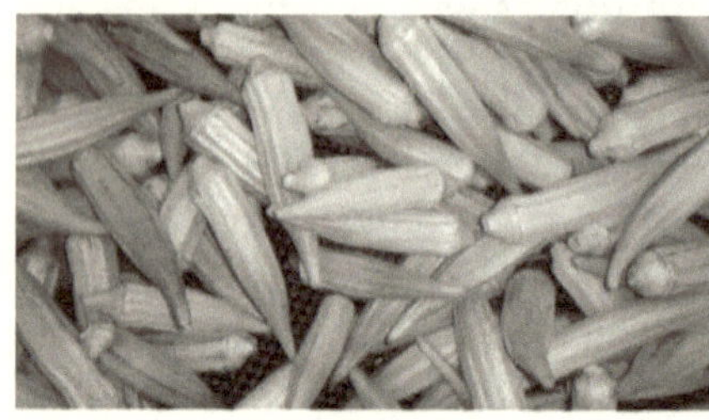

This is an annual plant in the temperate regions and perennial in the tropics. It is related to cotton, Hibiscus and Cocoa. The plants grow to a height of 5–6ft with palmate lobed leaves. The flowers are bisexual, large with 5 petals and sepals. The

Okra

fruit that is the vegetable is about 3–8 inches long with numerous black seeds. Very often, when used for culinary purposes, the fruit pods are harvested when they are tender and before the seeds have matured. **Health relevance:** The green fruits are highly mucilaginous and are recommended for treating intestinal diseases particularly irritable bowel syndrome. The fruits are rich in antioxidants, vitamins and minerals.

Plantain Banana *(Musa Paradisiaca)*: Kingdom: Plantae; Division: Angiospermae, Class: Monocotyledonae, Order: Zingiberales;

Family: Musaceae. Chromosome number, 2n = 22, 2n = 4x = 44, 2n = 5x = 55, 2n = 7x = 77, 2n = 8x = 88

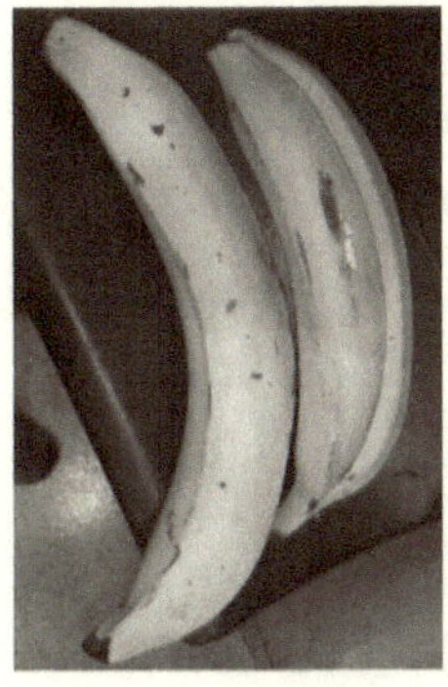

Plantain

Plantains are triploid hybrids of Banana formed naturally due to crossing of two wild banana species, *Musa acuminata* and *M. balbisiana*. As in the case of Banana, the plants have an underground stem from which the upright fleshy pseudostem arises, culminating in a crown of very large green leaves. Flowers are produced in an inflorescence wherein, the female flowers are located at the bottom of the inflorescence wheras; the male flowers are located in the top layer. Fruits develop after pollination and are seedless. The fruit-pulp is very starchy and is a major staple food in many African and South American countries. The unripe fruits are cooked and consumed as vegetable, as dried carbohydrate flour or as fried chips. The ripened fruit is consumed as an uncooked fruit or in various culinary preparations. The green skin is also cut into tiny pieces and cooked as a vegetable or in stir-fries. The skin is rich in minerals and phytochemicals. **Health:** Plantains are rich sources of Carbohydrates, fiber and potassium.

Tamarind *(Tamarindus indica)***: Kingdom: Plantae; Division: Angiospermae, Class: Eudicots; Order: Fabales; Family: Fabaceae/Caesalpineaceae). Chromosome number, 2n = 26.**

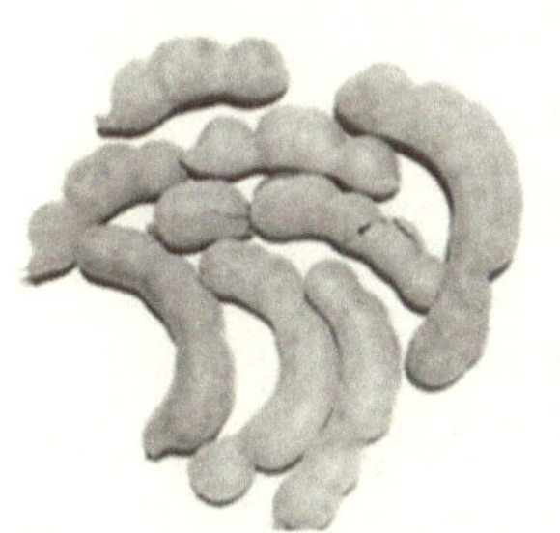

Tamarind

Tamarind trees are very robust tall evergreen legume trees that are grown mainly in the Indian sub-continent, Sri Lanka, South East Asia, China, Pacific islands, Mexico, Carribean islands, South and Central America, Florida in N. America as well as many tropical and subtropical countries. Trees grow essentially wild in East Africa, The trees provide shade and the fruits are used to prepare many different cuisines in Asia, Africa, Carribean islands, Mexico, South and Central America. Trees grow to a height of 50–60 ft with wide thick woody stems (about 2–3 ft diameter) with evergreen leaves on branches produced near the tree crown. Leaves are pinnately compound and have a sour tart taste, Fruits are pods with a brown crunchy skin containing brown pulp. Each pod contains 2–6 seeds, which are very hard. The fruit pulp is used as a component of many different foods. The seeds are very hard like stones but are nutritious. **Health:** Fruits contain Vitamin C and tartaric acid. Fruit pulp is used as a poultice on foreheads to control headaches. In Southern India, the leaves are steeped in boiling water that is then used to bathe aching limbs. Ingestion of tamarind is also effective in excretion of fluoride from water.

Tomato *(Lycopersicon esculentum)*: Kingdom: Plantae; Division: Angiospermae, Class: Eudicots; Order: Solanales; Family: Solanaceae; Genus and species: *Lycopersicon esculentum*. **Chromosome number, 2n = 24.**

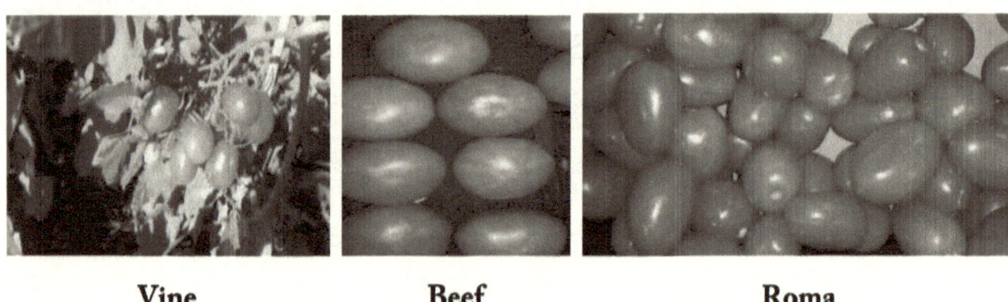

| Vine | Beef | Roma |

Tomato, like potato, originated in the Andes region of South America and spread worldwide. The plant is an annual day neutral plant and hence flowering throughout the growth period. The plants are herbaceous, soft stemmed, with compound, serrated, hairy leaflets. The plants may be determinate whereby the fruits are produced at the top after a level of bushy indeterminate growth. They produce many branches with a vine like growth producing fruits throughout the growing period. There are many cultivars of tomato ranging from grape tomato, cherry tomato, Compari, Roma, plum, pear and Beefsteak varieties. The fruits range from the very small sweet grape tomatoes about 0.5 inches in diameter to the large beefsteak that is about 4 inches in diameter. The fruit colors vary from buff white, pink, and purple, orange to dark red and even blue black. Some chocolate colored varieties have also been genetically produced recently. The most common color is red. **Health relevance:** Tomato fruits are rich in Vitamin C and antioxidants and contain the alkaloid Lycopene which is regarded as a very useful phytochemical for treating enlarged prostates (Benign prostate hyperplasia). Tomato leaves are rich in toxic solanine alkaloid.

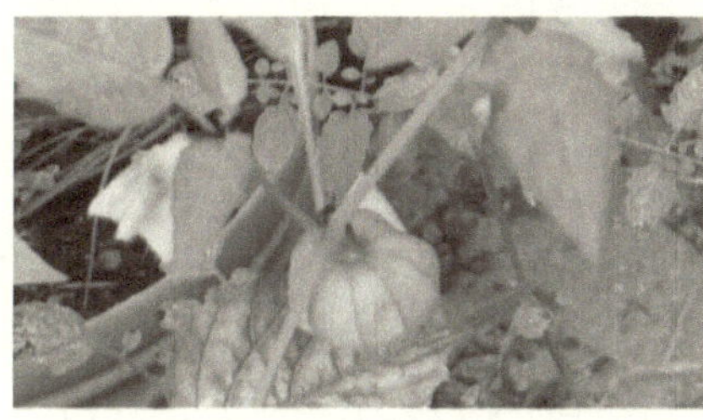

Tomatillo

Tomatillo *(Physalis philadelphica):* **Kingdom: Plantae; Division: Angiospermae, Class: Eudicots, Order: Solanales; Family: Solanaceae. Botanical name:** *Physalis philadelphica.* **Chromosome number, 2n = 24.** Tomatillos also known as Mexican husk tomato is a plant of the nightshade family bearing small, spherical and green or green-purple fruit of the same name. These plants are natives of Mexico and Central America but are now grown in North America and selected European countries. Fruits are similar to tomato but have a sheath of calyx covering the fruit. The calyx has to be removed before use. The fruits are yellow, red, green or purple. Plants are self-incompatible and need two different plants for pollination (Self-incompatibility genes). The fruits are sour tasting. **Health:** Tomatillos have dietary fiber, niacin, potassium, and manganese.

Table 13: Nutritional values of Fruit vegetables

Nutrient	Bitter Melon	Brinjal eggplant	cucumber fruit-veg	Moringa drumstick	Okra pod	Plantain raw	Pumpkin gourd	Zucchini squash	Tomato Ripe
Water, g	94.03	92.3	95.23	88.2	89.6	65.28	91.6	94.79	94.52
Protein, g	17	0.98	0.65	2.1	1.93	1.3	1	1.21	0.88
Total lipid (fat), g	1	0.18	0.11	0.2	0.19	0.37	0.1	0.32	0.2
Carbohydrate, g	0.17	5.88	3.63	8.53	7.45	31.89	6.5	3.11	3.89
Fiber, g	3.7	3	0.5	3.2	3.2	2.3	0.5	1	1.2
Sugar, g	2.8	3.53	1.67	1.48	15	2.76	2.5	2.63	
Calcium, mg	19	9	16	30	82	3	21	16	10
Iron, mg	0.43	0.23	0.28	0.36	0.62	0.6	0.8	0.37	0.27
Magnesium, mg	17	14	13	45	57	37	12	18	11
Phosphorus, mg	31	24	24	50	61	34	44	38	24
Potassium, mg	296	229	147	461	299	499	340	261	237
Sodium, mg	5	2	2	42	7	4	1	8	5
Zinc, mg	0.8	0.16	0.2	0.45	0.58	0.14	0.32	0.32	0.17
Vitamin C, mg	84	2.2	2.8	141	23	18.4	9	17.9	13.7
Thiamin, mg	0.04	0.039	0.027	0.053	0.2	0.052	0.05	0.045	0.037
Riboflavin, mg	0.04	0.037	0.033	0.074	0.06	0.054	0.11	0.094	0.019
Niacin, mg	0.4	0.649	0.098	0.62	1	0.686	0.6	0.451	0.594
Vitamin B-6, mg	0.043	0.084	0.04	0.12	0.22	0.299	0.061	0.163	0.08

Folate, DFE, μ	72	22	7	44	60	22	16	24	15
Vitamin B-12, μg	0	0	0	0	0	0	0	0	0
Vitamin A, μg	24	1	5	4	36	56	426	10	42
Vitamin A, IU	471	23	105	74	716	1127	8513	200	833
Vitamin E, mg	0	0.3	0.03	NA	0.27	0.14	1.06	0.12	0.54
Vitamin D, μg	0	0	0	0	0	0	0	0	0
Vitamin D, IU	0	0	0	0	0	0	0	0	0
Vitamin K	NA	3.5	16.4	NA	31.3	0.7	1.1	4.3	7.9
Fatty acids, g	NA	0.034	0.037	NA	0.03	0.033	0.052	0.084	0.028
Mono-unsat, g	NA	0.016	0.005	NA	0.02	0.102	0.013	0.011	0.031
Poly-unsat, g	NA	0.076	0.032	NA	0.03	0.003	0.005	0.091	0.083

Floral Vegetables

The flowers/florets/inflorescence of some plants are used as vegetables. Chief among these are Artichoke, Banana, Broccoli and Cauliflower.

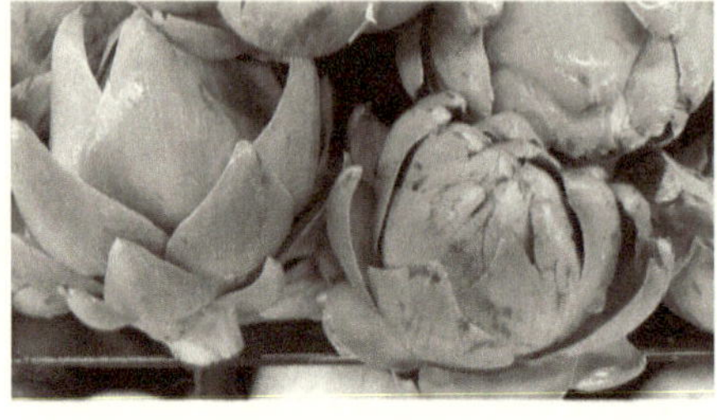

Artichoke

Artichoke or Globe artichoke *(Cynara cardunculus var. scolymus);* Kingdom: Plantae: Division: Angiospermae, Class: Eudicots; Order: Asterales; Family; Asteraceae. Chromosome number: 2n = 32

The edible vegetables are the flower buds in the flower head or inflorescence before they bloom. The flower head consists of many unopened flower heads in a cluster with many bracts. The plants are perennials growing to a height of 6 ft. with lobed large green leaves. The fleshy flower head is cooked by boiling in water. The Cynarin in the artichoke inhibits taste receptors and hence it renders even water to have sweet taste.

Health: Artichoke flower heads are rich in antioxidants. Artichoke reduces the risk of arteriosclerosis and reduces intensity of irritable bowel syndrome and helps overcome functional dyspepsia.

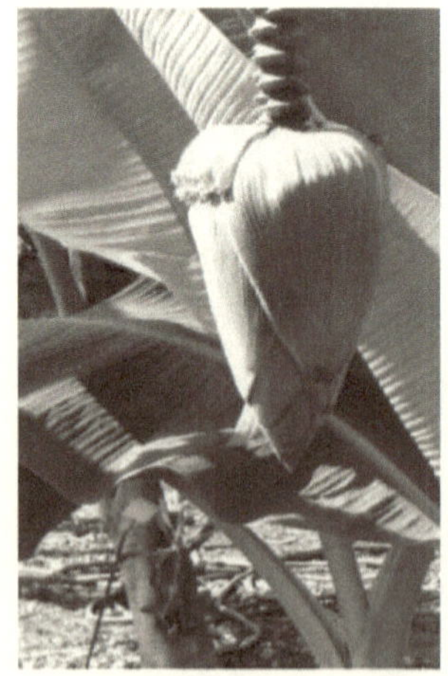

Banana Flower

Banana flower *(Musa* sp.): Kingdom: Plantae; Division: Angiospermae, Class: Monocotyledonae, Order: Zingiberales; Family: Musaceae.

The banana inflorescence with numerous flowers is also used as vegetable. The outer pink/brown colored bracts that cover the inflorescence are removed before the flowers inside are washed and cooked. A full description of the Banana plant is given under fruit vegetables and culinary fruits.

Broccoli: *(Brassica oleracea):* **Kingdom: Plantae: Division: Angiospermae, Class: Eudicots; Order: Brassicales; Family; Cruciferae; Genus and species:** *Brassica oleraceae.* **Other Names: Wild cabbage, Headless cabbage, Chinese broccoli, Biflorus. Chromosome number: 2n = 18.**

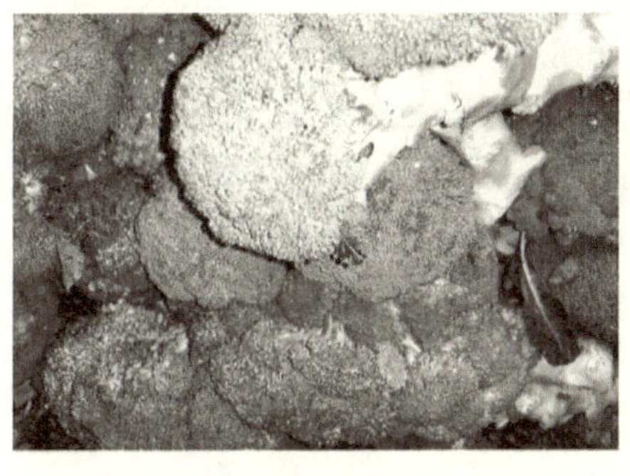

Broccoli

Broccoli is a member of the italic group of *Brassica oleraceae*. Broccoli is a stout thick stemmed plant in the Brassicaceae family that also includes cabbage, kale, Brussels sprouts, Mustard, and Chinese greens like bok choy. The plant can grow to height of 1 ft-8 ft. high. The flower head is the vegetable. The florets are green in color although selective breeding has resulted in varieties with purple flower heads. Arcadia broccoli, Early Dividend Broccoli, Gypsy broccoli, Patron Broccoli, and Premium broccoli are popular varieties. **Health relevance:** Broccoli is rich in vitamin C, selenium, antioxidants and phytochemicals with reported anticancer properties. It contains glucoraphanin that can be converted into sulfaraphane with anticancer properties. The vegetable also contains diindolylmethane and indole-3-carbinol that have anticancer properties. However, most of these health-promoting chemicals are lost by extensive boiled cooking. Nevertheless, these phytochemicals are retained after steam cooking, stir-frying or microwave cooking. Recent studies in 2015 at the University of Pittsburgh have shown that broccoli sprout extracts protect against development of mouth cancers and the researchers have coined the term "Green chemoprevention" for treatment protocols based on plants.

Cauliflower: (Brassica oleracea cultivar botritis): Kingdom: Plantae: Division: Angiospermae, Class: Eudicots; Order: Brassicales;

Family; Cruciferae; Genus and species: Brassica oleracea cultivar botritis, Chromosome number: 2n = 18

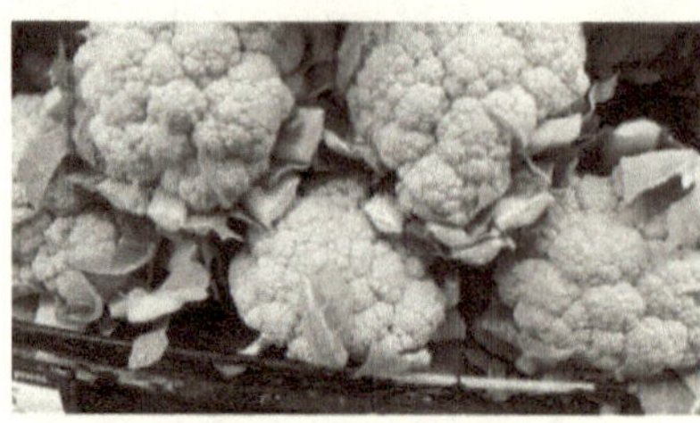

Green cauliflower

Cauliflower belongs to the same genus and species as Broccoli, Brussels sprouts, Cabbage and Kale. However, it is differentiated by being in the Botritis group. It is an annual seed bearing plant. Here, the flower head inflorescence, as a whole is the nutritional vegetable used for culinary purposes and in salads. There are four major groups of Cauliflowers namely: Italian, Northern European annuals, North West Biennial Europe and Asian. These groups differ from each other mainly with regard to being annual or biennial, harvest time and slight morphological differences. The most common varieties produce white heads but some varieties produce orange (Cheddar, Orange bouquet), green (Alverda, green goddess, Vorda), and purple heads (Graffiti, Purple cape). **Health:** Cauliflowers are rich in minerals, folic acid, fiber and many phytochemicals. The orange colored varieties are a rich source of carotene and the purple ones are a rich source of anthocyanin.

References

Briggs. W.H., Xiao, H., Shen, C., Parkin, K.L., and I.L. Goldman, (2000): Differential inhibition of Human Platelet Aggregation by selected Allium thiosulfinates. Journal of Agriculture and Food Chemistry 11: 5731-5735.

Allen, P. and C. Wyman, (1986): Glossary of oriental vegetables. Family Farm Series, Small Farm Center, Univ. of California, Davis

Bailey L.H. (1912), republished in 1975: Kohlrabi for stock feeding. In Cyclopedia of American Agriculture: Vol. IIcrops. Macmillan Publishing New York, p. 389-390 ISBN 0405067623

Block, E. (2010): Garlic and Other Alliums: The Lore and the Science. Royal Society of Chemistry, ISBN 0-85404-190-7

Cosgrove, D.R., Oelke, E.A., Doll, J.D., Davis, D.W., Undersander, D.J., and E.S. Oplinger: (1991): Jerusalem artichoke

Desa, Dian (1985): "Water purification with Moringa seeds."Waterlines 3 (4): 22–3. doi: 10.3362/0262-8104.1985.019.

Eddouks, M., Maghrani M; Zeggwagh, N.A; Michel JB (2005): "Study of the hypoglycaemic activity of Lepidium sativum L. aqueous extract in normal and diabetic rats." J Ethnopharmacol 97 (2): 391–395. doi: 10.1016/j.jep.2004.11.030. PMID 15707780

Englisch, W; Beckers, C; Unkauf, M; Ruepp, M; Zinserling, V (2000): "Efficacy of Artichoke dry extract in patients with hyperlipoproteinemia." Arzneimittel-Forschung 50 (3): 260–5. Doi: 10.1055/s-0031-1300196. PMID 10758778.minger, AH (1994) Foods & nutrition encyclopedia, Volume 1 CRC Press, 1994 ISBN 0-8493-8980-1 p. 750

Food and feed crops of the United States Interregional Research Project IR-4, IR Bul. 1 (Bul. 828 New Jersey Agr., Expt. Sta.)

Fu, I.M., C. Shennan, and G.E. Welbaum (1993.): Evaluating Chinese cabbage cultivars for high temperature tolerance. p. 570-573. In: J. Janick and J.E. Simon (eds.), new crops. Wiley, New York

Goldman, I.L. (2002): Recognition of fruits and vegetables as healthy: Vitamins and phytonutrients. HortTechnology 13: 252-258

Gopalakrishnan T.P. (2007): Vegetable Crops, New India Publishing, pp. 244–247. ISBN 9788189422417

Grubben, G.J.H. & Denton, O.A. (2004): Plant Resources of Tropical Africa 2 Vegetables PROTA Foundation, Wageningen; Backhuys, Leiden; CTA, Wageningen

Heiser, Jr., C.B. (1979): The gourd book, Univ. Oklahoma Press, Norman, OK…

http://healthremediesjournal.com/top-9-health-benefits-of-kale/?utm_source = kale&utm_medium = kale&utm_campaign = google

http://www.ncbi.nlm.nih.gov/pmc/articles/PMC3117318/

https://www.hort.purdue.edu/newcrop/ID-56/colecrops.html.

Native Sunflowers for Conservation Use in Montana and Wyoming

Janick, J. (2002): Herbals: The connection between horticulture and medicine. HortTechnology, 13(2): 229-238

Little Jr., Elbert L.; Roger G. Skolmen (1989): "Ulu, breadfruit" (PDF), United States Forest Service

National Research Council (2008): "Tamarind." Lost Crops of Africa: Volume III: Fruits. Lost Crops of Africa 3, National Academies Press. ISBN 978-0-309-10596-5

NDL/FNIC Food Composition Database Home Page," USDA.Gov

O'Hair, S.K. (1998): Cassava. Tropical Research and Education Center, University of Florida, https://www.hort.purdue.edu/newcrop/CropFactSheets/cassava.html

Prajapati, R.P., Kalariya, M., Parmar, S.K., and N.R. Sheth (2010): Phytochemical and pharmacological review of Lagenaria sicereria. J. Ayurveda Integr Med. 2010 Oct-Dec, 1(4): 266–272.

Qiang, Z.; Lee, S.O.; Ye, Z.; Wu, X.; Hendrich, S. (2012): "Artichoke Extract Lowered Plasma Cholesterol and Increased Fecal Bile Acids in Golden Syrian Hamsters." Phytotherapy Research 26 (7): 1048–1052. doi: 10.1002/ptr.3698. PMID 22183827

Silva, N., Mendes-Bonato, A.B., Sales, J.G., Pagliarini, M.S. (2011): Meiotic behavior and pollen viability in Moringa oleifera

(Moringaceae) cultivated in southern Brazil. Genet Mol Res. 2011, 10(3): 1728-32.

Singh, R.J., (2003): Plant cytogenetics, 2nd edition, CRC Press, Boaca Raton, pp385.

Smartt, J., and N.W. Simmonds, (1995): Evolution of crop plants. 2nd ed. Longman Scientific and Technical, New York

Susanne, S., Renner, Pandey, A.K., (2013): The Cucurbitaceae of India: Accepted names, synonyms, geographic distribution, and information on images and DNA sequence, PhytoKeys.s (20): 53–118. Published online 2013

Talalay, P. and J.W. Fahey, (2001): Phytochemicals from cruciferous plants protect against cancer by modulating carcinogen metabolism. J. Nutr. 131: 3027s–3033s.

Terry, L.A. (2011): Health promoting properties of fruit and vegetables, CAB International, Cambridge, Massachusetts, Pp 380.

Zohary D., and Hopf, M., (2000): Domestication of plants in the Old World 3rd Ed... Oxford: Oxford University Press. p.139

Winslow, S.R (2014): United States Department of Agriculture, natural resources conservation service, Plant Materials Technical Note No. MT-105: http://www.nrcs.usda.gov/Internet/FSE_PLANTMATERIALS/publications/mtpmctn12457.pdf

Chapter 10
Culinary Fruits

Although many vegetables are actually fruits by botanical definition, the term fruit used here refers to those fruits that are used to prepare Jams, preserves, fruit juices, salads and as desserts. These include apples, banana, black berries, blue berries, guava, grape fruit, lychee, mango, oranges, peaches, pears, pine apple, raspberries, strawberries,, and ripe plantain. All these supply various antioxidants, carotenoids, sugar, vitamins, minerals and phytochemicals that are useful for preventing disease and maintaining good health. Since most fruit trees are sprayed with fungicides and pesticides, the fruits may contain residues of these toxic chemicals and hence the fruits have to be thoroughly washed or the skin which contains biologically useful phytochemicals have to be peeled off before consumption. Many health conscious consumers choose to turn to fruits grown organically so that they can get the full health benefits of the concerned fruits. In this section, the important facets of fruit trees and fruits are described below.

Apple *(Malus domestica)*: Kingdom: Plantae; Division: Angiospermae, Class: Eudicots; Order: Rosales; Family: Rosaceae; Genus and species: Malus domestica. Chromosome number, n = 17, 2n = 34, 3n = 51

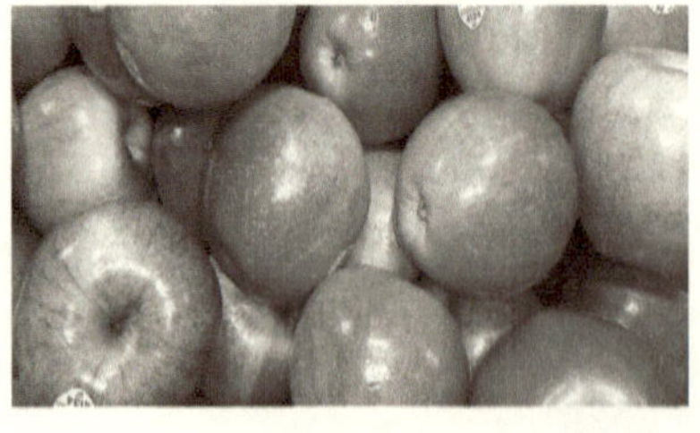

Apples

Apple fruits botanically known as *Malus domestica* a member of the Rose family are among the most important culinary fruits. Apple plants are deciduous trees, which are about 6 ft-15 ft. high. Leaves of the tree are simple, glabrous, with serrated margins. Apple blossom flowers, which are 12 inches wide, are borne on inflorescences and are fragrant and white or pink in color. There are many varieties of apple, such as Washington red, Jonathan Gold, Gala, Golden delicious, red delicious, Granny Smith, Fuji, Bramley, Pink lady, Macintosh etc. Fruits may be small, medium or large and may be green, red, golden yellow, pink or variegated in color. The skin contains flavonoids, carotene and the polyphenols quercetin and catechin as well as procyanidins and ursolic acid that help in maintaining good colon health. The pulp after removing the skin is rich in sugars and fiber. However, the skin of commercial apples may have residual pesticides and fungicides which are sprayed on the plants to prevent loss of crop due to diseases and hence it is safer to peel the skin before eating and in turn this causes loss of beneficial phytochemicals present on the skin. **Health:** Apples contain proteins that may cause allergic symptoms in some people. Inflammation of the mouth, throat and sores are common symptoms of allergy. Such individuals are also allergic to many nuts and pollen. Apple seeds contain small amounts of highly toxic cyanogenic glycosides that are converted to hydrogen cyanide. However, the seeds have a thick seed coat that is not digested if consumed whole but, if the seed is cut while ingesting, it can release the toxin. Fortunately, one has to ingest very large numbers of injured apple seeds to have any toxic consequences.

Asian Palmyra palm/Sugar palm/Toddy Palm, (*Borassus flabellifer*): Kingdom: Plantae, Division: Angiospermae, Class: Monocotyledonae, Order: Arecales/Palmales, Family: Aricaceae/Palmaceae.

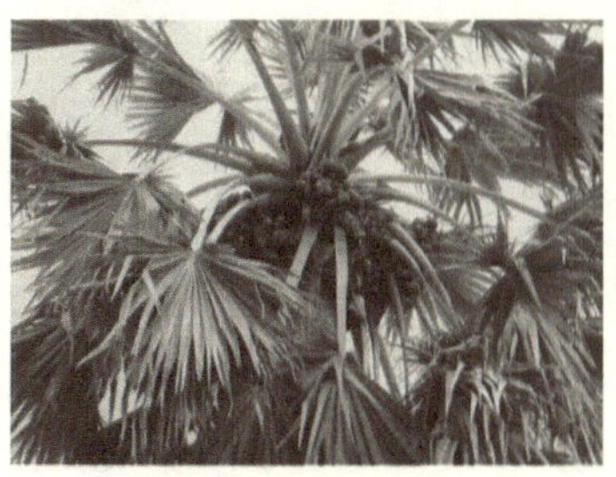

Palmyra Palm

The Palmyra palm is a long-lived tall tree (100 ft) that grows in Southern India, Sri Lanka, Myanmar, Thailand, Malaysia and other South East Asian counries. It grows well in arid and semi-arid regions. Leaves are very large, Bluish-green, strong about the size of an umbrella (9 ft across). Leaves form a canopy. The stem shows scars of old leaves that have fallen off. Fruits are produced in clusters and are about 7–9 inches in diameter. Fruits have a black husk inside which are found the edible jelly-like portion covered by a thin skin. The edible fruit contains a sweet liquid. The edible fruit is called Nongu in Tamil, Panam Nongu in Malayalam, Taad faali in Gujarathi, Siwalan in Javanese etc. The sap from the inflorescence can be tapped to obtain a sweet juice that can be fermented to produce the alcoholic palm-toddy or can be concentrated to produce the sugary molasses-like Palm sugar. **Health:** Fruit and fruit fluids are rich in minerals and glucose. They are quite refreshing especially in the summer.

Banana/Plantain (Musa sp): Kingdom: Plantae, Division: Angiospermae, Class: Monocotyledonae, Order: Zingiberales, Family: Musacee, Genus and species: *Musa acuminata (cultivated fruit banana),* **M.** *paradisiaca,* **M.** *balbisiana (wild banana),* **M.** *Sapientum* **(syn: M.paradisiaca). Cultivated banana, n = 11, 2n = 22, 3n = 33, 4n = 44. Plantains: 3n = 33.**

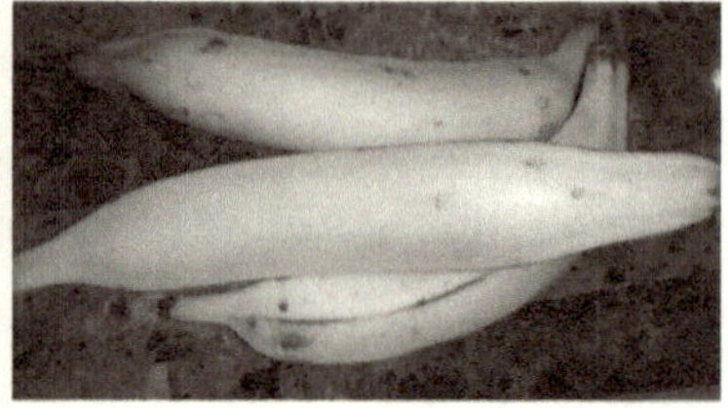

Plantains

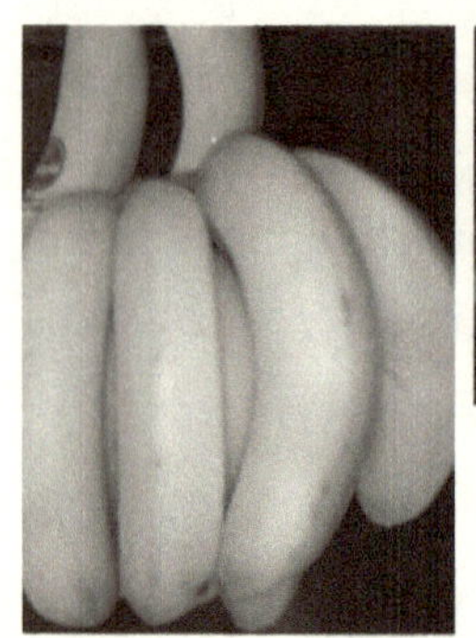

Banana

All currently cultivated varieties are hybrids of the diploid *M. acuminata* and *M.balbisiana.* The former are referred to as the A chromosome group banana and the latter as the B group banana. The hybrids are either triploids (AAB, ABB,) or tetraploids (AABB, AAAB, ABBB). There are also AA, BB, AAA, BBB, AAAA, BBBB diploids, triploid and tetraploids. Thus, these chromosomal combinations enable the generation of several distinctive varieties of bananas.

The banana also known as plantain plants are monocotyledonous, herbaceous, flowering plants, growing to a height of about 10 ft – 25 ft with underground stems called "corms" from which fibrous roots arise for anchoring the plants and absorbing nutrients and water from the soil. The underground stems also give rise to above ground pseudo stems from which large spirally arranged leaves with long petioles and large leaf blades arise. These leaves at maturity are about 3–8 ft long by 2 ft wide with a petiole and blade. The leaf blades or laminas have a central thick mid rib and parallel veins. The leaf petioles enlarge at the base to form a sheath covering the central soft pseudo stem. The large leaf blades are used as biodegradable plates for serving and eating food. Although, the wild varieties produce seeds in fruits, the cultivated varieties that are all hybrids produce parthenocarpic seedless fruits in tiers of large bunches. Each individual fruit can range in size from 3 inches long to more than a foot long depending on the variety. The pulpy edible parts of fruits are covered by a thick rind that has to be removed before consumption. The rinds range in color from green, yellow, purple and red. After they ripen, they are yellow in most edible varieties. Generally, the varieties referred to as banana are smaller. They are mostly consumed after they are ripened but the unripe fruits can also be cooked as a vegetable. The varieties referred to as plantains, are mostly used for cooking and frying when they are raw but these are also edible as ripened fruits before and after cooking. Bananas and plantain bananas represent important sources of food for millions of people in tropical/subtropical world. They are cooked, fried, chipped, dried and or served as dessert food. Apart from the fruit, the central pseudostem, inflorescence, and unripe banana skin are also used as vegetables. The unripe and ripe fruits are rich in carbohydrates, potassium and vitamin B6. The banana rind skin contains antioxidants. The peel has the ability to absorb metals and hence powdered banana peel has been tried as a cleanup agent to remove nuclear and heavy metal industrial contamination of soils. Additional descriptions of the botany of Banana and plantain can be found in the section on fruit-vegetables.

Health relevance: Apart from its nutritive value as a source of carbohydrates and dietary fiber, it is considered good as a source of potassium. There are unverified claims of its use in cancer prevention.

Banana peels contain lutein. It is an antioxidant reported to prevent damage to eyes due to UV irradiation. The peels are also said to ease depression. Researchers in Taiwan discovered that banana peel extract could ease depression because of its effect on serotonin that is a neurotransmitter in the brain responsible for balancing mood and emotions.

Berries: Blackberries, Black currants, Blueberries, Loganberries, Raspberries, Strawberries are collectively referred to as berries. All are juicy colored fruits with multiple fruits developed from small flowers in an inflorescence. However, botanically speaking berries are defined as a simple fruit with a fleshy pericarp containing seeds produced from the ovary of a single flower and so the botanical definition includes fruits like banana and grapes in the term berry. Here, we will bring together under berries all those that are referred to as berries in common usage and not botanical usage.

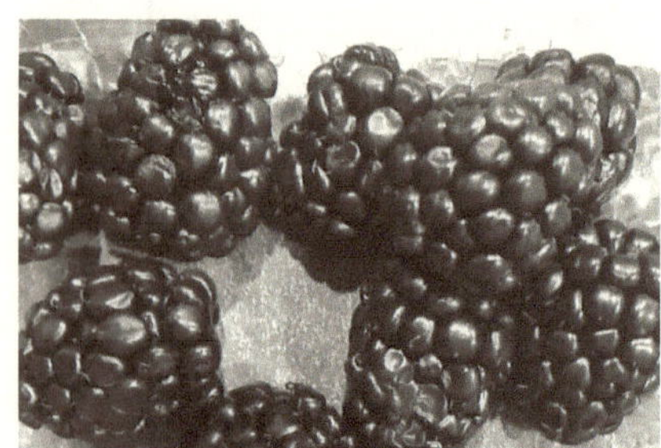

Blackberries

Black berries *(Rubus laciniatus and R. ursinus* – American black berries; *Rubus armeniacus* (Himalayan Blackberry) and *Rubus laciniatus* (Evergreen Blackberry): Kingdom: Plantae, Division: Angiospermae, Class: Eudicots; Order: Rosales, Family; Rosaceae. Chromosome number, n = 17. Ploidy ranges from 2n - 12n.

Blackberries are perennial plants that typically bear biennial stems ("canes") from the perennial root system. During the first year (primo cane), the plant grows with elongated stems known as canes and a collection of stems form a bramble. The canes produce palmate compound leaves with 5–7 leaflets. During the second year, the primo cane becomes a floricane wherein the leaf buds produce flowering laterals with a few small leaflets. The flowering laterals produce racemosa inflorescence that contains small flowers that after pollination develop into multiple fruits with small drupelets. These multiple fruits ripen and exhibit a black glabrous color. **Health:** Blackberry seeds contain oil rich in omega-3 (alpha-linolenic acid) and omega-6 fats (linoleic acid) as well as protein, dietary fiber, carotenoids, ellagitannins and ellagic acid. Blackberries contain, many anti-oxidants, polyphenolic compounds such as ellagic acid, tannins, ellagitannins, quercetin, gallic acid, anthocyanins, and cyanidins. Some reports suggest that the fruits may have anti-cancer potential.

Blueberries *(Vaccinium sp.)*: Kingdom: Plantae, Division: Angiospermae, Class: Eudicots, Order: Ericales, Family: Ericaceae, Genus and species: Northern high bush blueberry *(V. corymbosum)*, Alaskan blueberry *(V. alaskaense)*, Lowbush blueberry (V. angustifolium), Northern blueberry *(V. boreale)*, New Jersey blueberry *(V. caesariense)*, Hillside blueberry (*V. constablaei*), Evergreen blueberry *(V. darrowii)*, Elliott blueberry (*V. elliottii*), Southern blueberry *(V. formosum)*, Black highbush blueberry *(V. fuscatum)*, Hairy fruited blueberry *(V. hirsutum)*, Shiny blueberry *(V. myrsinites)*, Sour top velvet leaf or Canadian blueberry *(V. myrtilloides)*, cyan fruited blueberry *(V. operium)*, Dryland blueberry *(V. pallidum)*, Upland highbush blueberry *(V. simulatum)*, Southern blueberry *(V. tenellum)*, Rabbiteye blueberry (*V. ashei/V. virgatum*), and Korean blueberries *(V. koreanum)*. Chromosome numbers are, n = 12. 2n = 24, 4n = 48, 6n = 72. In addition, there are many amphidiploid varieties.

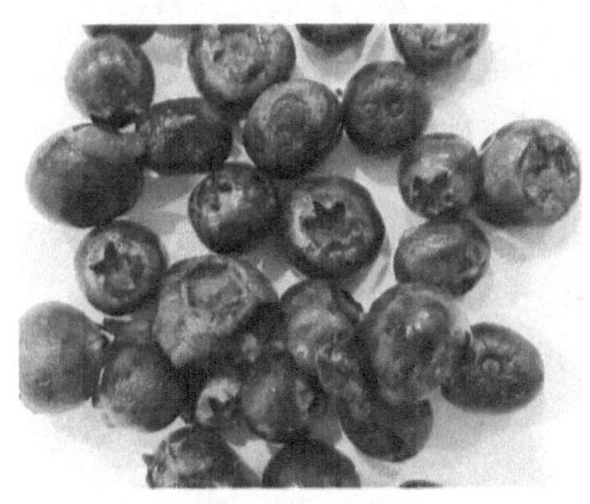

Blueberries

Blue berry plants are perennial shrubs. Leaves are ovate or lanceolate; flowers are white pink or red. Fruit is a dark bluish purple berry and covered with a waxy coating. Fruits are sweet with degree of sweetness varying depending on variety. Fruits are generally ready for harvest from June – August. **Health:** Blueberries are rich in anthocyanins, polyphenols, resveratrol and micronutrients. Blueberry supplementation is believed to reduce risk of cardiovascular disease, cancer and other metabolic diseases.

Boysenberry *(Rubus ursinus X R. ideus):* Kingdom: Plantae; Division: Angiospermae Class: Eudicots Order: Rosales; Family: Rosaceae. N = 7, 2n = 14. Ploidy levels ranged from 2n - 12n.

Boysenberries are hybrids of raspberries, Logan berries, American dewberries and black berries. The berries are aggregate berries similar to the parents. Fruits are red to black.

Dewberries (Rubus aboriginum): Kingdom: Plantae; Division: Angiospermae, Class: Eudicots Order: Rosales; Family: Rosaceae. Chromosome number, 2n = 28

Dewberries are dioecious plants that produce purple-black aggregate fruits on trailing brambles. They are used as table fruits as well as made into jams and jellies.

Loganberry *(Rubus ursinus X R. ideus):* Kingdom: Plantae; Division: Angiospermae Class: Eudicots; Order: Rosales; Family: Rosaceae. Chromosome number, 2n = 42

The Logan berry plant is a cross between the hexaploid (6n) black berry – *R. ursinus* and the diploid (2n) raspberry – *R. ideus.* Fruits are pink-red and are very similar to the berries of raspberries and black berries.

Raspberries *(Rubus sp):* Kingdom: Plantae; Division: Angiospermae, Class: Eudicots; Order: Rubiales; Family: Rubiaceae. Chromosome number: 2n = 14, 3n = 21.

There are many species of Raspberry. Raspberry plants are bushy canes with thorns. There are some new thornless varieties generated by genetic crossing. Fruits are golden yellow or deep pink or blue black. **Health:** Raspberry fruits are rich in Vitamin C with a low glycemic index. They have high quantities

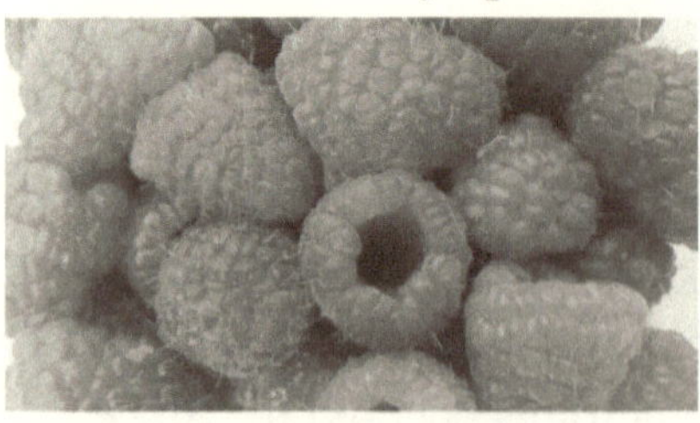

Raspberries

of Flavanoids, beta-carotene, anthocyanin and dietary fiber. They are rich in flavonoids, tannins, polyphenols, anthocyanin and carotene. Because of the low glycemic index, they are a good source of fruit for diabetic patients.

Strawberry *(Fragaria sp):* Kingdom: Plantae; Group: Angiospermae, Class: Eudicots; Order: Rosales Family: Rosaceae Genus: Hybrid: Fragaria sp. Fragaria × ananassa. N = 7. Polyploids ranged from 2n-8n. Most large size berries are 8n.

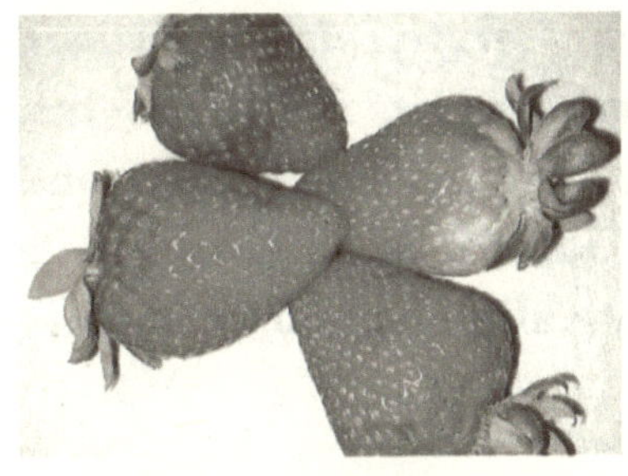
Strawberries

There are at least 20 different species of strawberries that range from diploid species with 14 chromosomes to decaploid (10 n) species with 70 chromosomes. There are 10 sets of 7 different chromosomes. Cultivated strawberry plants are hybrids that are grown currently by plastic culture. Herein, plastic sheets are laid over raised soil bunds and plants grown in nurseries are planted in holes that are pierced through the plastic sheets. The plants that are herbaceous in nature form runners with trifoliate leaves. Individual flowers are about ½–¾" across when they are fully open. They can be pistillate, staminate or perfect. Staminate flowers are the least common. Each flower has 5 white petals 5 green sepals and 5 green sepal-like bracts. Each pistillate flower has a dome shaped cluster of pistils at its center that is greenish yellow or pale yellow. Each staminate flower has 20–35 stamens with pale yellow filaments and yellow anthers. Each perfect flower has a dome shaped cluster of pistils at its center and a ring of surrounding stamens. The blooming period occurs from late spring to early summer lasting about 3–4 weeks. Afterwards the flowers are replaced by fruits when growing conditions are favorable otherwise they abort. These fruits are up to ½" long and across; they are globoid or globe-ovoid in shape becoming bright red at maturity. Small seeds are scattered across the surface of these fruits in sunken pits. The persistent sepals and sepal like bracts are appressed to the upper surface of these fruits. The fleshy interior of these fruits has a sweet-tart flavor and they are edible. The fruit is formed not from the ovary but from the flower receptacle. Each fruit thus formed, encloses several tiny seeds. Fruits are red in color generally and are sweet and luscious.

Garden strawberries contain flavonoids, anthocyanin, phenolic acids, polyphenols and tannins. Some people are allergic to strawberries and exhibit hives, hay fever and oral symptoms. The allergen Fra a1 is said to be the cause of allergy.

Citrus sp: *(Oranges, Limes, lemons, grapefruits, Kumquat, Tangerines, And Tangelo): Kingdom: Plantae, Division:* **Angiospermae, Class: Eudicots, Order: Sapindales, Family: Rutaceae, Genera and species: Citrus sp... Basic chromosome number of all Citrus sp is 2n = 18. However, cultivated citrus sp are all polyploids including allopolyploids.**

Citrus fruits refer to oranges, limes, lemons, grapefruit, pomelo, tangerines, clementines and many other hybrids. Citrus plants in general are small shrubs or trees about 5–15 ft. tall with spiny stems and aromatic simple leaves. Citrus flowers are fragrant, bisexual with 5 petals and sepals. The fruits are globose or slightly elongated with leather like rind with oil glands containing citrus oils. The endocarp is segmented into liths containing juice vesicles. The following are some of the important commonly consumed edible citrus fruits.

1. **Grape fruit** (C. sinensis X C. maxima)**: Chromosome number: X = 9, 2n = 18, 3n = 27, 4n = 36**

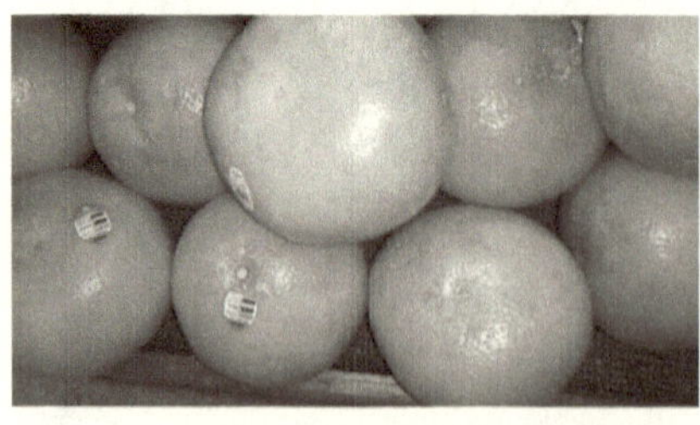

Grape Fruit

These are hybrid citrus plants producing a large globular fruit that may have white, pink, or ruby-red fruit segments. The trees are evergreen and grow to about 15–20 ft tall with glossy dark green leaves. Grapefruits contain large concentrations of Naringin and furano coumarins that interfere with many drugs especially statins and beta blocking blood pressure medications. Drinking grape juice along with, before or soon after taking prescription drugs can have serious consequences due to interference in availability of the prescribed dose of the drug. Tangelo, Ugli, Minneola are hybrids of grapefruit.

2. Kumquats *(C. japonica):* 2n = 18

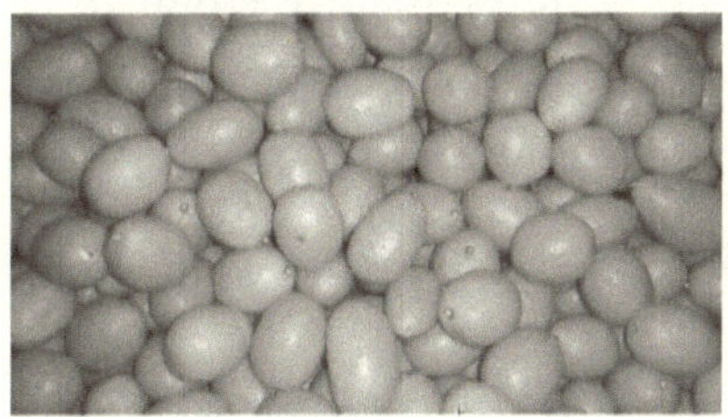

Kumquats

These are small trees related to orange trees grown in China, Japan, Korea, Viet Nam, Thailand, Nepal and India. Currently they have been introduced into other South Asian countries including, Chile in South America, Florida, California, Nevada, Arizona in the United States. There are many different varieties: Round Kumquat (Murumi), Oval (Nagami), Jiangsu (Fukushi), Centennial (variegated derived from Nagami). The trees are evergreen short trees or shrubs and there are many different varieties. The edible fruits are dark orange in color and are somewhat small about the size of tangerines. The Skin and fruits contain essential oils including citronella, limonene, citronellal and alpha pinene. **Health:** Good source of vitamin C.

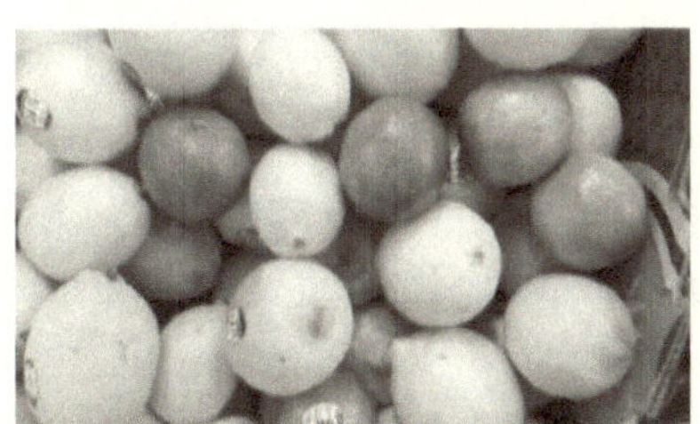

Lemons & Limes

3. Lemon *(C. Limon):* n = 9.

Lemons are evergreen trees producing yellow ellipsoidal fruits that contain about 6% citric acid that gives it the sharp sour taste.

4. Limes *(Citrus sp):* Limes are a collection of different types all of which produce a round green fruit that is rich in vitamin C. Collectively, they refer to: Australian desert lime (C. *glauca*), Australian finger lime (C. *australasica*), Australian round lime (C. *australis*), Kaffir lime (C. *hystrix*), Mexican lime/Bar tenders lime (C. *aurantifolia*), and Sweet lime (C. *limetta*). Besides there are certain other fruits that are also called limes but are not citrus limes. They are wild lime (Adelia ricinella), Spanish lime (*Melicoccus bijugatus*) and Limequat (Hybrid of lime and kumquat).

5. Sathukudi/Mousambi *(C. limetta):* This is a vary commonly consumed citrus fruit in India especially by people recovering from health conditions due to its health benefits by providing vitamin C. In India, the fruits are often called as oranges. The plants are small trees with thorny stems. The trees are evergreen growing in near semi-arid conditions. The fruits are globose with lemon-green skin.

6. Sweet oranges *(Citrus aurantium):*

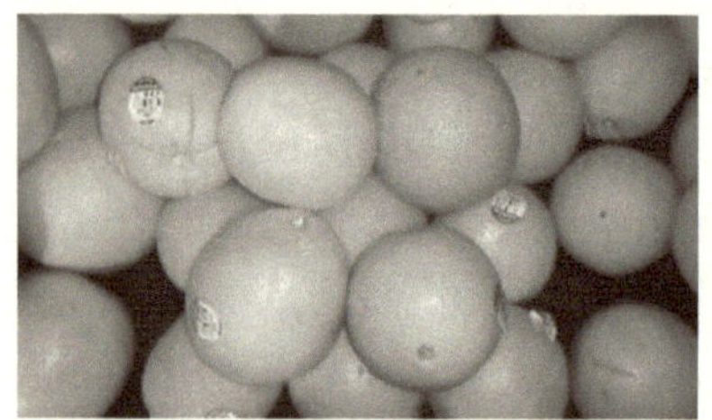

Sweet Oranges

The common sweet orange, navel and blood oranges are different hybrid varieties of oranges. They are trees grown widely all over the world. The main edible products are the fruit segments and juice. Orange blossom honey and orange blossom water are prized by-products from orange groves.

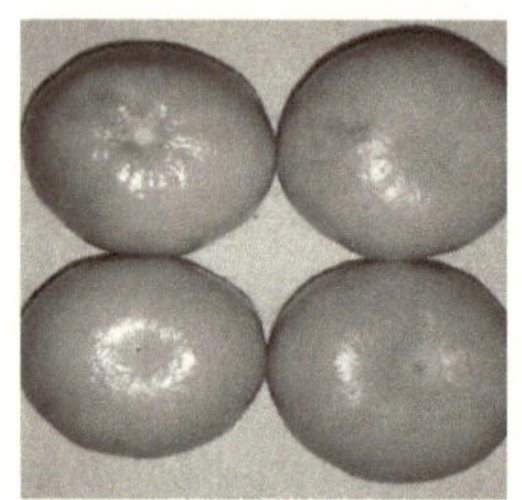

Tangerine

7. Tangerines *(C. tangerina):*

Tangerine trees are also evergreen trees. The fruits are smaller than the sweet oranges. The fruit segments contain the pebbly juice vesicles. The fruits are rich in beta-carotene, folates and vitamin C besides potassium and magnesium minerals.

8. Tangelo *(C. X tangelo):* Tangelos are hybrids of C. reticulata X C.maxima or *C. paradasi).* The fruits are small with a tufted knob-top. Minneolas are also a variety of tangelos as are honey bell tangelos. The outer skin is a deep orange color. Fruits are sweet and are rich source of vitamin C. Unlike grapefruit, tangelos do not contain significant amounts of furocoumarins and hence are not a significant problem for those taking prescription statin drugs for cholesterol control.

9. Buddha's hand, *(Citrus medica var. sarcodactylis),* is an unusual type of citrus. It is not globose but has finger like projections. It is also edible but does not contain juice or pulp.

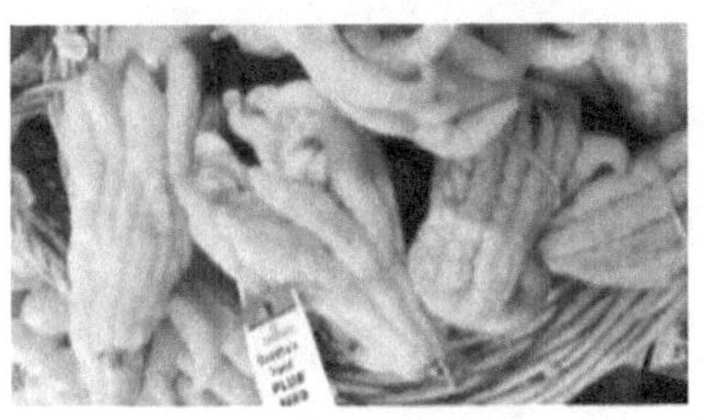

Buddha's Hand

10. Ugli *(Citrus reticulata X C. Paradisi):*

The Ugli is a cross between grapefruit and Mandarin orange. The plants are mainly grown in Jamaica in the Caribbean islands. The fruits have deformed appearance which is reflected in the name "Ugli." Fruits are juicy and sour-sweet.

Ugli

Another member of the citrus group is called Citron or Citrus apple *(Citrus medica).* It is not used as a culinary fruit but is used to make pickles (Narthangai) in India. The plant grows in Southern India, Morocco, Syria and other middle eastern countries as well as in Puerto Rico in the Carribean USA.

Health relevance of Citrus fruits: The fruits contain Vitamin C, citric acid, flavonoids and limuloids. Citrus fruits supply Vitamin C and hence prevent scurvy disease. Citrus juices reduce development of kidney stones by forming the soluble calcium citrate instead of insoluble calcium oxalate that can crystallize and form kidney stones. Thus, drinking citrus juice helps to prevent formation of kidney stones. However, certain citrus fruits like grape fruits and bitter orange contain polyphenolic compounds that interact with cholesterol lowering Statin and close to 80 + prescribed drugs.

Cranberries, **(***Vaccinium* *oxycoccus/V.eryhthrocarpum/ V.macrocarpon):* **Kingdom: Plantae; Division: Angiospermae; Class: Eudicots Order: Ericales; Family: Ericaceae. 2n = 12. Most are hexaploid 6n = 72.**

Ripe cranberry fruits are deep red berries with a sour acidic taste. The berries are borne on creeping shrubs/vines about 7 ft long. Flowers

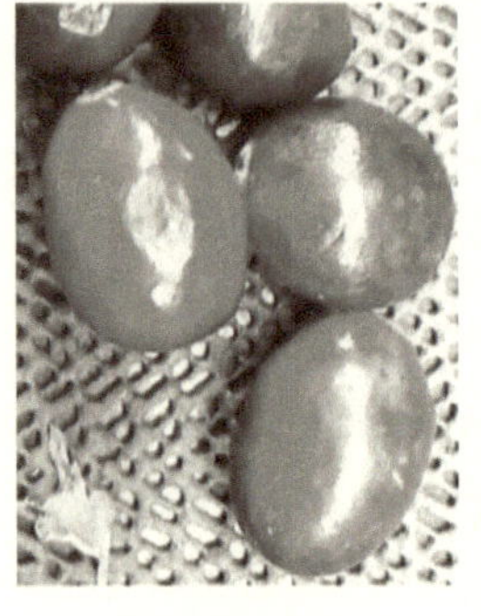

Cranberries

with reflexed petals exposing the style and stamens are pollinated by bees. Plants are related to blue berries and Huckleberries. The fruits are used to make sauces and juices. **Health**: Cranberries are rich in Vitamin C, polyphenols, flavones and anthocyanins. The fruit juices and extracts are reported to prevent adhesion of the E. coli bacterial pilus to the walls of urinary tracts thus, preventing urinary infections. The fruits and extracts in capsule form are being marketed as anti-urinary tract infection agents. However, some studies dispute these claims.

Custard Apple, (*Annona cherimoya*); Sugar apple (*Annona squamosa*), African custard apple (*A. senegalensis*); Pond apple (*A. glabra*), Pawpaw (*Asimina triloba*), Soursop (*A. muricata*), Atemoya (*AnnonaX Atemoya*; hybrid of *A. cherimola X A. sqamosa*): Kingdom: Plantae; Group: Angiospermae, Magnoliids; Order: Magnoliales; Family: Annonaceae. 2n = 18

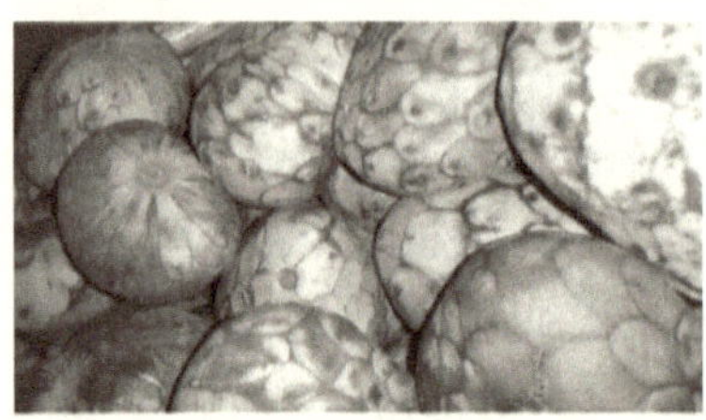

Custard Apple

There are 7 closely related species with edible fruits belonging to the Annonaceae family. All are evergreen trees growing in tropical/subtropical climatic conditions. Of these, African custard apple is endemic to Africa and the Pond/Alligator apple found in Florida have only a minor role as edible fruits. The other five, especially Custard and Sugar apple are consumed globally. In all cases, one fleshy, ovate to spherical fruit is produced per flower. Each fruit consists of many individual small fruits or syncarps, with one syncarp and seed per pistil. Seeds are bean-like with tough coats; the seed kernels are toxic. **Health:** Leaves and seeds contain the neurotoxin Annonacin. Annonacin has been identified as the cause of certain neurodegenerative diseases. Annonacin has been shown to have anti-cancer activities in laboratory experiments and limited animal studies. However, Annonacin has not been approved for human use. The seed extracts are powerful insecticides.

Dates: *(Phoenix dactylifera):* **Kingdom: Plantae; Division: Angiospermae Monocotyledonae Family: Palmales Family: Palmaceae Genus and species: Phoenix dactylifera. 2n = 36.**

Date palm trees grow tall to a height of 70–80 ft. At the crown of the stem, the plant produces several compound leaves that are about 13–20 ft. long with spiny petioles and pinnate leaflets that are a foot or more long. The plants are dioecious with separate male and female plants. The flowers are wind pollinated. Ripe dates contain about 80% sugar. The remainder consists of protein, fiber and trace elements including boron, cobalt, copper, fluorine, magnesium, manganese, selenium and zinc. **Health relevance:** The low glycemic index of dates is of particular use for diabetics.

Dragon fruit *(Hylocereus undatus/H. tricostatus):* Kingdom: Plantae; Division: Angiospermae Eudicots, Order: Caryophyllales Family: Cactaceae, Other synonums: Cactus angularis, Cereus triangularis, C. tricostatus.

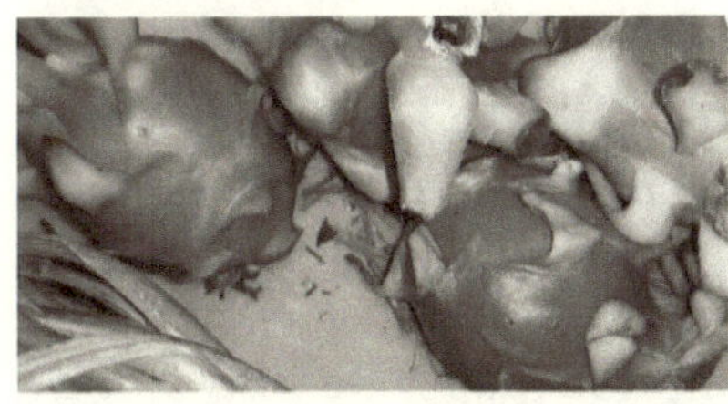
Dragon Fruit

These cacti are found in Australia, South East Asia, Central and South America. The cacti are referred to as Pitahya. The fruits that may be red or golden colored are eaten raw along with seeds. Fruit juice is also made into wine. The fruits are commonly sold in Vietnam and are now available in fruit and vegeatable stores in many countries.

Figs *(Ficus carica):* Kingdom: Plantae; Division: Angiospermae; Class: Eudicots; Order: Caricales; Family: Moraceae; Genus: Ficus carica.

Fig plants are natives of the Middle East and Western and Southeastern Asia and grown now in most parts of the temperate regions. It is a deciduous tree growing to a height of 20–35 ft. The leaves are three or five lobed, palmate. The inflorescence is a syconium containing many unisexual flowers. The whole inflorescence develops into the fruit. A small hole allows the fig wasp *Blastophega psenes* to enter and pollinate the flowers iside the swollen syconium. The edible fruit consists of the mature syconium containing numerous one seeded fruits or druplets. The fruit is 3–5 centimetres 1.2–2.0 in long with a green skin sometimes ripening towards purple or brown.. *Ficus carica* has milky sap laticifer. The sap of the fig's green parts is an irritant to human skin. Persistent or common figs have all female flowers that do not need pollination for fruiting; the fruit can develop through parthenocarpic means. There are several varieties of figs namely: Black Mission with blackish purple skin and pink colored flesh; Kadota with green skin and purplish flesh; Calimyrna with greenish yellow skin and amber flesh; Brown Turkey with purple skin and red flesh. The variety Adriatic is the variety most often used to make fig bars **Health relevance:** Fruits are rich in antioxidants. Has low sugar and hence suitable for consumption in limited quantities by diabetics. Nutritional value is given in Table.

Grapes *(Vitis vinifera)*: Kingdom: Plantae; Division: Angiospermae, Class: Eudicots; Order: Vitales; Family: Vitaceae Genus and species: 2n = 38. Polyploids and aneuploidy are cultivated.

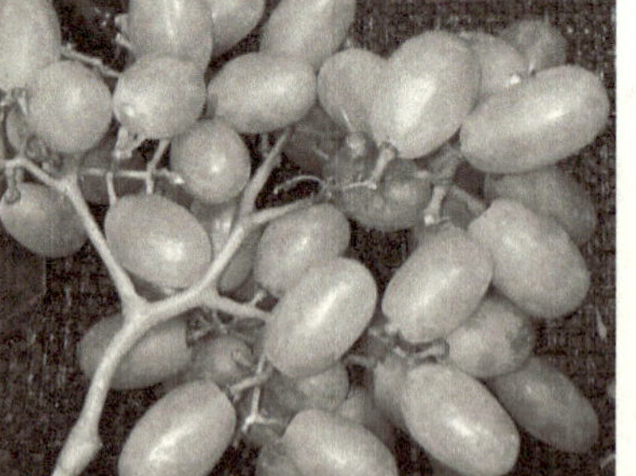

Grapes

The common grapevine *Vitis vinifera* has many varieties. In addition to this species, there are other species such as Concord *(V. lambrusca),* wild grapevine of North America *(V.riparia);* muscadine grape *(V.rotundifolia);* Asian grape. *(V. Amurensis).* In general, grapes are classified into table grapes meant for consumption as fruit or for making grape juice and wine grapes meant for making wine and related alcoholic beverages. Table grapes are green, red or black and many new varieties such as the proprietary Moon drop grapes are generally seedless and large whereas wine grapes are small with thick skin and high sugar content. Raisins are dried grapes.

The common grapevine is a native of the Mediterranean region including central Europe, southwestern Asia including western Iran, North Africa and Portugal. It is now grown in almost all parts of the world including South and N. America, Australia, India and China. The plants are vines growing to a height of 30–40 yards. They have thick vines with flaky bark. The leaves are palmate with lobes. Flowers are hermaphrodite in the cultivated *V. vinifera* but in the sub species *sylvestris* male and female flowers are found on separate plants (Dioecious), the fruits grow in bunches and are called berries. The fruits range from green, dark purple, brown and black. The berries have a waxy coating and may have thick or thin skins. There are many seedless varieties such as Thompson, Reliance, Black – Monukka, Venus and Benjamin. Seedless varieties tend to have less of the potential health benefits compared to the seeded varieties. The lack of seeds does not cause any planting problems since grapevines are propagated by vegetative cuttings. **Health:** Grapes are rich in Polyphenols particularly anthocyanins, flavonols, Resveratrol and many other phytochemicals that have great cardiovascular health benefits. Drinking wines – red in particular, seem to cause reduced platelet aggregation, increased vasodilation and decreased angiotensin activity. Grape seed oil is used in the cosmetic industry due to its perceived skin care benefits. Grapes and grape products are toxic to dogs due to resultant renal failure. Grape seed extract derived from the ground-up seeds of red wine grapes is now used to treat a number of diseases mainly related to cardiovascular conditions.

Guava: Kingdom: Plantae; Division: Angiospermae; Class: Eudicots; Order: Myrtales; Family: Myrtaceae; Genus and species: *Psidium guajava*. Chromosome number, n = 11, 2n = 22, 3n = 33. Both diploids and triploids are found in nature.

Guava fruits grow on small trees grown mostly in Mexico, Central and South America, Indian subcontinent, Malaysia, Thailand, Indonesia, 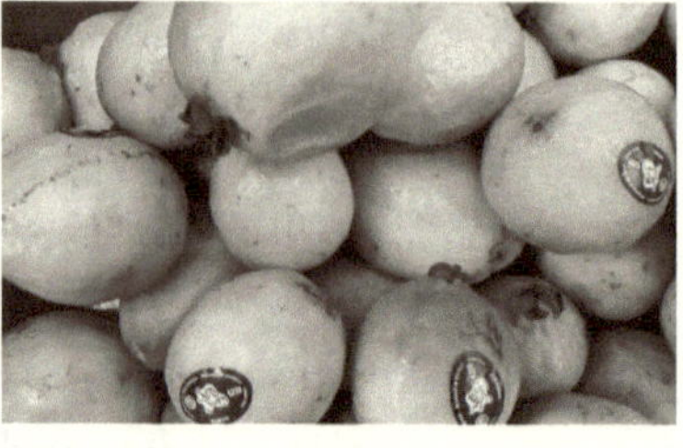China and several other tropical and subtropical countries. They have glabrous simple leaves that contain various phytochemicals that are considered to have medicinal value. Fruits are round to oval about 2.5 inches in diameter. Fruits are green or yellow when ripe and the

Guava

juicy pulp inside may be white or pink-red depending on the variety. Fruits are rich in gallocatechin, guaijaverin, leucocyanidin and amritoside and contain high levels of pectin. Fruits are rich in Vitamin C, carotenoids and polyphenols. **Health relevance:** The high soluble fiber content of Guava fruits helps relieve constipation. Guava leaf has been used as a folk remedy for diabetes. Guava leaf inhibits the increase in the plasma level of blood sugar. Guava leaf is believed to inhibit histamine release from cells and hence ingestion of leaf powders is considered to relieve allergic symptoms.

Indian Gooseberry/Amla (*Embelica officianalis*): **Indian gooseberry** (*Emblica officinalis/Phyllanthus emblica*): **Kingdom: Plantae; Division: Angiospermae, Class: Eudicots, Rosids, Order: Malphigiales; Family: Phyllanthaceae, Genus:** Phyllanthus. **Chromosome number, Polyploids varying from 98–104, considered to be 14 xs. Haploid x = 7.**

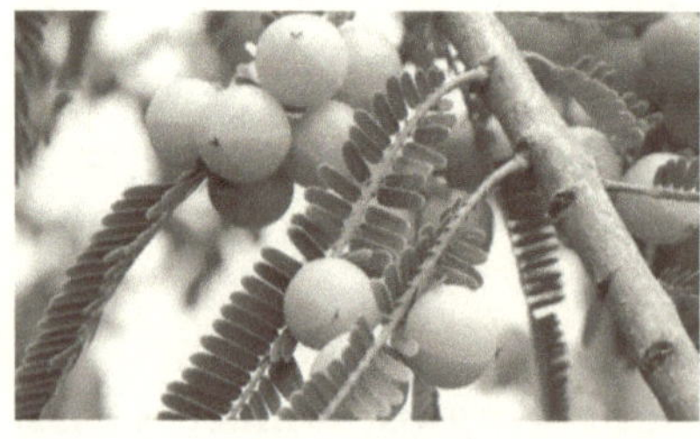This plant also known as, Amla or Amalika in India is a deciduous tree of the family Phyllanthaceae. It is known for its edible fruit that in addition to being a good source of vitamin C is well known for its medicinal properties.

Indian Gooseberry

The Amla tree is a deciduous tree with simple pinnate leaves. The edible fruit is greenish-yellow with six vertical stripes wherein each striped area represents a segment of the fleshy fruit.

The seed inside the fruit has a hard shell and is brownish in color. The fruit upon wounding quickly turns brown to black due to polyphenol oxidase activity. The fruits are sour tasting and are used to prepare pickles after steeping in salt water and or adding spices. It is not a table fruit. **Health:** All parts of the plant but especially the fruits are prescribed for various illnesses by practioners of both Indian traditional Ayurvedic, Unani and Siddha medicine as well as Chinese traditional medicine. The fruits are components of the ancient Ayurvedic rejuvenative medicine known as Chavanaprash. The fruits in any form or formulation are considered a very good medicine for digestion, enhance bowel movement, alleviate asthma, stimulate hair growth and remove toxins from blood. Chinese traditional medicine also recognizes the usefulness of the berries for throat infections and other ailments. Some modern studies indicate that the fruits or fruit extracts reduced pancreatitis in rats and recovery of the pancreas after pancreatitis attacks. There are also reports that the fruits can help control of diabetes and ameliorate diabetic neuropathy. The fruits are also anti-oxidants.

Jackfruit *(Artocarpus heterophyllus/A.integrifolia):* **Kingdom: Plantae, Division: Angiospermae, Class: Eudicots, Order: Rosales, Family: Moraceae. Chromosome number, 2n = 56**

Jackfruits are large evergreen perennial trees that grow in many tropical and sub-tropical climates. The fruits are used as a vegetable after cooking, the ripe fruits as dessert and culinary source and seeds are used in various dishes. **Health:** Fruits are a rich source of vitamin C, soluble fiber and minerals. Seeds contain carbohydrates and proteins.

Jambol/Jamun/Java plum/Black-plum *(Syzygium cumina/ Syzygium jambolanum/Eugenia jambolana):* **Kingdom: Plantae, Group: Angiospermae, Class: Eudicots, Order: Myrtales Family: Myrtaceae. Chromosome number, 2n = variously recorded as 22, 42–44, 44, 66.**

Jambul plants are natives of the Indian sub-continent, Sri Lanka, Malaysian archipelago and Indonesia. The Indian subcontinent is referred to as Jambudvipa (island of Jambu) in ancient Vedic texts of India. The plant has been introduced into other countries in Africa and

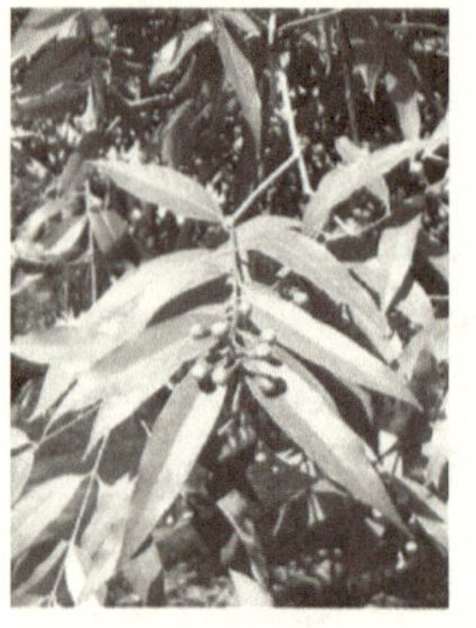

Sourth Asia and in Florida in N. America. It is a slow growing species with dense foliage of leathery leaves and is often planted as a shade tree in hot climates. It can reach heights of up to 30 m and can live more than 100 years. The edible fruits are rich in Flavanoids. Fruits are oblong or ovoid and become black upon maturity. The flesh of the fruit is very pinkish purple. A variant variety produces white fleshy fruits. **Health:** Leaves, bark, fruit pulp and seeds are used in Ayurvedic preparations for lowering blood pressure, controlling diabetes. The fruits are rich in Carotene the precursor of Vitamin A and are rich in vitamin C, anthocyanin and many anti-oxidants.

Jambol

Kiwi Fruits, (Actinidia sp.): Kingdom: Plantae; Division: Angiospermae, Class: Eudicots; Order: Ericales; Family: Actinidiaceae;Genus and species; *A.kolomicta; A. melanandria; A. polygama; A. purpurea, A. deliciosa; A. chinensis; A. coriaceae; A. arguta.* **Chromosome number, X = 29, 2n = 58. Many are hexaploid 6n = 174.**

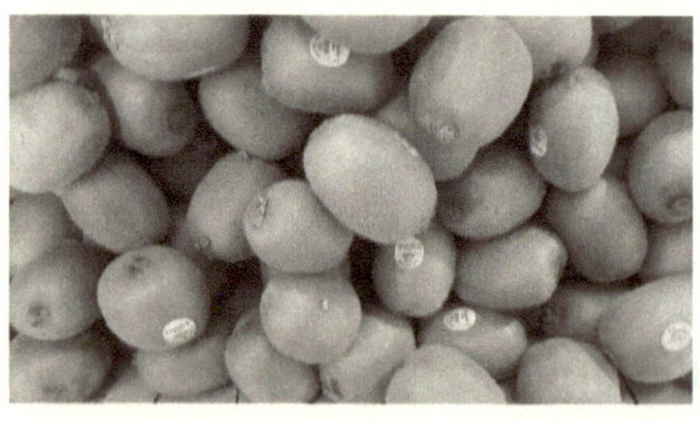

The plant is a native of China from where it spread to New Zealand and got its English name from there since Kiwi is the native bird of New Zealand. The fruit trees are grown in China, New Zealand, Italy, Chile and many regions with a mild climate. The Kiwi plant is a vine and there are separate male and female plants that are usually grown together to enable pollination. Fruits have a Khaki colored fuzzy skin. They contain vitamin C and K and the rich green pulp is full of antioxidants including carotene as well as the proteolytic enzyme actinidain and oxalate crystals. **Health relevance:**

Kiwi

The fruits contain oxalate crystals and the enzyme actinidain that can be allergic. People with a tendency to form Kidney stones could be susceptible if they consume kiwi juice or eat substantial amounts of the delicious fruit. Experimental studies show that Kiwi fruits prevent platelet aggregation and thereby act like blood thinning agents.

Loquat/Japanese or Chinese plum *(Eriobotrya japonica)*: Kingdom: Plantae; Division: Angiospermae, Class: Eudicots; Order: Rosales; Family: Rosaceae. Chromosome number, 2n = 34, 4n = 68

Loquats with over 500 cultivars are natives of China but are grown in many sub-tropical climes including Florida and southern states in the United States. Plants are evergreen shrubs or short trees growing to height of 10–20 ft. Loquat fruits grow in clusters and are slightly ovate and about the size of an egg. The fruits are yellowish pink or orange with a reddish tinge. The succulent flesh inside is white or slightly yellow with a single almond shaped seed. The fruits are slightly sour/tangy. Fruits are rich in pectin and sugar. Fruits are used to make various jams and jellies and for making specific alcoholic beverages. The seeds have a hard shell but the contents are poisonous due to cyanogenic glycosides. **Health:** Loquat fruit syrup is used in Chinese medicine as a demulcent and cough medicine. In Japan, dried leaves are used to treat skin conditions such as psoriasis.

Longan *(Dimocarpus longan)*: Kingdom: Plantae; (Division): Angiosperms; (Division): Class: Eudicots; Order: Sapindales; Family: Sapindaceae; Genus: *Dimocarpus. Chromosome number*

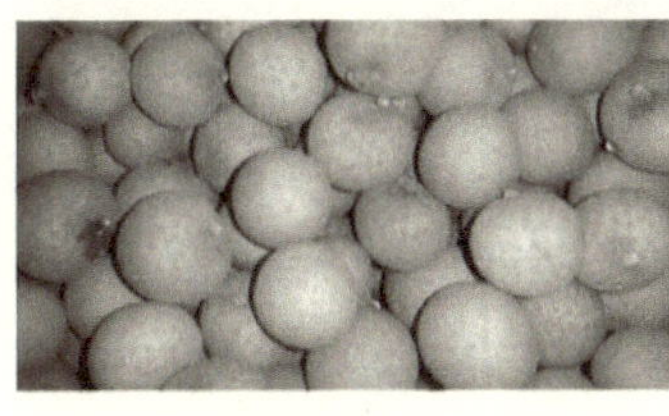

Longan

Longan is an evergreen tree belonging to the soapberry family that grows to a height of about 20 ft. It is related to lychee and rambutan of the same family. It is a native of South Asia and produces edible fruits. The fruit is sweet, juicy with succulent white flesh. Fruits are eaten fresh or after drying. Fruits are rich in Vitamin C. **Health:** Good nutritional value.

Litchi/Lychee *(Litchi chinensis)*: Kingdom: Plantae; Division: Angiospermae, Class: Eudicots; Order: Sapindales; Family: Sapindaceae. Chromosome number, 2n = 30.

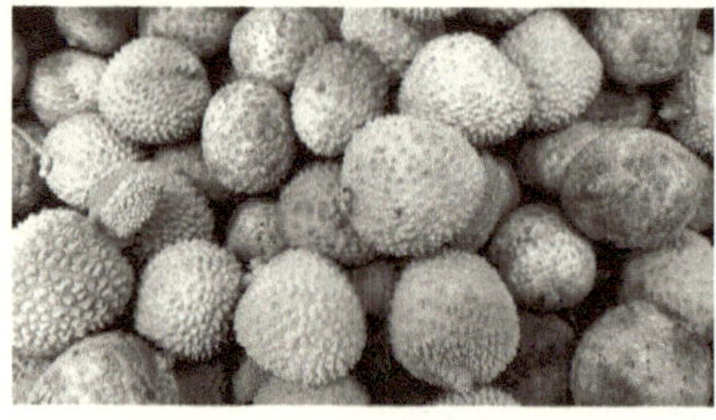

Litchi

There are three sub species namely: 1. *L. Chinensis sub sp. Chinensis* that is the only commercially cultivated plant with several cultivars, 2. *L. Chinensis sub sp. Javensis* that is cultivated locally in Malay Peninsula and Indonesia, 3. *L. Chinensis sub sp. Philippinensis* that is not cultivated but grows wild in the Philippine islands.

The lychee fruit is a fragrant oval-globular fruit with a translucent whitish flesh and pink-red skin. The fresh juice from the fruit has a very aromatic refreshing smell. The plants are natives of China but are now grown in most sub-tropical climatic conditions in many other countries. Plants are evergreen trees growing about 50 ft tall. Flowers are borne in panicles. **Health:** Fruits are rich in Vitamin C and sugar. Polyphenols and anthocyanins are other constituents. Studies conducted in India by the Centers for disease control (CDC-USA) indicated that consumption of large numbers of litchi fruits has been correlated with induction of non-inflammatory encephalopathy in children in North India and Vietnam. It is known that litchi fruits contain the phytotoxic α-(methylenecyclopropyl) glycine an analog of the neurotoxic L-amino acid hypoglycine.

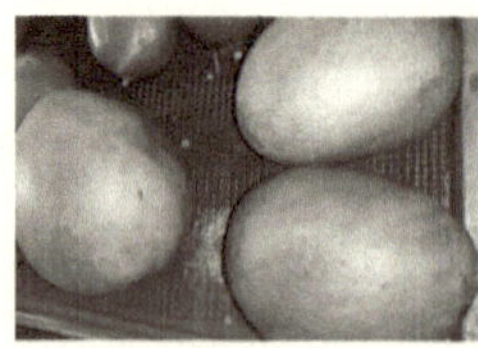

Mango

Mango *(Mangifera indica)*: Kingdom: Plantae; Division: Angiospermae, Class: Eudicots; Order; Sapindales; Family: Anacardiaceae; Genus and species: *Mangifera indica*. Chromosome number, 2n = 40.

The cultivated edible mango known as Indian mango is cultivated mainly in tropical countries. There are many varieties of this species.

Fruits may be globose, oval or tiny green. The latter are used mainly for making pickles. Plants range from dwarf types about 10 ft. tall to those

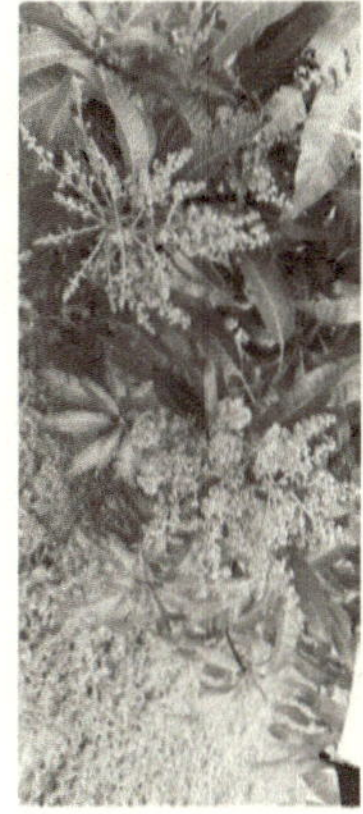

that may grow to a height of 100 ft. or more with spreading branches. The leaves are long about 6 "to 12" long, glabrous and aromatic. Small flowers are borne on inflorescence panicles. Table fruits are yellow, orange, red or green and contain a pulpy edible fruit enclosing a fibrous big sclerified pit enclosing a single seed. Mango fruits contain many phytochemicals including polyphenols, quercetin, kaemferol, gallic acid, caffeic acid, catechins and alpha and beta-carotene, lupeol and the unique xanthoid Mangiferin. **Health:** Mango oils resins and leaf extracts may cause severe allergic reactions including anaphylactic reactions in susceptible individuals

Mango leaves-flowers

Mangosteen/Monkey fruit Garcinia mangostana/Gambogia gemmigutta L.: Kingdom: Plantae; Division: Angiospermae Class: Eudicots; Order: Malphigiales; Family: Lusciaceae/Guttiferae Genera: Gambogia; species: Many: **Malabar Tamarind/Kudam puli/ Kodukka puli** *(G. gemmi-gutta)*; **Button Mangosteen** *(G. prainiana)* **Lemon drop mangosteen. Chromosome number is variable. Reported to be 2n = 56, 76, 88–90, 96, 120–130. Confusion probably due to different ploidy level of accessions tested.**

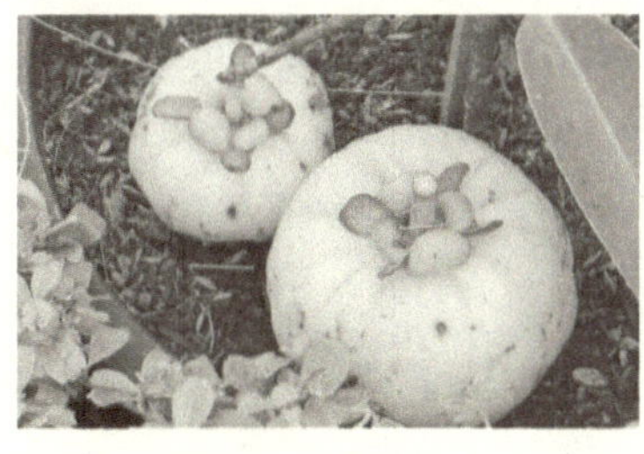

Although there are about 300 species of **Garcinia** or related genera, the two best-known species of Mangosteen are the purple mangosteen *G. mangostana* and the Malabar tamarind *G. gemmigutta*. The plants are natives of the Indonesian/ Malaysian archipelago but are grown

Mangosteen

extensively in South Asia and tropical South America and Africa. The fruits of these plants have become popular in folk lore and popular press because of their supposed property of appetite suppression and weight reduction. The mangosteens are tropical evergreen tall trees. The fruits are pot shaped with an inedible exocarp rind and spongy endocarp that is white in color. The edible endocarp is segmented or divided into lozenges with each segment enclosing an almond sized seed.

The rind exocarp contains polyphenols, and xanthanoids like mangostin. The edible flesh of the fruit is sweet, has a pleasant aroma, and contains much smaller quantities of antioxidants, polyphenols and mangostin. Commercial preparations contain whole fruit extracts including exo and endo carp or only the dried powder from the exocarp. The chemical compound hydroxycitric acid (HCA) found in the fruit is an appetite suppressant. The effect of Mangosteen extracts on weight loss is unclear. Most reports of its effectiveness are either from studies on animals or anecdotal particularly through television and popular media. However, hydroxyl citric acid that is a component of these fruits is reported to cause testicular degeneration. **Health claims:** Popular use as a weight reduction fruit based on anecdotal and some animal studies but yet to be proven by controlled human studies. The fruit and rind extracts have been in use in native cultures for treating constipation, removing worms and parasites from the intestine and skin infections. The American Cancer Society does not endorse mangosteen products as a potential treatment for cancer. The hydroxycitric acid in Mangosteen is known to cause testicular degeneration.

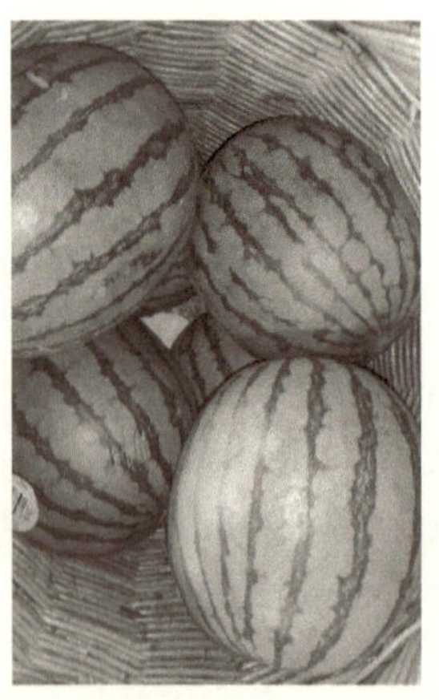

Watermelon

Melons *(Cucumis melo and Citrullus lanatus)*: Kingdom: Plantae; Division: Angiospermae, Class: Eudicots, Eudicots; Order: Cucurbitales; Family: Cucurbitaceae. Chromosome number, 2n = 24.

Cucumis melo includes different varieties known variously as Muskmelon, honeydew, Crenshaw, Casaba, cantaloupe, Persian melon, Santa Claus melon and Christmas melon. The watermelon *(Citrullus lanatus)* is also a melon but of a different species. All the different melons exhibit somewhat similar characteristics. They are all vines that spread on the ground. They have lobed leaves of different sizes producing fruits of different colors and sizes. All have high levels of water and are good sources of electrolytes. Since the fruits touch the soil, the fruits should be washed and the skin removed in order to prevent ingestion of harmful bacteria like salmonella or E. coli that may be attached to the skin.

Mulberries: Black mulberry *(Morus nigra)*, Red Mulberry *(M. Rubra)*, White mulberry (M. Alba): Kingdom: Plantae; Division: Angiospermae, Class: Eudicots; Order: Rosales; Family: Moraceae. Chromosome number, 2n = 308.

Mulberry trees are large deciduous trees which grow in temperate climatic conditions in North and South America, Australia, China, India, other South Asian countries, Europe and Africa. Mulberry trees are host to the silkworm *Bombyx mori*. The trees can be monoecious (separate male and female flowers in same tree) or dioecious (separate male and female trees). Plants are highly branched with glabrous simple leaves. Flowers are borne in inflorescences known as catkins. The fruits are small multiple fruits, which look similar to black berries and raspberries. Fruits may be green, red, black or white upon maturity. The white variety has a milder taste. Fruits are rich in anthocyanins. **Health claims:** The rich anthocyanin content of fruits is beneficial for cardiovascular health. The stem, leaves as also fruits contain resveratrol that may have cardio protective effects. Nevertheless, the experimental results are inconclusive and do not verify the initial claims on cardio-protection made by the supplements industry.

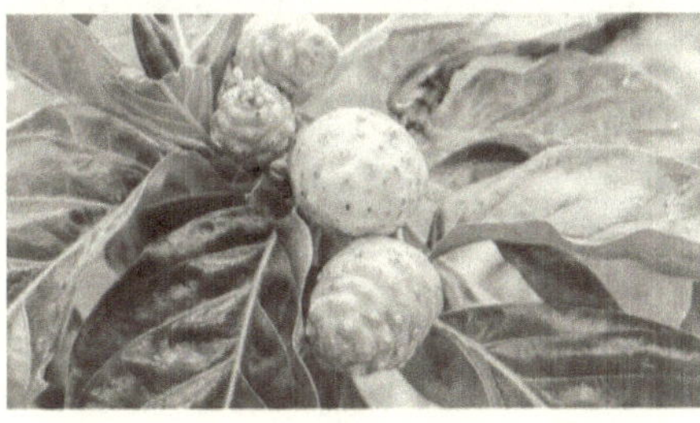

Noni

Noni/Indian Mulberry/Beach mulberry/Cheese fruit *(Morinda citrifolia):* Kingdom: Plantae; Division: Angiospermae, Class: Eudicots; Order: Gentianales; Family: Rubiaceae. Chromosome number, 2n = 44.

Noni trees are cultivated for their fruit that is reputed to have multiple health benefits. The fruits and fruit juice are popular products in health food stores. The plants grow to a height of about 30 ft and are cultivated in Australasia, India and rest of South East Asia, Pacific-Polynesian islands and in many tropical countries. The fruits are multiple fruits that are green turning to near white as they ripen. They have a strong cheesy aroma. The fruits are referred to as famine food since they are eaten as staple foods under famine conditions in Polynesia and Australasia. **Health claims:** The fruits contain moderate amounts of carbohydrates, vitamins and minerals. They do contain multiple phytochemicals that are believed to confer various health benefits including: chemoprevention of cancer, hepato-protection (prevents liver disease), treats gout and protects the cardiovascular system against oxidative damage. However, most of these claims are anecdotal and have yet to be verified by controlled clinical trials.

Passion fruit/Maracujá *(Passiflora edulis)*: Kingdom: Plantae; Division: Angiospermae, Eudicots; Order: Malphigiales; Family: Passifloraceae; Genus and species: *Passiflora edulis; P. edulis var flavicarpa*. Chromosome number, 2n = 12, 2n = 18.

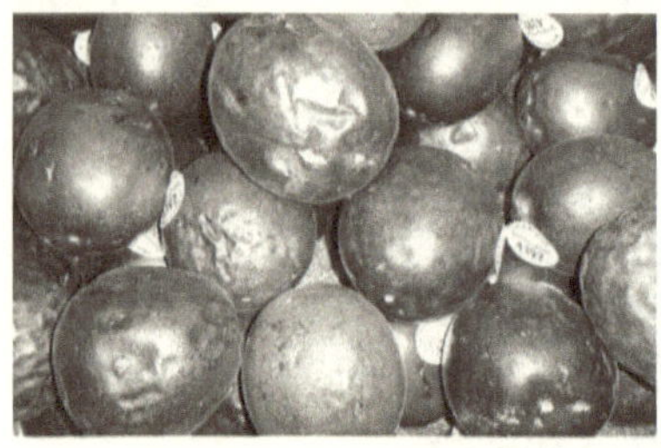

Passion fruit

The plant is a vine grown in South America, Central America, and Caribbean islands, Africa, Southern Asia, Israel Australia, New Zealand, Hawaii and United States. The fruits may be the size of a lemon in *P.edulis* or as large as a grapefruit in the *flavicarpa* variety. The fruits contain Beta-carotene, dietary fiber, Potassium and Iron. **Health claims:** It is rich in polyphenols particularly lycopene and may be of help in reducing blood pressure and in control of benign prostate hyperplasia. Passiflora plant extracts are also mild sedatives and is a component of some sleep medications marketed by the supplements industry.

Papaya *(Carica papaya)*: Kingdom: Plantae; Division: Angiospermae, Class: Eudicots; Order: Brassicales; Family: Caricaceae. Chromosome number is 2n - 18.

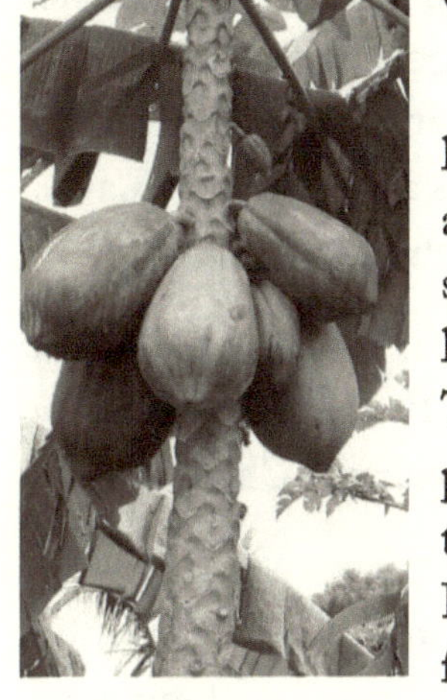

Papaya

Papaya trees are large trees with large palmate leaf blades held on long petioles that are spirally arranged on the crown of the stem. The stem has a scarred appearance where the older leaves were located and had fallen off when the plant grew up. The plants are dioecious (separate male and female plants). The plants can change their sex from male to female and vice-versa due to induced stress. Flowers appear in the leaf axils and develop into fruits after pollination and fertilization. Each fruit contains multiple black mucilaginous seeds. The fruits contain beta-carotene, anthocyanin and polyphenols. The fruits are also rich in the proteolytic enzyme papain. The stem leaves and unripe fruits contain latex that can irritate the skin. **Health:** Excessive consumption can result in the yellowing of skin and soles of feet in a harmless condition called carotenemia. The high content of papain in the fruit acts as good digestive aid and this property is used in the tenderizing of meat.

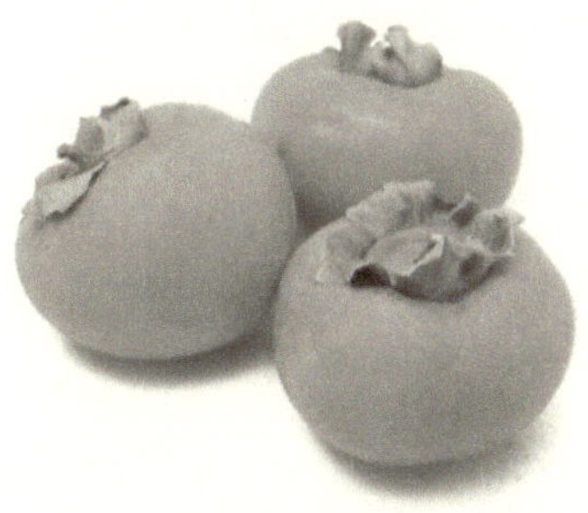

Persimmon

Persimmon *(Diospyros sp.)*: Kingdom: Plantae; Division: Angiospermae, Class: Eudicots, Order: Ericales; Family: Ebenaceae. Chromosome number, 2n = 90.

There are many species of *Diospyros* namely: 1 *D. kaki* (Asian persimmon, Japanese persimmon); 2 *D. lotuses* (date-plum); 3 *D. virginiana* (American persimmon); 4 D. digyna (black persimmon); 5 *D. discolor* (Philippines); 6 *D. peregrina* (Indian persimmon), and 7. *D.texana* (Texas persimmon), The most widely cultivated species is the Asian Persimmon *D. kaki*. Fruits are produced in short trees. The fruits are yellow-orange to red. The fruits are spherical, ovoid or pumpkin-like and are about 0.5 inches to 4 inches in diameter and look like a tomato. The fruits may be astringent with high tannin content as in *D.texacana* or the non-astringent chocolate persimmon. Consuming large quantities of persimmons causes a gum like formation (bezoars) in the intestine that can block evacuation of stools.

Pineapple *(Ananas comosus)*: Kingdom: Plantae; Division: Angiospermae, Class: Eudicots, Order: Bromiales; Family: Bromeliaceae; Genus and species: *Ananas comosus*. Chromosome number, 2n = 50.

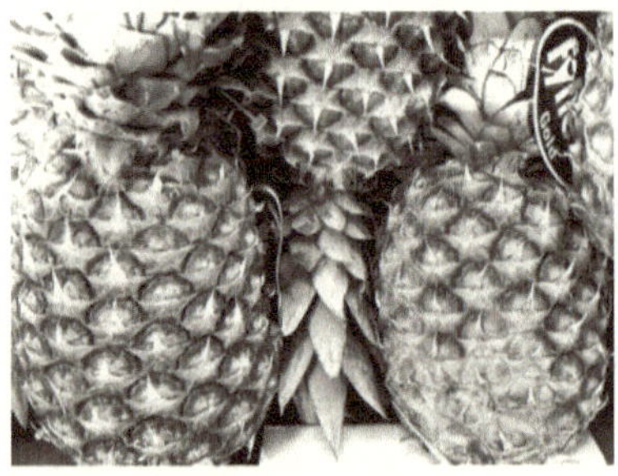

Pineapple

Pineapple plants are perennials with a tough waxy stem and long thick leaves with spiny margins. About 200 flowers are produced in a bunchy spike like inflorescence. Flowers are trimerous and when the ovaries from each flower develop into fruits, the entire individual fruits fuse to produce the edible football sized fruit. The eyelike structures seen on the fruits are the individual fruits that have fused to produce the compound fruit.

Health: Pineapple fruits contain manganese, vitamin C and the proteolytic enzyme Bromelain. Supplement Capsules and tablets containing Bromelain are prescribed for treating certain digestive disorders by practitioners of alternative medicine.

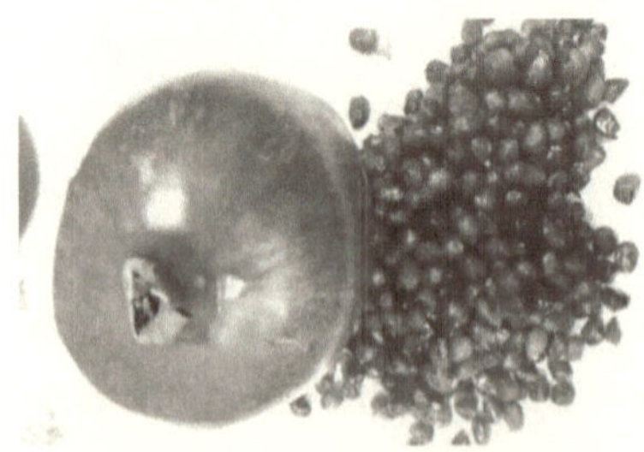

Pomegranate, pulp seeds

Pomegranates *(Punica granatum)*: Kingdom: Plantae; Division: Angiospermae, Class: Eudicots; Order: Myrtales Family: Lathyraceae; Genus and species: Punica granatum. Chromosome number, 2n = 16.

Pomegranates are shrubby trees growing to heights of 10–12 ft. high with spiny branches, glabrous leaves and bright red flowers. The edible fruits are oval-globose about the size of an orange/grapefruit with a very thick leathery outer skin that may be red or yellow in color. Inside are numerous pulpy seeds that may be bright red or pinkish white in color. The seeds are embedded in a white spongy pulp.

Health: The rind, bark and the pulpy seeds are used for treating gastrointestinal diseases and the pomegranate juice is considered very useful to prevent heart diseases. The rind made into a paste is used to stop nosebleeds and hemorrhoids by Ayurvedic medical practitioners in India. The fruits are rich in Vitamin K that accounts for the ability to stop bleeding. The fruits are also a rich source for flavonoids, polyphenols and anthocyanins. Modern laboratory and clinical research have shown that pomegranate juice reduces blood pressure, inhibits viral infections and buildup of dental plaque. However, the FDA does not yet endorse pomegranate juice as a supplement for health benefits claimed by health food supplement manufacturers. Clinical trials are ongoing for the beneficial effects of pomegranate juice for treating prostate cancer, prostatitis, diabetes, lymphoma, viral infections, atherosclerosis, coronary artery disease, kidney disease, memory maintenance, erectile dysfunction and osteoporosis. Thus, pomegranate is being visualized as a magic bullet for good health but controlled studies are needed to prove these potential benefits.

Quince *(Cydonia oblonga):* **Kingdom: Plantae; Division: Angiospermae, Class: Eudicots; Order; Rosales; Family: Rosaceae. Chromosome number, 2n = 34.**

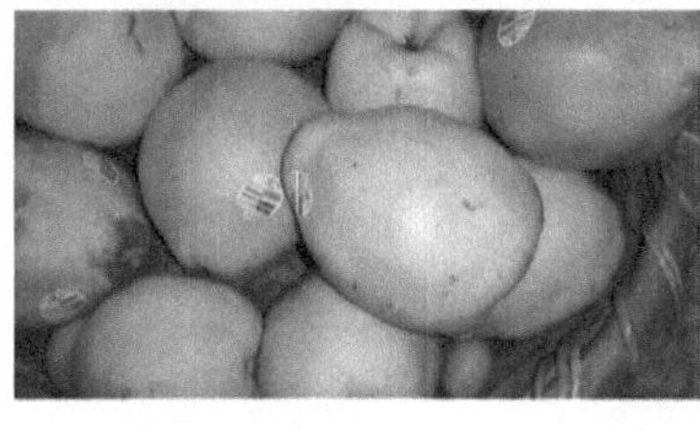

Quince

The quince is a small deciduous tree that bears a pome fruit, similar in appearance to a pear. It is bright golden-yellow when mature. The cooked fruit is used as food. The tree grows 5 to 8 meters (16 to 26 ft) high and 4 to 6 meters

(13 to 20 ft) wide. The fruit is 7 to 12 centimetres (2.8 to 4.7 in) long and 6 to 9 centimetres (2.4 to 3.5 in) across. It is grown in Turkey, Iran, Uzbekistan, Tajikistan, Himalayan regions in India and other Southwest Asian countries as well as in South America and warmer regions of Europe. Leaves are dense with hairs and are arranged in an alternate fashion on the stem. The fruits are yellow when ripe. The fruits are generally not eaten fresh but are processed by cooking and adding to various culinary preparations including Quince wine. **Health:** Like most fruits, quince are rich in Vitamin C and A.

Rambutan *(Nephelium lappaceum):* **Kingdom: Plantae; Division: Angiospermae, Eudicots; Order: Sapindales; Family: Sapindaceae. Chromosome number, 2n = 22**

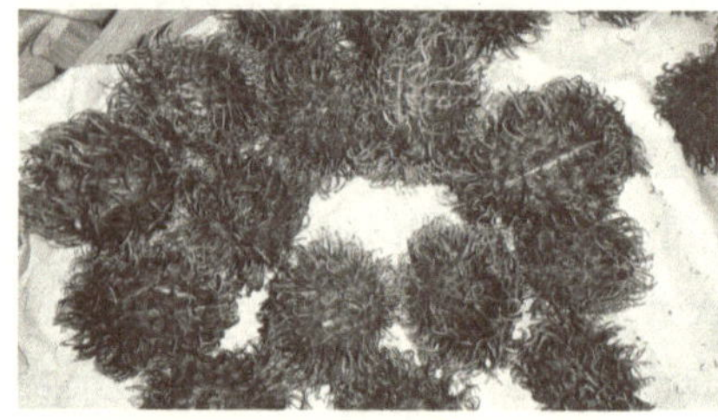

Rambutan

Rambutan is a tropical evergreen tree mainly grown in the Malay Archipelago, Indonesia and South East Asia (mainly Viet Nam, Cambodia, Thailand, and Laos). Plants are now cultivated in tropical Carribean islands and Central America. Trees are either staminate (male) or pistillate (female) and occasionally a few trees produce both male and female flowers on same plant. The fruits are produced in clusters and are oval or globular in shape with a flexible spiny leathery skin. The seeds are covered by a white fleshy aril. Fruits are aromatic and are sweet. **Health:** No specific health benefits other than nutritive value have been ascribed.

Rose Apple/Malabar plum *(Syzygium jambos/Myrtus Jambos):* **Kingdom: Plantae, Division: Angiospermae, Class: Eudicots, Order: Myrtales Family: Myrtaceae. Chromosome number, 2n = 28, 33, ~44, 46, ~54 and 66.**

The plants are shrubby short trees grown in India, Malaysian archipelago, South East Asia,

Carribean islands, some parts of Mexico, Central America and in South central Florida, USA. In India, it is widely grown in the state of Kerala where it goes by the name Champakka. The plants bear fragrant flowers and fruits with a thin Skin, It looks very similar to guava. Fruits are red or beige with a tinge of rose depending on the variety. Fruits are very rich in vitamin C.

Sapota/Zapota/sapodilla *(Manilkara zapota/Achras sapota):* **Kingdom: Plantae; Division: Angiospermae, Class: Eudicots; Order: Ericales; Family: Sapotaceae; Genus and species:** *Manilkara zapota/ Achras sapota.* **Chromosome number, 2n = 26**

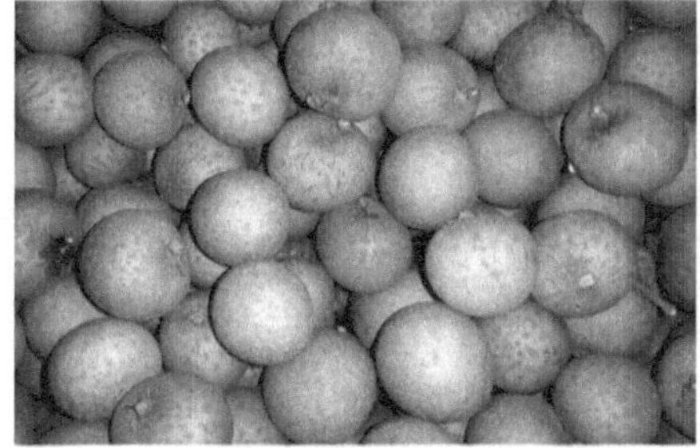

Sapota

The plant is a tree growing to a height of 30–90 ft. tall with a wide trunk. It produces glabrous ovate leaves. The fruits are globose/ ellipse about the size of a lemon. It has a thin brown skin enclosing a brownish fleshy pulp fruit rich in sugars. The seeds are black with a hard shell. Seeds are not edible. **Health:** Leaf extracts have shown cholesterol-lowering properties. The fruits are a rich source of sugars but have no other known medicinal value.

Star fruit/Carambola *(Averrhoa carambola):* **Kingdom: Plantae; Division: Angiospermae, Class: Eudicots; Order: Oxalidales; Family: Oxalidaceae. Chromosome number, 2n = 24 or 26.**

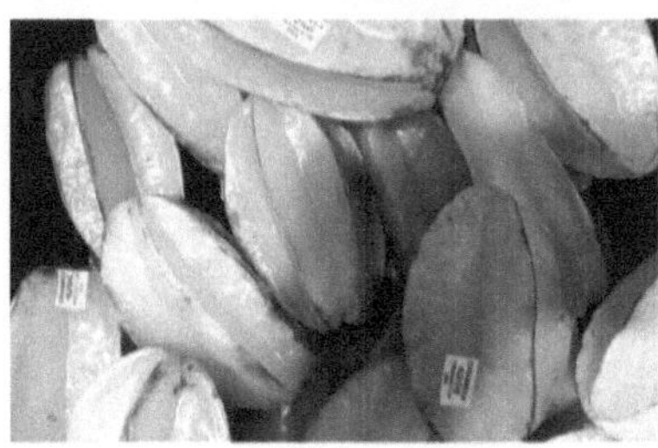

Star Fruit

The fruits have a star shape when cross-sectioned. The fruits are 4–6 inches long, have a greenish – yellow appearance with 4–5 longitudinal ridges running down the sides. The fruits are glabrous. There are two different varieties namely a larger sweet one and a smaller sour one. The entire fruit in either case is edible. The fruits are popular in South East Asia, Australia (Queensland), China, Pacific islands, parts of Africa, Carribean islands, Florida in the USA and in Latin America. They are grown commercially in all these areas. The plants are perennial evergreen small trees with pinnate compound leaves and pinkish-white perfect flowers in panicles. **Health:** The fruits have both anti-oxidant and anti-microbial properties. Carambola juice is a potent inhibitor of cytochrome P 450 and consumption of carambola can inhibit absorption of statin drugs and benzodiazapine tranquilizers. Cytochrome-P450 is a superfamily of hundreds of closely related hemeproteins found throughout the phylogenetic spectrum, from animals, plants, fungi, to bacteria. They include numerous complex monooxygenases (mixed function oxygenases). In animals, these P-450 enzymes serve two major functions: (1) biosynthesis of steroids, fatty acids, and bile acids, (2) metabolism of endogenous and a wide variety of exogenous substrates, such as toxins and drugs (biotransformation). Thus, inhibition of this system can have serious consequences. The Star fruit contains a neurotoxin-caramboxin as well as oxalic acid that are both harmful for proper kidney function. Eating Carambola fruits or drinking its juice can trigger serious reactions (sometimes fatal) in individuals on Kidney dialysis or kidney disease. In view of the above, great care should be exercised in consuming large quantities of this fruit.

Stone fruits: Kingdom: Plantae; Division: Angiospermae, Class: Eudicots; Order: Rosales Family: Rosaceae. Genera and Species: Prunus persica **(Peach),** *Prunus amygdalus* **(Almonds),** P. *avium* P. *cerasus* **(Cherries),** *Pyrus* **sp (Pear),** *Prunus domestica* **(Plum),** *Prunus armeniaca* **(Apricot),** *Prunus persica var nectarianum* **(Nectarine).** *Chromosome number,*

All stone fruits are deciduous trees belonging to the Rose family. The peach is classified with the almond in the subgenus Amygdalus distinguished from the other subgenera by the corrugated seed shell. Peach and nectarine trees grow to a height of about 12 ft-30 ft. and have lanceolate leaves. Flowers have 5 sepals and petals and are white or pink in color.

Almonds *(Prunus amygdalus/P.dulcis/Amygdalus communis):*

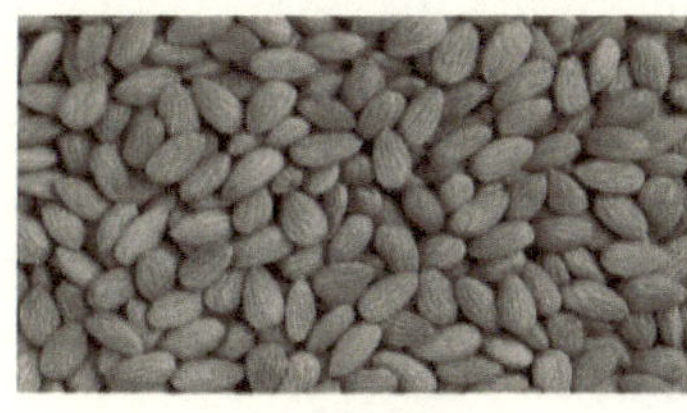

Almonds

Almonds are also members of the stone fruit group. The almond fruit known as a drupe contains an outer hull that is not fleshy but green and leathery and a hard shell endocarp that houses the edible seed. The seeds have an outer brown-colored seed coat. Inside the seed coat are the two cotyledons that are rich in almond oil, protein and other nutrients. **Health:** The domesticated sweet almond is safe to eat and is nutritionally very beneficial. However, the wild varieties *Prunus dulcis var. amara* and those derived from it are bitter to taste and contain amygdalin that is converted to Hydrogen cyanide upon crushing. A single seed is enough to cause death. Since almond seeds are susceptible to infection by the fungus *Aspergillus* and thus may contain the toxin aflatoxin, all almonds produced and sold in the USA have to be pasteurized before sale. Some individual seeds from sweet almonds may also be slightly bitter and hence not safe for consumption if bitter.

Peaches and Nectarines *(Prunus persica):* Chromosome number = 2n = 2x = 16

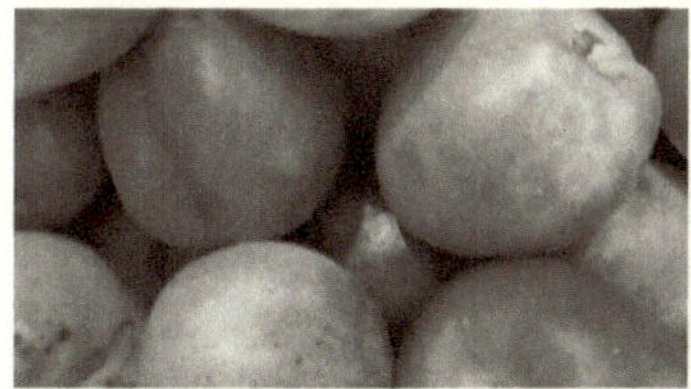

Nectarine

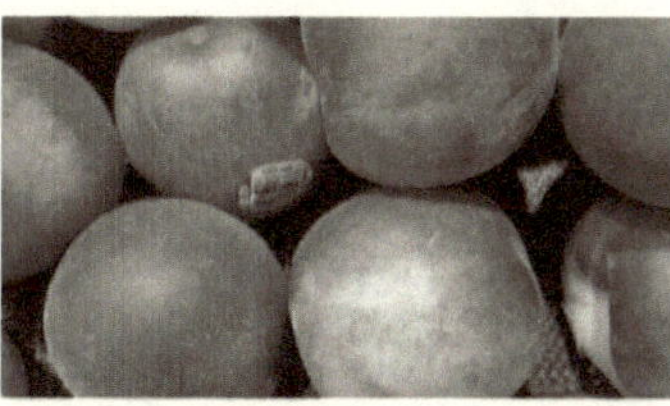

Peaches

Peaches and nectarines are both different varieties of *P. Persica.* They differ from each other by the absence of fuzz in the fruits of nectarines compared to peaches that have fuzz. Both peaches and nectarines are classified into those that cling to the stone seed-clingstones and those that don't-free stones. The fruit pulp is either white or yellow. The fruits contain a single hard stone-like seed. Peacherines are hybrids from crossing peaches and nectarines. Peaches and nectarines contain phenolic compounds chlorogenic acid, catechin and epicatechins, cyanidins, ellagic acid. The yellow varieties also have anthocyanins. **Health:** Some people develop allergies to peaches and nectarines. The seeds contain cyanogenic glycosides which if eaten can cause serious illness.

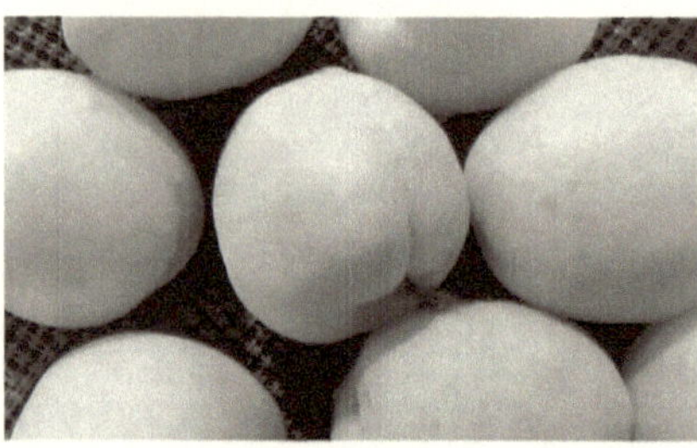
Apricots

Apricots and Plums *(Prunus armeniaca, Prunus sp.)*: Chromosome number, n = 8, 2n = 2x = 16.

Both apricots and plums belong to the genus *Prunus*. They are classified into three group's namely old world plums, new world plums and armeniaca plums. The latter are apricots. Plum fruits have a waxy coating. Apricot fruits are smaller and yellow in color. Greengage plums are green. Mirabelle plums are yellow. Victoria plums are pink-rose. Satsuma plums are red and Damsun plums are bluish-black. Dried plums are called prunes. Plums/prunes are traditionally used to relieve constipation since they contain dietary fiber and sorbitol.

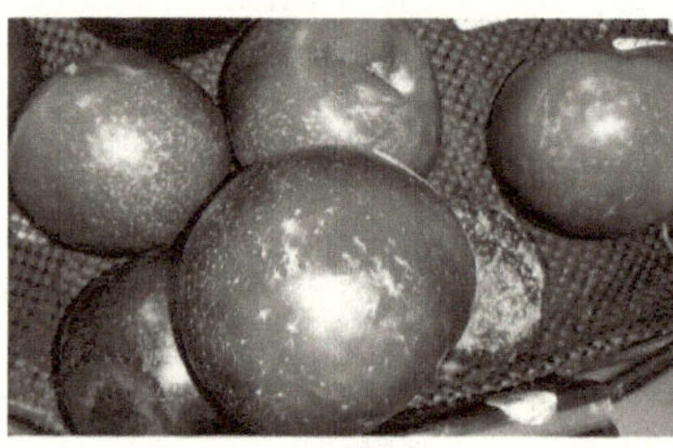
Plum

Apricots and plum seeds both have high concentrations of cyanogenic glycosides and hence are toxic. Practitioners of alternative medicine prescribe a drug known as laetrile extracted from apricot seeds to treat cancers but controlled research through modern medicine have failed to reveal any anticancer effects to laetrile. The National Institute of Health (NIH) and American Cancer Society does not endorse Laetrile or apricot pits as anti-cancer agents.

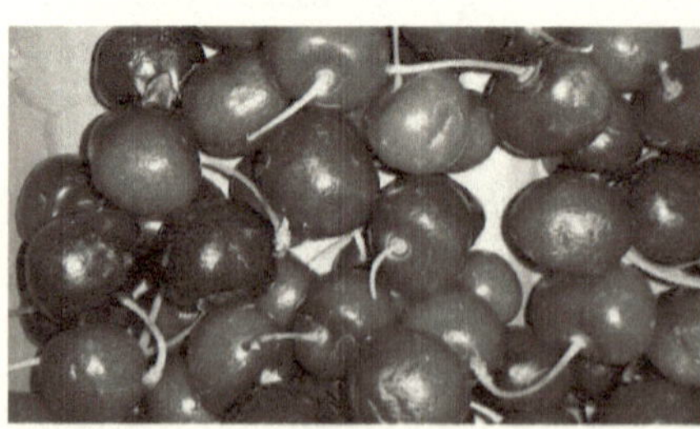
Cherry

The cherry fruits (Chromosome number, 2n = 16) are of two types namely sweet cherry (*P. avium*) and sour cherry *P. cerasus*. All other edible cherries are derived from one or the other of these two. The fruit is generally small, globular and glabrous. They have reddish pulp or in the case of Rainier varieties, the pulp may be white. Cherries have high content of anthocyanins and flavonoids. Some studies indicate that they have anti-inflammation and anti-gout properties.

White Sapote/Mexican apple *(Casimiroa edulis):* **Kingdom: Plantae; Division: Angiospermae, Class: Eudicots; Order: Sapindales; Family: Rutaceae; Chromosome number, 2n = 30.**

White sapote also known as Mexican apple is a tropical evergreen tree in the same family as citrus. It is grown for its fruit in Mexico, Central America and some Southern Carribean islands. The fruits are oval drupes. In certain varieties, they have a green inedible skin with white fruit pulp and in certain others a yellow skin with light yellow flesh. The fruits contain 1–5 seeds. The seeds have narcotic properties. The fruit contains many phytochemicals of which two namely Zapotinin and zapotin have been investigated for anti-carcinogenic properties. **Health:** The seed extracts and the flavone Zapotin have shown marked anti-cell proliferation activity when tested on colon cancer HT-29 cell lines indicating possible use as a chemo preventive and chemotherapeutic agent for colon cancer. Other studies have shown that Zapotin has similar anti-cancer activities in leukemic cell lines-Hl 60, HeLa cells, liver cells Hep-G2 and bladder cancer cells T 24. Eating fruit and seeds cause drowsiness and hence the seed extracts and Zapotin have been tested to show anti-anxiolytic activities. There is also a report that the seeds have aphrodisiac properties.

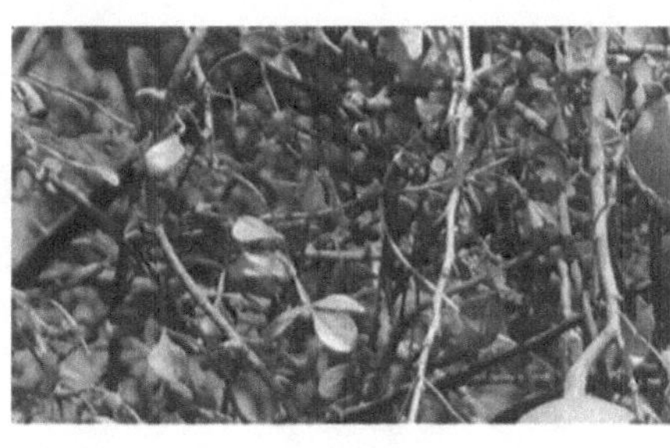

Bael

Bael/Bengal quince/golden apple/Vlangai *(Aegle marmelos):* **Kingdom: Plantae; Division: Angiospermae, Class: Eudicots; Order: Sapindales; Family: Rutaceae; Genus and Species:** *Aegle marmelos.* **Chromosome number, 2n = 18.**

This is a plant that grows as a tree in semiarid regions in India, Pakistan, Sri Lanka, Thailand and other subtropical regions in Asia. The plant produces trifoliate glabrous leaves. The fruits have a woody shell containing a brownish pulpy edible flesh. The pulp contains vitamin C and the phytochemical Angeline that is gaining popularity as an anabolic supplement. **Health relevance**: In the Ayurvedic system of alternative medicine, this fruit finds several and frequent therapeutic uses in different forms and recipes. They are prescribed for treatment of a number of diseases such as gastro intestinal diseases, piles, oedema, jaundice, vomiting, obesity, pediatric disorders, gynecological disorders, urinary complaints and as a rejuvenative. The phytochemical aegiline, which is found in the fruit, is reported to have anti-hyperlipidemic and anti-glycemic properties. It is gaining use as a supplement in health food stores.

Wood Apple/Elephant Apple/Monkey Fruit/Curd fruit *(Limonia acidissima)*: Kingdom: Plantae; Division: Angiospermae, Class: Eudicots; Order: Sapindales; Family: Rutaceae. Chromosome number, 2n = 18.

The plant *Limonia acidissima* is also called Wood apple although it is quite a different plant from *Aegle marmelos*. This plant is also called variously as monkey fruit, elephant apple and curd fruit. The plant is a monotypic genus that grows in the Indo-Malay region. *Limonia acidissima* is a large tree growing to 9 metres (30 ft) tall, with rough, spiny bark. The leaves are pinnate, with 5–7 leaflets, each leaflet 25–35 mm long and 10–20 mm broad, with a citrus-scent when crushed. The fruit is a berry 5–9 cm diameter, and may be sweet or sour. It has a very hard rind that can be difficult to crack open, and contains sticky brown pulp and small white seeds. The fruit looks similar in appearance to fruit of the other wood apple Bael (*Aegle marmelos*). **Health:** The fruits are rich in beta-carotene. The Ayurvedic system of India recommends the fruit for relieving digestive issues. Some reports suggest that the fruit pulp acts as a mosquito repellant.

Table 14 – Nutritional profile of culinary fruits (1)

Metabolite	Apple	Apricot	Banana Fruit	Blue berries	Black berries	Cherries Sweet	Fig Dry	Dry Date Common	Grape American	Grape Europe
Water, g	85.56	86.35	74.91	84.21	88.15	82.25	30.1	20.53	81.3	80.54
Protein-g	0.26	1.4	1.09	0.74	1.39	1.06	3.3	2.45	0.63	0.72
Total lipid (fat), g	0.17	0.39	0.33	0.33	0.49	0.2	0.93	0.39	0.35	0.16
Carbohydrate, g	13.81	11.12	22.84	14.49	9.61	16.01	63.9	75.03	17.15	18.1
Fiber	2.4	2	2.6	2.4	5.3	2.1	9.8	8	0.9	0.9
Sugar	10.39	9.24	12.23	9.96	4.88	12.82	47.9	63.35	16.25	15.48
Calcium, mg	6	13	5	6	29	13	162	39	14	10
Iron, mg	0.12	0.39	0.26	0.28	0.62	0.36	2.03	1.02	0.29	0.36
Magnesium, mg	5	10	27	6	20	11	68	43	5	7
Phosphorus, mg	11	23	22	12	22	21	67	62	10	20
Potassium, mg	107	259	358	77	162	222	680	656	191	191
Sodium, mg	1	1	1	1	1	0	10	2	2	2
Zinc, mg	0.04	0.2	0.15	0.16	0.53	0.07	0.55	0.29	0.04	0.07
Vitamin C, mg	4.6	10	8.7	6	21	7	1.2	0.4	4	3.2
Thiamin, mg	0.017	0.03	0.031	0.28	0.02	0.027	0.09	0.052	0.092	0.069
Riboflavin, mg	0.026	0.04	0.073	6	0.026	0.033	0.08	0.066	0.057	0.07
Niacin, mg	0.091	0.6	0.665	12	0.646	0.154	0.62	1.274	0.3	0.188
Vitamin B-6, mg	0.041	0.054	0.367	77	0.03	0.049	0.11	0.165	0.11	0.086

Metabolite	Apple	Apricot	Banana Fruit	Blue berries	Black berries	Cherries Sweet	Fig Dry	Dry Date Common	Grape American	Grape Europe
Folate, DFE,	3	9	20	1	25	4	9	19	4	2
Vitamin B-12, µg	0	0	0	0.16	0	0	0	0	0	0
Vitamin A, µg	3	96	3	3	11	3	0	0	5	3
Vitamin A, IU	54	1926	64	54	214	64	10	10	100	66
Vitamin E, µg	0.18	0.89	0.1	0.57	1.17	0.07	0.35	0.05	0.19	0.19
Vitamin D µg	0	0	0	0	0	0	0	0	0	0
Vitamin D, IU	0	0	0	0	0	0	0	0	0	0
Vitamin K, µg	2.2	3.3	0.5	19.3	19.8	2.1	15.6	2.7	14.6	14.6
Fatty acids, g	0.028	0.027	0.112	0.028	0.014	0.038	0.14	0.032	0.114	0.054
Monounsat, g	0.007	0.17	0.032	0.047	0.047	0.047	0.16	0.036	0.014	0.007
Polyun sat, g	0.051	0.077	0.073	0.146	0.28	0.052	0.35	0.019	0.102	0.048
Trans fat	0	0	0	0	0	0	0	0	0	0
Cholesterol, mg	0	0	0	0	0	0	0	0	0	

Note: Apple is average of red and golden delicious as well as gala, Fuji and granny smith varieties

Table 15 – Nutritional profile of Culinary fruits (2)

Metabolite	Guava	Jack	Jambul	Kiwi	Mango	Mango	Nectarine	Peach	Pear	Plum	Quince
	Pink	Fruit	JavaPlum			steen	Yellow	Yellow			
Water	80.8	73.5	83.13	82.4	83.46	87.59	88.87	84	87.2	83.8	
Protein-g	2.55	1.72	0.72	1.02	0.82	0.5	1.06	0.91	0.36	0.7	0.4
Total lipid (fat), g	0.95	0.64	0.23	0.28	0.38	0.4	0.32	0.25	0.14	0.28	0.1
Carbohydrate, g	14.32	23.3	15.56	15.8	14.98	15.6	10.55	9.54	15.2	11.4	15.3
Fiber	5.4	1.5	0.6	1.4	1.6	5.1	1.7	1.5	3.1	1.4	1.9
Sugar	8.92	19.1	12.3	13.66	7.89	8.39	9.75	9.92			
Calcium, mg	18	24	19	17	11	5.49	6	6	9	6	11
Iron, mg	0.26	0.23	0.19	0.21	0.16	0.17	0.28	0.25	0.18	0.17	0.7
Magnesium, mg	22	29	15	12	10	13.9	9	9	7	7	8
Phosphorus, mg	40	21	17	25	14	9.21	26	20	12	16	17
Potassium, mg	417	448	79	315	168	48	201	190	116	157	197
Sodium, mg	2	2	14	3	1	7	0	0	1	0	4
Zinc, mg	0.23	0.13	0.08	0.09	0.12	0.17	0.17	0.1	0.1	0.04	
Vitamin C, mg	228.3	13.7	14.3	161	36.4	7.2	5.4	6.6	4.3	9.5	15
Thiamin, mg	0.067	0.11	0.006	0	0.028	0.054	0.034	0.024	0.01	0.03	0.02
Riboflavin, mg	0.04	0.06	0.012	0.07	0.038	0.054	0.027	0.031	0.03	0.03	0.03
Niacin, mg	1.084	0.92	0.26	0.23	0.669	0.286	1.125	0.806	0.16	0.42	0.2
Vitamin B-6, mg	0.11	0.33	0.038	0.08	0.119	0.041	0.025	0.025	0.03	0.03	0.04

Metabolite	Guava	Jack	Jambul	Kiwi	Mango	Mango	Nectarine	Peach	Pear	Plum	Quince
	Pink	Fruit	JavaPlum			steen	Yellow	Yellow			
Folate, DFE,	49	24	0	31	43	31	5	4	7	5	3
Vitamin B-12, µg	0	0	0	0.08	0	0	0	0	0	0	0
Vitamin A, µg	31	5	3	1	54	NA	17	16	1	17	2
Vitamin A, IU	624	110	23	1082	35	332	326	25	345	40	
Vitamin E, µg	0.73	0.34	1.4	0.9	0.77	0.73	0.12	0.26			
Vitamin D µg	0	NA	0	0	0	0	0	0			
Vitamin D, IU	0	NA	0	0	0	0	0	0			
Vitamin K µg	2.6	NA	6.1	4.2	2.2	2.6	4.4	6.4			
Fatty acids, g	0.272	0.2	0	0.07	0.092	0	0.025	0.019	0.02	0.02	0.01
Monounsat, g	0.087	0.16	0	0.02	0.14	0.088	0.067	0.08	0.13	0.036	
Polyun sat, G	0.401	0.09	0	0.11	0.071	0.113	0.086	0.09	0.04	0.05	
Trans fat, g	0	0	0	0	0	0	0	0	0	0	
Cholesterol, mg	0	0	0	0	0	0	0	0	0	0	0

Avg of red delicious, golden, Gala, granny smith, and Fuji varieties.

a Value based on analyses of Tommy Atkins, Keitt, Kent, and/or Haden cultivars of Mango.

Table 16 – Nutritional profile of culinary fruits: Citrus and melon

Metabolite	Grape Fruit	Lemon	Lime	Orange All types	Tangerine	Cantaloupe Melon	Casaba Melon	Honeydew melon	Water melon
Water	90.89	88.98	88.3	86.75	85.17	90.15	91.85	89.82	91.45
Protein–g	0.63	1.1	0.7	0.94	0.81	0.84	1.11	0.54	0.61
Total lipid (fat), g	0.1	0.3	0.2	0.12	0.31	0.19	0.1	0.14	0.15
Carbohydrate, g	8.08	9.32	10.5	11.75	13.34	8.16	6.58	9.09	7.55
Fiber	1.1	2.8	2.8	2.4	1.8	0.9	0.9	0.8	0.4
Sugar	6.98	2.5	1.69	9.35	10.58	7.86	5.69	8.12	6.2
Calcium, mg	12	26	33	40	37	9	11	6	7
Iron, mg	0.09	0.6	0.6	0.1	0.15	0.21	0.34	0.17	0.24
Magnesium, mg	8	8	6	10	12	12	11	10	10
Phosphorus, mg	8	16	18	14	20	15	5	11	11
Potassium, mg	139	138	102	181	166	267	182	228	112
Sodium, mg	0	2	2	0	2	16	9	18	1
Zinc, mg	0.07	0.06	0.11	0.07	0.07	0.18	0.07	0.09	0.1
Vitamin C, mg	34.4	53	29.1	53.2	26.7	36.7	21.8	18	8.1
Thiamin, mg	0.036	0.04	0.03	0.087	0.058	0.041	0.015	0.038	0.033
Riboflavin, mg	0.02	0.02	0.02	0.04	0.036	0.019	0.031	0.012	0.021
Niacin, mg	0.25	0.1	0.2	0.282	0.376	0.734	0.232	0.418	0.178
Vitamin B-6, mg	0.042	0.08	0.04	0.06	0.078	0.072	0.163	0.088	0.045
Folate, DFE,	10	11	8	30	16	21	8	19	3
Vitamin B-12, µg	0	0	0	0	0	0	0	0	0
Vitamin A, µg	46	1	2	11	34	169	0	3	28
Vitamin A, IU	927	22	50	225	681	3382	0	50	569

Metabolite	Grape Fruit	Lemon	Lime	Orange All types	Tangerine	Cantaloupe Melon	Casaba Melon	Honeydew melon	Water melon
Vitamin E, mg	0.13	0.15	0.22	0.18	0.2	0.05	0.05	0.02	0.05
Vitamin D µg	0	0	0	0	0	0	0	0	0
Vitamin D, IU	0	0	0	0	0	0	0	0	0
Vitamin K	0	0	0.6	0	0	2.5	2.5	2.9	0.1
Fatty acids, g	0.014	0.039	0.02	0.015	0.039	0.051	0.025	0.038	0.016
Monounsat, g	0.013	0.011	0.02	0.023	0.06	0.003	0.002	0.003	0.037
Polyun sat, G	0.024	0.089	0.06	0.025	0.065	0.081	0.039	0.059	0.05
Trans fat	0	0	0	0	0	0	0	0	0
Cholesterol, mg	0	0	0	0	0	0	0	0	0

Grapefruit, raw, pink and red and white, all areas Oranges all commercial varieties

Table17 – Nutritional profile of culinary fruits (3)

Metabolite	Mulberries Black	Papaya	Passion fruit	Persimmon	Pineapple	Pomegranate	Rasp berries	Sapota	Star fruit	Strawberries
Water	87.68	88.06	72.93	80.32	86	77.93	85.75	64.87	91.38	90.95
Protein-g	1.44	0.47	2.2	0.58	0.54	1.67	1.2	1.45	1.04	0.67
Total lipid (fat), g	0.39	0.26	0.7	0.19	0.12	1.17	0.65	0.46	0.33	0.3
Carbohydrate, g	9.8	10.82	23.38	18.59	13.1	18.7	11.94	32.1	6.73	7.68
Fiber	1.7	1.7	10.4	3.6	1.4	4	6.5	5.4	2.8	2
Sugar	8.1	7.82	11.2	12.53	9.85	13.67	4.42	20.14	3.98	4.89
Calcium, mg	39	20	12	8	13	10	25	18	3	16
Iron, mg	1.85	0.25	1.6	0.15	0.29	0.3	0.69	0.78	0.08	0.41
Magnesium, mg	18	21	29	9	12	12	22	11	10	13
Phosphorus, mg	38	10	68	17	8	36	29	26	12	24
Potassium, mg	194	182	348	161	109	236	151	454	133	153
Sodium, mg	10	8	28	1	1	3	1	7	2	1
Zinc, mg	0.12	0.08	0.1	0.11	0.12	0.35	0.42	0.19	0.12	0.14
Vitamin C, mg	36.4	60.9	30	7.5	47.8	10.2	26.2	0.19	34.4	58.8
Thiamin, mg	0.029	0.023	0	0.03	0.08	0.067	0.032	23	0.014	0.024
Riboflavin, mg	0.101	0.027	0.13	0.02	0.03	0.053	0.038	0.013	0.016	0.022
Niacin, mg	0.62	0.357	1.5	0.1	0.5	0.293	0.598	0.116	0.367	0.386
Vitamin B-6, mg	0.05	0.038	0.1	0.1	0.11	0.075	0.055	1.432	0.017	0.047
Folate, DFE,	6	37	14	8	18	38	21	0.72	12	24
Vitamin B-12, µg	0	0	0	0	0	0	0	0	0	0
Vitamin A, µg	1	47	64	81	3	0	2	7	3	1
Vitamin A, IU	25	950	1272	1627	58	0	33	143	61	12

Metabolite	Mulberries Black	Papaya	Passion fruit	Persimmon	Pineapple	Pomegranate	Rasp berries	Sapota	Star fruit	Strawberries
Vitamin E, mg	0.87	0.3	0.02	0.73	0.02	0.6	0.87	2.11	0.15	0.29
Vitamin D µg	0	0	0	0	0	0	0	NA	0	0
Vitamin D, IU	0	0	0	0	0	0	0	NA	0	0
Vitamin K, µg	7.8	2.6	0.7	2.6	0.7	16.4	7.8	NA	0	2.2
Fatty acids, g	0.027	0.081	0.059	0.02	0.01	0.12	0.019	0.169	0.019	0.015
Monounsaturated	0.041	0.072	0.086	0.037	0.01	0.093	0.064	0.102	0.03	0.043
Polyunsaturated, g	0.207	0.058	0.411	0.043	0.04	0.079	0.375	0.097	0.184	0.155
Trans fat	0	0	0	0	0	0	0	0	0	0
Cholesterol, mg	0	0	0	0	0	0	0	0	0	0

Pineapple: Avg of 80% sweet Var and 20% other; Pomegranate Based on samples of California Wonderful variety.

References

Appel, L.J., et al., (2005): Effects of protein, monounsaturated fat, and carbohydrate intake on blood pressure and serum lipids: results of the OmniHeart randomized trial. JAMA, 2005, 294(19): p. 2455-64.

Arawwawala M., Thabrew, L, Arambewela, L., Handunnetti, S., (2010): Anti-inflammatory activity of Trichosanthes cucumerina Linn. In rats, J Ethnopharmacol., 2010 Oct 5, 131(3): 538-43. Doi: 10.1016/j.jep.2010.07.028. Epub 2010 Jul 21.

Around the World with Brassicas, http://www.fastplants.org/pdf/activities/around_world.pdf

Chang CT, Chen YC, Fang JT, Huang CC (2002): "Star fruit (Averrhoa carambola) intoxication: an important cause of consciousness disturbance in patients with renal failure." Ren Fail 24 (3): 379–82. Doi: 10.1081/JDI-120005373. PMID 12166706

Chang JM, Hwang SJ, Kuo HT; et al. (2000): "Fatal outcome after ingestion of star fruit (Averrhoa carambola) in uremic patients." Am J Kidney Dis 35 (2): 189–93. Doi: 10.1016/S0272-6386(00)70325-8. PMID 10676715

Desai, B.B., and Sanunke, D.K. (1991): Fruits and vegetable, In Foods of Plant origin; Production, Technology and Human Nutrition, Eds. Salunkhe, D.K.M and Deshpande, S.S. Pp301-412. Van Nostrand, Reinhold, New York, Pp 499

Duckworth, R.B. (2013): Fruit and Vegetables, Elsevier, pp330

Fritsch, R.M., and Friesen, N. (2002): Evolution, domestication and taxonomy. Book Chapter, Allium crop science, recent advances, 2002 CABI Publishing (H ISBN 0851995101), http://www.cabi.org/cabebooks/ebook/20083015158

Fruits of Vietnam, FAO corporate document repository. http://www.fao.org/docrep/008/ad523e/ad523e02.htm

Heslop-Harrison, P. (2007): Article from European Cytogenetics Newsletter 20, 2007. http://www.le.ac.uk/bl/phh4/openpubs/bananacytogenetics.htm

https://www.nutsforlife.com.au/resources/nuts-images/

http://www.hsph.harvard.edu/nutritionsource/what-should-you-eat/vegetables-and-fruits/

http://www.med.umich.edu/umim/food-pyramid/fruits_and_vegetables.html

J.S. Heslop-Harrison and T.T., Schwarzacher, (2007): Domestication, Genomics and the Future for Banana. Annals of Botany Volume 100, Issue 5Pp. 1073-1084.

Julia F. Morton (1987): "Carambola." In Julia F. Morton, Fruits of warm climates. pp. 125–128.

Kavanaugh, C.J., P.R. Trumbo, and K.C. Ellwood, (2007): The U.S. Food and Drug Administration's evidence-based review for qualified health claims: tomatoes, lycopene, and cancer. J Natl Cancer Inst, 2007. 99(14): p. 1074-85.

Li, T.S.C. (2008): Vegetables and Fruits: Nutritional and Therapeutic Values. CRC Press, pp. 1–2. ISBN 978-1-4200-6873-3

Lin, S., Sharpe, R.H., and Janick, J. (1999): "Loquat: Botany and Horticulture." Horticultural Reviews 23: 235–236.

Magness, J.R., G.M. Markle, C.C. Compton (1971): Food and feed crops of the United States. Interregional Research Project IR-4, IR Bul. 1 (Bul. 828 New Jersey Agr, Expt. Sta.,)

Marcelo Guerra, Andrea Pedrosa, Ana Emília Barros e Silva, Maria Tereza Marquim Cornélio, Karla Santos and Walter dos Santos Soares Filho

(1997): Chromosome number and secondary constriction variation in 51 accessions of a citrus germplasm bank. On-line version ISSN 1678-4502, Braz. J. Genet., vol.20 no.3 Ribeirão Preto Sept. 1997, http://dx.doi.org/10.1590/S0100-84551997000300021   http://dx.doi.org/10.1590/S0100-84551997000300021.

Moscone E.A., Scaldaferro M.A.; Grabiele M; Cecchini nm; Sánchez garcía, Y; jarret, R.; Daviña J.R., Ducasse, D.A.,; Barboza G.E; Ehrendorfer, F., (2007): the evolution of chili peppers (capsicum – solanaceae): a cytogenetic perspective, I: VI International Solanaceae Conference: Genomics Meets Biodiversity, SHS Acta Horticulturae 745, DOI: 10.17660/ActaHortic.2007.745.5.

Rubatzky, V.E., Yamaguchi, M. (1997): Alliums, Family: Alliaceae (Amaryllidaceae) (World Vegetables, pp 279-332. Springer pp755, 10.1007/978-1-4615-6015-9_17, Print ISBN 978-1-4613-7756-6, Online ISBN, 978-1-4615-6015-9

Sapota: http://www.cabi.org/isc/datasheet/34560.

Syzygium cumini (PROSEA): in Plant resources of South East Asia: http://uses.plantnet-project.org/en/Syzygium_cumini_ (PROSEA).

Chapter 11

Nuts

As per scientific definition, a nut is a fruit with a hard shell containing one to two seeds wherein, the shell does not break open to release the

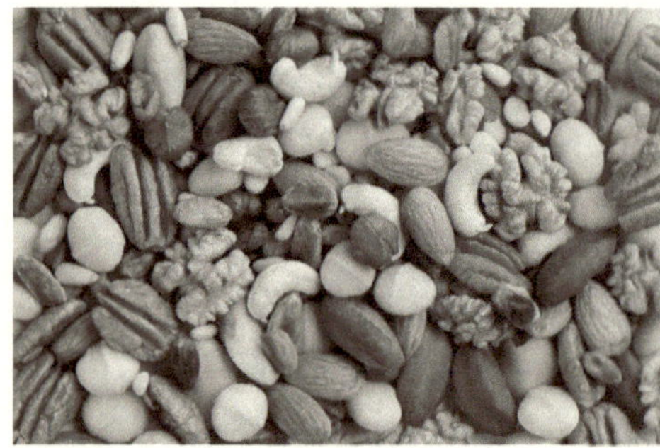

Mixed nuts

seed. However, many edible nuts do not fit this definition. The popular definition of a nut is any large oily kernel found within a shell and used in food. Many commonly used nuts such as walnuts, almonds; pistachios, are not true nuts in the restrictive botanical sense but are indeed culinary nuts based on usage. Various culinary nuts are important sources of nutrition and are consumed as snacks in various food preparations including some drinks. While many nuts like Almonds, Brazil nuts, Cashew nuts, Chestnut, Coconut, Filibert, Hazelnut, Macadamia, peanut, Pecan, Pistachio, Pinenuts and Walnuts are the most commonly used dietary nuts; there are many others that are important sources of nutrition for various indigenous people. The following nuts are not so common but are important nutritional sources: Acorn nuts *(Quercus Lithocarpus)*, American beech *(Fagus grandifolia)*, European beech *(Brosimum alicastrum)*, Chinese chestnuts *(Castanea mollissima)* Sweet chestnuts *(Castanea sativa)*; Johnstone River Almond *(Elaeocarpus bancroftii)*; Kurrajong *(Brachychiton spp).*; Malabar chestnut *(Pachira aquatica)*; Mongongo *(Ricinodendron rautanenii)*; Palm nuts

(Elaeis guineensis); Paradise nut *(Lecythis usitata);* Karuka *(Pandanus spp),. Planted karuka (Pandanus julianettii); Wild karuka (Pandanus brosimos); Red bopple nut (Hicksbeachia pinnatifolia);* Yellow walnut *(Beilschmiedia bancroftii);* Monkeypuzzle nut *(Araucaria araucana);* Bunya nut *(Araucaria bidwillii);* Peanut tree Bush nut *(Sterculia quadrifida);* Chilgoza pine *(Pinus gerardiana),* Pekea nut or butternut of Guiana *(Carioca nuciferum);* Gabon nut *(Coula edulis);* Burrawang nut *(Macrozamia communis),* Cycads *(Macrozamia spp).;* White walnut *(Juglans cinerea);* Black walnut *(Juglans nigra)* Bread Nuts *(Artocarpus camansi);* Jack nuts *(Artocarpus heterophyllus);* Bush mango *(Irvingia gabonensis);* Pili nuts *(Canarium ovatum);* Canarium nut *(Canarium harveyi C.indicum or C. commune);* Australian cashew nut *(Semecarpus australiensis).*

Nuts contain many essential vitamins and minerals as well as protein, fats, fiber and carbohydrates. Several studies have revealed that the inclusion of nuts as a part of the daily dietary regimen prevents the likelihood of congestive heart diseases since they help to lower serum LDL (Low-density lipids) cholesterol. This cardio protective effect is attributed to the presence of Omega-3-fatty acids, presence of antioxidants and low glycemic index of many edible seeds like Almonds Walnuts etc. However, this cardio protective role does not extend to all seeds.

The botany and medical relevance of the common dietary nuts are described below.

Almonds *(Prunus amygdalus)*: Kingdom: Plantae; Division: Angiospermae, Class: Eudicots Order: Rosales; Family: Rosaceae; Genus and species; Prunus amygdalus/ dulcis. Chromosome number, 2n = 16

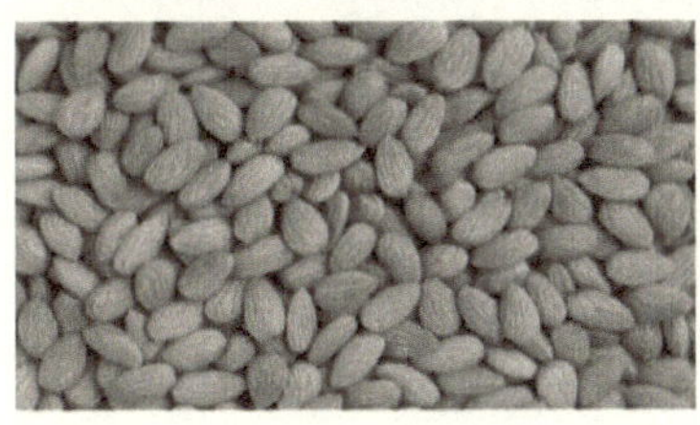

Almonds

Plants are deciduous trees about 12 ft-35 ft. tall with simple leaves having a serrated margin. Flowers are white or rosy pink with 5 petals. Fruits are called drupes not nuts with a thick leathery green exocarp enclosing the seed covered by a hard-pitted shell. The shell has to be cracked open to reveal the edible almond.

Almond seeds are generally sweet but some species like *P. dulcis var amara* are bitter, as are seeds from some individual trees. Bitter almonds yield hydrogen cyanide and so consumption of even small amounts of bitter almonds can cause severe health problems including death.

Brazilnuts *(Bertholletia excelsa)*: Kingdom: Plantae; Division: Angiospermae, Class: Eudicots Order: Ericales; Family: Lecithidaceae; Genus and species: *Bertholletia excelsa.* Chromosome number, 2n = 24.

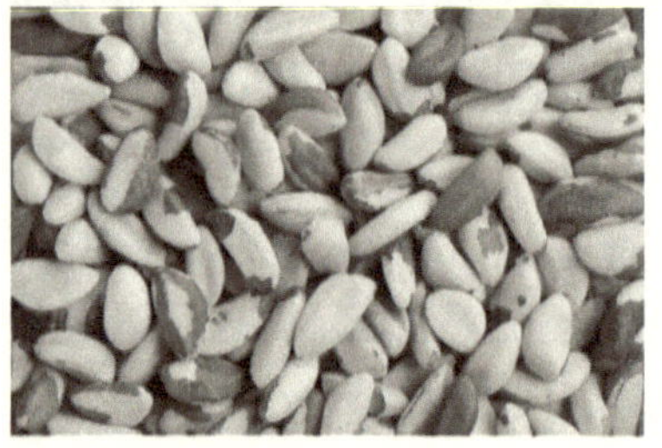

Brazil nuts

The Brazil nut is a large tree reaching 50 m (160 ft) tall and with a trunk 1 to 2 m – or 3 to 7 ft. in diameter making it among the largest of trees in the Amazon rainforests. It may live for 500 years or more and according to some authorities often reaches an age of 1000 years. Plant leaves are deciduous, alternate, simple, entire or crenate, oblong 20–35 cm or 7.9–13.8 in long and 10–15 cm or 3.9–5.9 in breadth. The flowers are small, greenishwhite, in panicles 5–10 cm or 2.0–3.9 in long. Each flower has a two-part deciduous calyx, six unequal creamcolored petals and numerous stamens united into a broad hoodshaped mass. The fruit takes 14 months to mature after pollination of the flowers. The fruit itself is a large capsule resembling a coconut endocarp in size and weighing up to 2 kg or 4.4 lb. It has a hard woody shell, which contains eight to 24 triangular seeds 4–5 cm or1.6–2.0 in long. The "Brazil nuts" are packed like the segments of an orange.

Health: Nutritionally, Brazil nuts are a good source of some vitamins and minerals. Brazil nuts are perhaps the richest dietary source of selenium. Recent research suggests that proper selenium intake is correlated with a reduced risk of both breast cancer and prostate cancer.

However, these findings are inconclusive. Other investigations into the effects of selenium on prostate cancer have also been inconclusive. Brazil nuts have one of the highest concentrations of phytic acid at 2 to 6% of dry weight. Phytic acid can prevent absorption of some nutrients mainly iron. Brazil nuts contain small amounts of radium. Radium, is a radioactive element, It is not retained by the body and may not be causing any mutations. Still, this is a matter of concern. According to Oak Ridge Associated Universities, the presence of radium is not because of elevated levels of radium in the soil but due to "the very extensive root system of the tree which reaches out deep into soil and absorbs any radium present normally and concentrates it in the plant. Brazil nuts like many nuts are allergenic.

Cashew nuts *(Anacardium occidentale)*: **Kingdom: Plantae; Division: Angiospermae Class: Eudicots; Order: Sapindales Family: Anacardiaceae. Chromosome number, 2n = 42.**

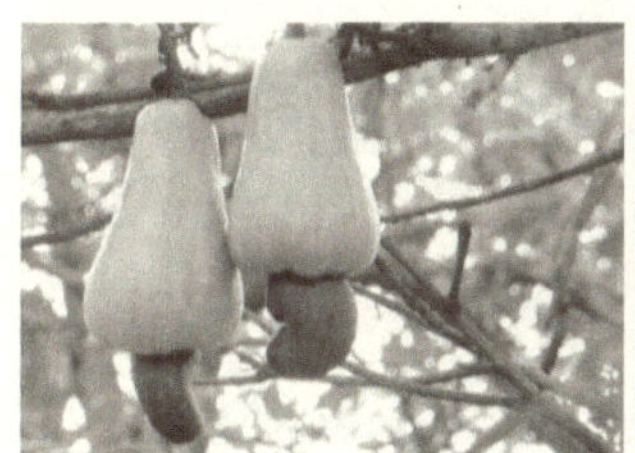

Cashew Fruit-nut

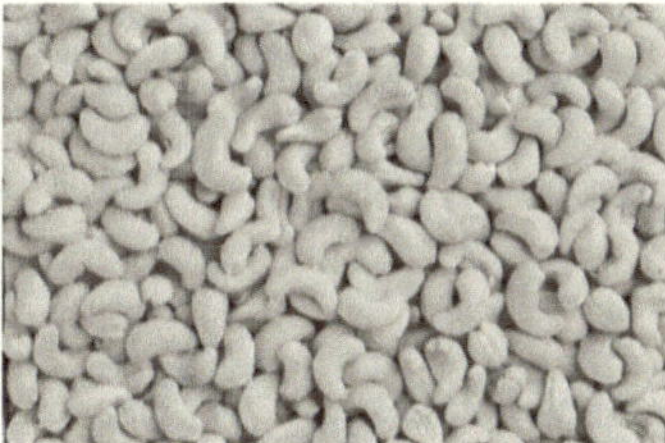

Cashewnut

The cashew tree is a tropical evergreen that produces the cashew nut and the cashew apple. The normal variety grows to a height of 40 ft. but the dwarf cashew growing up to 20 ft. has proved more profitable with earlier maturity and higher yields. The leaves are spirally arranged and are leathery, elliptic to obovate with smooth margins. The flowers are produced in a panicle or corymb, each flower is small, pale green at first then turning reddish with five slender acute petals. The fruit of the cashew tree is an accessory fruit sometimes called a pseudocarp or false fruit. What appears to be the fruit is an oval or pear-shaped structure a hypocarpium that develops from the pedicel and the receptacle of the cashew flower. The cashew apple is edible and has a strong "sweet" smell and a sweet taste. The pulp of the cashew apple is very juicy but the skin is fragile making it unsuitable for transport. The cashew apple fruit juice is fermented to produce a highly aromatic wine called feni.

The true fruit of the cashew tree is a kidney shaped drupe that grows at the end of the cashew apple. The drupe develops first on the tree and then the pedicel expands to become the cashew apple. Within the true fruit is a single seed, which is the cashew nut. The seed is surrounded by a double shell containing an allergenic phenolic resin (anacardic acid) a potent skin irritant chemically related to the better known allergenic oil urushiol which is also a toxin found in the related poison ivy. Properly roasting cashews destroys the toxin but it must be done outdoors as the smoke that is not unlike that from burning poison ivy contains urushiol droplets that can cause severe sometimes life-threatening reactions by irritating the lungs. People who are allergic to cashew urushiols may also react to mango or pistachio that is also in the Anacardiaceae family. Cashews as with other tree nuts are a good source of antioxidants. Alkyl phenols in particular are abundant in cashews. **Health:** Cashews contain soluble oxalates and people with a tendency to form kidney stones may need moderation and medical guidance.

Chestnuts (*Castanea sativa*): Kingdom: Plantae; Division: Angiospermae; Class: Eudicots; Order: Fagales; family: Fagaceae; Genus: Castanea. European Sweet Chestnut: (Castanea sativa), Chromosome number, 2n = 24.

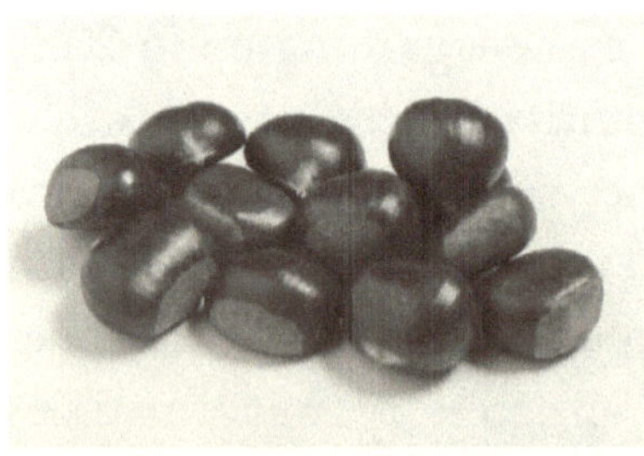

Chestnuts

Asian species are divided into Japanese chestnut (*Castanea crenata*), Chinese chestnut (*C. mollissima*) and (*C. henrii*), and Seguins chestnut also from China (*C. seguinii*). American chestnuts are Eastern American Chestnut (*Castanea dentate*), Allegheny Chinkapin or Dwarf cherstnut (Castanea pumila), Southern states Chestnuts *C. alnifolia, C. ashei, C. floridana and C. paupispina*).

Depending on the species, chestnuts may be shrubs or trees. Japanese and Chinese species tend to be multilayered and spreading whereas, the European and American species tend to grow erect with massive trunks. Chestnut plant leaves are simple, ovate or lanceolate with serrate edges. Flowers are unisexual, clustered into catkins. Fruits are enclosed in paired or clustered capsules called burr, which burst open at maturity to reveal the fruit. The fruit is usually brown in color, flattened on both sides and has two skins. The outer skin is hard husk/hull and the inner skin is a pellicle adhering to the seed. The seed has two nutritionally rich edible cotyledons that contain no cholesterol and very little fat and are gluten free. The edible cotyledons are rich in Vitamin C but this vitamin is lost upon heating while being prepared for edibility by boiling. The complete nutritional value of Chestnuts is given in Table.

Coconut *(Cocos nucifera):* Kingdom: Plantae; Division: Angiospermae; Class: Monocotyledonae; Order: Arecales; family: Arecaceae. Chromosome number,

The nuts are important source of vegetable oil. Botany and other details are given in the section on Oil seeds.

Hazelnuts (*Corylus* sp.): Kingdom: Plantae; Division: Angiospermae, Class: Eudicots Order: Fagales Family: Betulaceae; Genus and Species: *Corylus heterophylla,* C. *cornuta,* C. *Yunnan,* C. *sieboldiana,* C. *wangii,* C. *fargesii,* C. *jacquemontii.* **Chromosome number, 2n = 22 or 28.** The Filibert nut s is derived from the related C. *maxima* and the nuts are very similar to hazel nuts and are often confused with it.

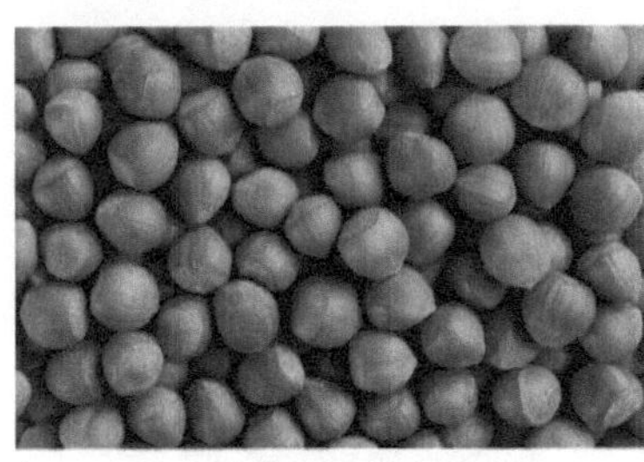

Hazel nuts

Hazel nuts are closely related to filibert. The plants are deciduous trees or large shrubs with simple rounded leaves with double serrate margins. The flowers are produced very early in spring before the leaves and are monoecious with singles catkins. The male catkins are pale yellow and 5–12 cm long and the female ones are very small and largely concealed in the buds with only the bright red 1 to 3 mm long styles visible. The fruits are nuts 1–2.5 cm long and 1–2 cm diameter surrounded by a husk which partly to fully encloses the nut. The nut is also known as a cobnut. The seed has a thin dark brown skin. **Health:** Pollen causes allergies. Seeds are rich in protein and unsaturated fats.

Macadamia *(Macadamia integrifolia):* Kingdom: Plantae; Division: Angiospermae, Class: Eudicots; Order: Family: Proteaceae; Other Species: *M. integrifolia M. jansenii M. ternifolia M. tetraphylla.* Chromosome number, n = 14, 2n = 28.

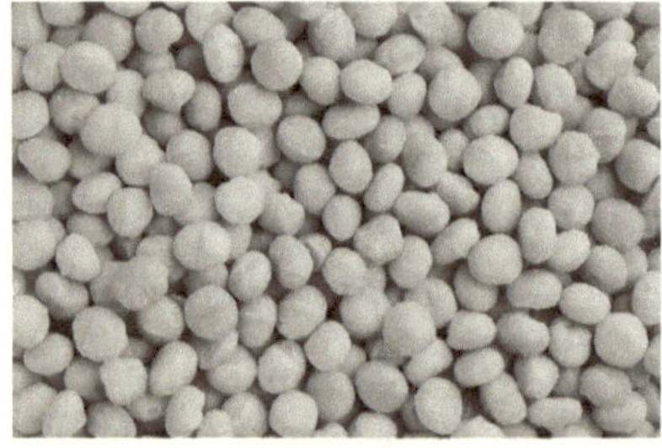
Macadamia

It is a species of trees indigenous to Australasia, Hawaii and pacific islands. This species is a small tree; the leaves have toothed-margins and are 7 to 15 cm in length. The flowers are white or pinkish followed by woody rounded fruits that are 2 to 3.5 cm in diameter. The seeds contain high amounts of monounsaturated fats and palmitoleic acid. The high fat content makes it a product used in the cosmetic industry. **Health:** The seeds contain cyanogenic glycosides that can be leached out during processing. The seeds are also allergenic. However, they have other nutritional benefits.

Peanuts *(Arachis hypogea): Botany and other aspects have been described earlier.* Chromosome number, 2n = 20.

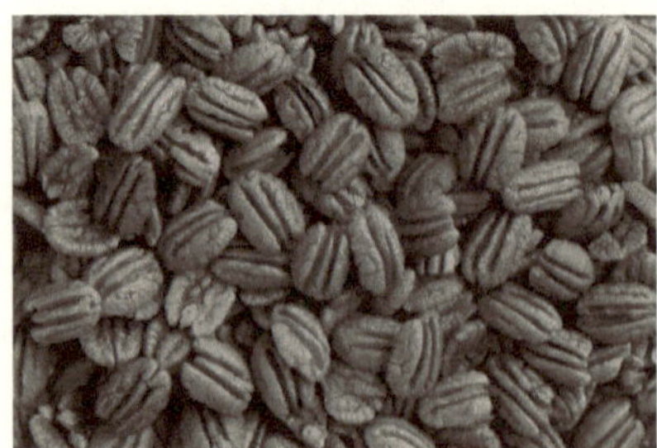
Pecans

Pecans *(Carya illinoinensis):* Kingdom: Plantae; Division: Angiospermae, Class: Eudicots; Order: Fagales Family: Juglandaceae, Genus and Species: *Carya illinoinensis.* Chromosome number, 2n = 32.

Pecans are large deciduous trees, growing to a height of about 60–130 ft. with a girth of the trunk of 6–7 ft. The trees are related to hickory and are native to Mexico and Southern United States. The pecan plant leaves are pinnate with about a dozen leaflets. The nut is really a fruit with a single stone surrounded by a husk. When the husk splits, it releases the edible nut. The seeds are brown in color and have nutty buttery flavor. Pecan trees as old as 300 years still bear fruits nuts. Pecans are rich in omega-6-fatty acids and protein. **Health relevance:** The addition of a handful of pecan nuts to food each day lowers LDL cholesterol. Pecans may also delay age related nerve degeneration.

Pistachio nuts *(Pistacia Vera):* **Kingdom Plantae; Division: Angiospermae, Class: Eudicots Order: Sapindales; Family: Anacardiaceae; Genus and species:** *Pistacia Vera.* **Chromosome number, 2n = 28. Triploids, tetraploids present.**

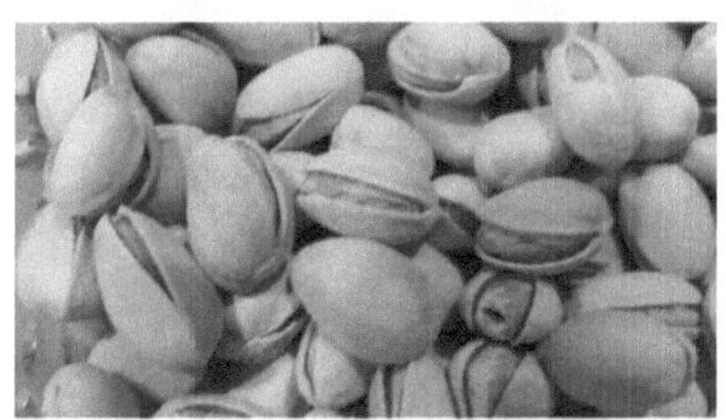

Pistachio

This plant, which belongs to the same family as cashewnut, is grown mainly in Iran, Syria, Lebanon, Turkey, Greece Egypt, India, Afghanistan, Italy, Israel, Uzbekistan and California USA. The plants are bushy and grow up to 10 meters-33 ft. tall. It has deciduous pinnate leaves 10–20 centimeters 4–8 inches long. The plants are dioecious with separate male and female trees. The flowers are apetalous, unisexual, and borne in panicles. The plants are highly salt tolerant and grows well in saline soil. The plants do not grow well in highly irrigated soil and as such, they are excellent plants to grow in arid and semiarid regions. The fruit is a drupe containing a nut. The fruit has a tough outer shell that splits open to release the edible seed. Each pistachio tree produces about 50 kg of nuts every two years. **Health relevance:** The seeds contain urushiol that causes allergic reactions. Pistachio nuts can lower LDL cholesterol. The nuts are good substrates for the fungus *Aspergillus* that in turn produces the toxin Aflatoxin and hence care should be taken while eating the nuts. Bitter tasting nuts must be avoided.

Walnuts *(Juglans regia):* **Kingdom: Plantae; Group: Angiospermae, Class: Eudicots; Order: Fagales; Family: Juglandaceae; Genus and Family:** *Juglans regia* **(English walnut),** *J. Nigra* **(Black walnut);** J. *cinerea* **(Butternut). Chromosome number, 2n = 32.**

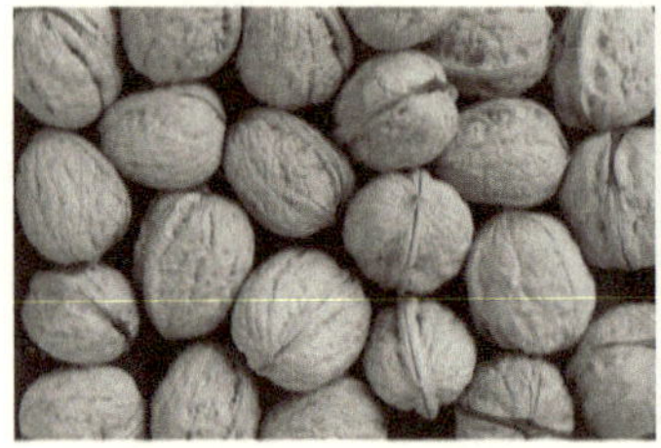

Walnut in shell

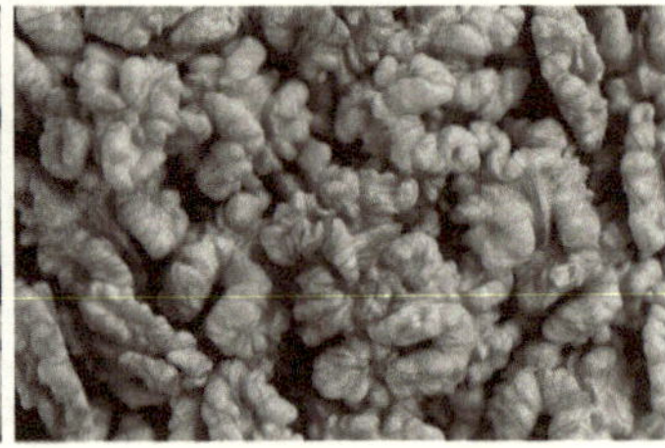

Walnut

Walnut trees are deciduous trees about 30–130 Ft. Tall with pinnate leaflets. The 21 species in the genus range across the north temperate southeast Europe to Japan and more widely in southeast Canada west to California and south to Argentina. The walnuts are stone fruits with a single bi-segmented kernel seed. The shelled walnuts are covered by a thin seed coat that is rich in antioxidants. **Health relevance:** The nuts are rich in antioxidants, monounsaturated and polyunsaturated fats rich in alpha lineolic acid. Although, walnuts are touted to have anticancer properties, the American Cancer Society concluded that there is no scientific basis for this claim. Traditional Chinese medical practitioners prescribe a diet rich in walnuts for good kidney health, Asthma and strong joints. The antioxidant content as well as lineolic acids are considered good for cardio protection.

Table: 18 – Important nutrient profile of various edible nuts

NUTS	Carbohydrate g	Fiber g	Protein g	Sugars g	Sat fat g	Mono unsat g	Poly unsat g	Trans Fat g	Cholesterol g
Almonds	21.55	12.5, g	21.15	4.35	3.802	31.551	12.329	0.015	0
Brazil, dry	11.74	7.5	14.32	2.33	16.13	23.879	24.399	NA	0
Cashewnuts, raw	30.19	3.3	18.22	5.91	7.783	23.797	7.845	NA	0
Chestnut-China, raw	49.07	NA	4.2	NA	0.164	0.581	0.288	NA	0
Chestnut-Japan, dry	81.43	NA	5.25	NA	0.183	0.65	0.322	NA	0
Chestnut-Europe, Unpeeled	45.54	NA	2.42	NA	0.425	0.78	0.894	NA	0
Hazelnut/Filibert	16.7	9.7	14.95	4.34	4.464	45.652	7.92	NA	0
Macadamia, raw	13.82	8.6	7.91	4.57	12.06	58.877	1.502	NA	0
Peanuts, all types	16.13	8.5	25.8	4.72	6.279	24.426	15.558	0	0
Pecans	13.86	9.6	9.17	3.97	6.18	40.801	21.614	NA	0
Pine nuts, dry	13.08	3.7	13.69	3.59	4.899	18.764	34.071	NA	0
Pistachio nuts, raw	27.51	10.3	20.27	7.66	5.556	23.82	13.744	0	0
Sunflower nuts, dry	20	8.6	20.78	2.62	4.455	18.528	23.137	NA	0
Walnuts-Black, dry	9.58	6.8	24.06	1.1	3.483	15.442	36.437	NA	0
Walnuts-English, dry	13.71	6.7	15.23	2.61	6.126	8.933	47.174	NA	0

References

Alasalva, C, Shahidi, F, (2008): Tree Nuts: Composition, Phytochemicals, and Health Effects (Nutraceutical Science and Technology), CRC. p., 143.

Duorte, O., Paull, R.E., (2015): Exotic fruits and nuts of the new world, CABI, Wallingford, oxfordshire, U.K. pp332.

http://www.mayoclinic.org/diseases-conditions/heart-disease/in-depth/nuts/art-20046635

Preedy, V., Watson, R.R., and V. Patel (2011): *In,* Nuts and Seeds in Health and Disease Prevention, 1st Edition. Academic Press, Elsevier publishers, p1232

Ramsay, H.P., (1963): Chromosome numbers in the Proteaceae): Australian Journal of Botany 11(1) 1 – 20

Ros, E. (2010): Health Benefits of Nut Consumption. Nutrients, 2010 Jul; 2(7): 652–682. PMCID: PMC3257681.

Sabaté J., Salas-Salvadó J., Ros, E. (2006): Nuts, nutrition and health outcomes. Br. J. Nutr. 2006, 96: S1–S102. [PubMed]

Chapter 12
Beverage Plants

Liquid beverages are consumed along with food or separately both as sources of energy stimulation and hydration. The most important beverages consumed are Tea, coffee and cocoa besides fruit and vegetable juices as well as various carbonated drinks. Among these tea, coffee and cocoa are all derived from plant sources and are consumed worldwide. The following are brief descriptions of the botany and biology of these three plants.

Coffee (*Coffea arabica, C.robusta, C.liberica*): kingdom: Plantae; Division: angiospermae, Class: Eudicots order: Gentianales, family: Rubiaceae; genus and species: *Coffea arabica, C. Ro busta, C. liberica*. Chromosome number, 2n = 22, 4n = 44, 6x = 66 and 8x = 88.

Coffea arabica is a plant that was indigenous to Ethiopia but is now grown in Southern India, Eastern Africa, Brazil, Central America and Java Island in Indonesia, Hawaii and Columbia and is the main

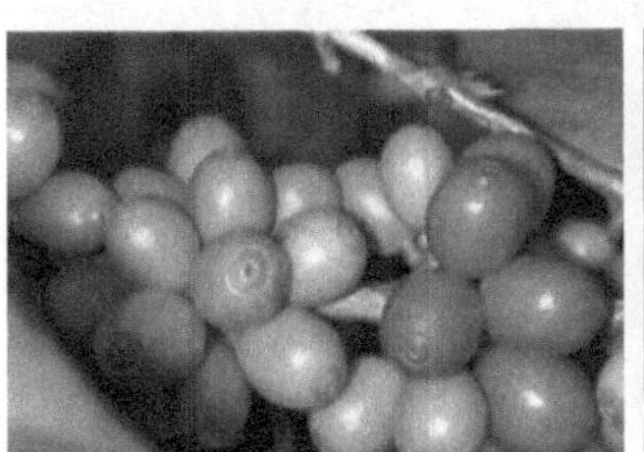

Coffee plant

Coffee berries

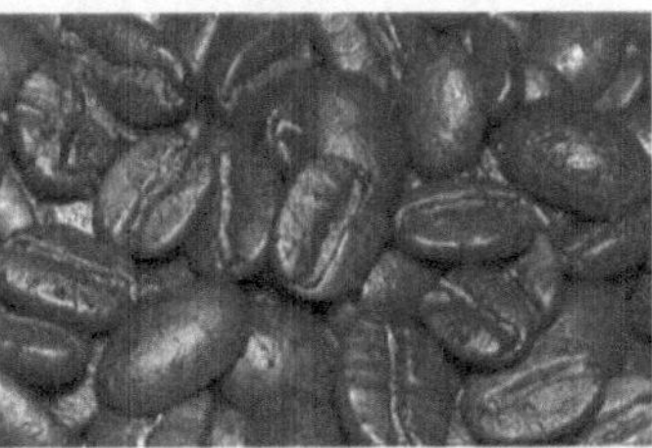

Coffee beans

type of coffee. *Coffea robusta* grows in Indonesia, West Africa, Brazil, and Vietnam and the bean is mainly used to make instant coffee. *Coffea liberica* grows mainly in Liberia, Ivory Coast and Malaysia and makes up a small percentage of coffee. Plants grow to a height of 25 to 40 feet and have extensive branching, producing glabrous opposite simple leaves that are elliptic to ovoid. Flowers are white and grow in clusters. The fruit is a drupe containing two seeds but some varieties contain a single seed known as a pea. Berries with a single seed are called as pea berries. Seeds are covered with membranes known as the parchment coat and silver skin. Each tree can produce 1 pound to 10 pounds of dried beans.

Coffee contains caffeine that is a stimulant and also contains monoamine oxidase inhibitors that contribute to psycho activity. Coffee is broken down into theobromine and theophylline by the liver enzymes. **Health relevance:** coffee may have potential health benefits. Although there are reports suggesting beneficial effects in preventing cancer, these reports have not been substantiated. There are also some studies that suggest that drinking excessive coffee can lead to risk of dementia, Parkinson's disease, heart disease, diabetes and Alzheimer's disease. Lately, there are many reports regarding the beneficial effects of green coffee. High levels of coffee consumption can lead to overstimulation of the vascular system. Over drinking of coffee can also lead to poor absorption of iron. Anxiety and other psychosomatic effects may result from excessive coffee consumption.

Chocolate/Cacao *(Theobroma cacao):* **Kingdom: Plantae; Division: Angiospermae, Class: Eudicots, Order: Malvales; Family: Malvaceae. Other names: kakaw; K'ichekagaw cacahuati – meso American languages. Chromosome number, 2n, 2x = 20.**

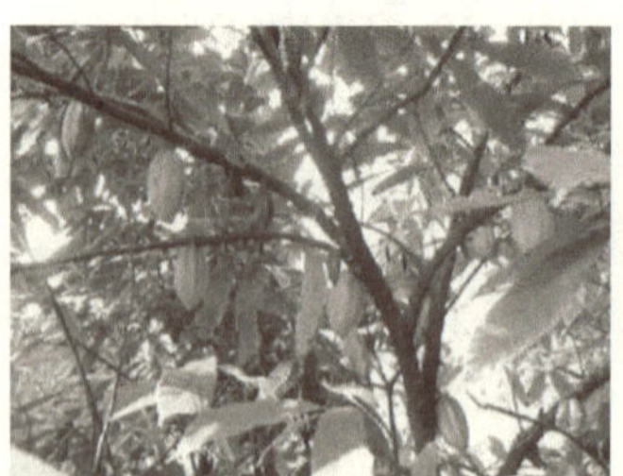

Cacao

Cacao plants are natives of the meso American region but are now grown in many parts of the world in Africa, Southeast Asia including India, New Guinea and other regions in addition to the meso American region. Cacao plants are small trees about 20 feet high with large oblong leaves about a foot long. The flowers are produced in clusters directly on short stocks on the stem. Flowers are small bisexual with five sepals, five petals and five stamens and five ovary chambers. The fruits are yellow to orange oblong with 10 ribs containing about 20 to 60 seeds. The fruits are called pods and the seeds are commonly called beans. The seeds are embedded in a white pulp within the fruit. While the seeds are the main source of chocolate cocoa, the pulp may be used for preparing various drinks and jellies or maybe fermented to produce an alcoholic beverage. The seeds are also rich in protein and contain various polyphenolic alkaloids that are antioxidants. The polyphenols include anthocyanins, isoflavones, flavanones, flavonols, flavan-3-ols, catechins, epicatechins, proanthocyanidins, and flavones. Many different studies show that cocoa and chocolates possess remarkable cardio protective properties by reducing the risk of heart attack and stroke by reducing blood pressure and decreasing the oxidation of low-density lipoprotein's-LDL and clumping of platelets. Additionally, cocoa and chocolate consumption seems to improve cognitive functions. It is also considered to have anti-inflammatory properties. Many brands of commercially available chocolates contain substantial amounts of milk fats and sugar that can mitigate the good effects of consuming chocolates and cocoa. Chocolate also contains caffeine that can act as a stimulant and hence might impair sleep pattern if consumed in large amounts. In order to achieve the beneficial effects of cocoa, chocolates must contain at least 70% cocoa. Consuming pure cocoa without adding sugar or with sugar substitutes in drinks and other foods would be a better choice for getting the benefits of cocoa consumption. **Health relevance:** The high levels of antioxidants in cocoa are believed to have cardio protective health benefits.

Tea *(Camellia/Thea sinensis)*: Kingdom: Plantae; Division: Angiospermae, Class: Eudicots; Order: Ericales; Family: Theaceae;

Genus and species: *Camellia sinensis var sinensis* **Chinese tea** *C. sinensis var assamica Assamese*–**Indian tea. Chromosome number, 2n, 2x = 30**

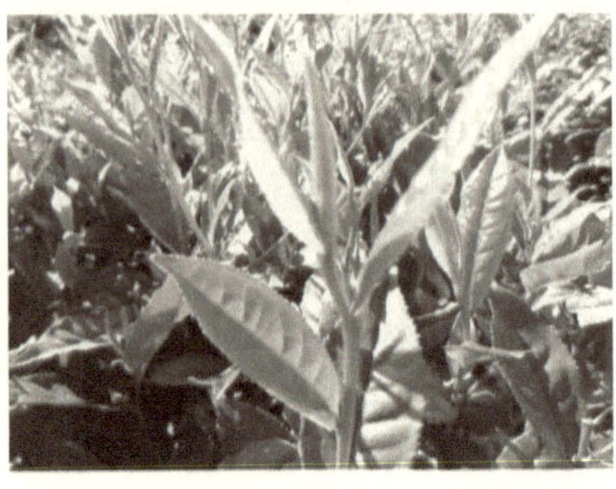

Tea-India

It is an evergreen tree that grows to a height of 50 ft but is usually pruned to a height of 6 ft in order to aid in plucking of the leaves. It grows in the cooler tropical and subtropical countries chiefly China, India, SriLanka, Cambodia, Kenya and Uganda. Some varieties grow in the United Kingdom, Vancouver Island in Canada and Washington State in USA as well as in Tasmania Australia. Tea plants require high rainfall and acid soils and grow in the higher elevations. The Assam type is characterized by larger glabrous leaves whereas the Chinese varieties have smaller leaves and the Cambodian varieties have leaves of intermediate sizes. Only the young tender 3 leaves known as flushes are plucked for processing. Older leaves are deeper green. Different leaf ages produce differing tea qualities since their chemical compositions are different. Tea of poorer quality can be obtained by processing older leaves. Green tea, White tea, yellow tea, and black tea are some of the types of tea that are produced from tea leaves using different processing methods. In addition, Darjeeling Tea and Nilagiris tea are other types of tea produced from tea plants grown in Darjeeling and Nilgiris in India.

Flowers of the tea plant are yellow white with 7 to 8 petals and are produced in the axils of leaves. The flowers are aromatic with a pleasant smell. Seeds of the tea plant contain the oil that can be used for cooking and flavoring. The leaves contain antioxidants catechins, flavonoids, theonine, caffeine, theobromine and theophyllins. **Health relevance:** there are reports that suggest that drinking tea confers protection from cancers. Drinking both green and black tea may protect against development of cardiovascular disease. The catechins in tea have anti-inflammatory and neuroprotective properties.

Sugar and Sugar Substitutes

Cane sugar, sugarbeet and maple sugar are three of the most important plant sources for sucrose or sugar for human consumption. There are also a few plants that provide sugar substitutes that are valuable for diabetic and prediabetic individuals as substitutes for sugar. High levels of consumption of sugar are linked to the high incidence of diabetes and other health problems. In view of this, the search for sugar substitutes mainly from plant sources is an ongoing project. The following describes briefly the botany and biology of plants that are the main sources of sugar and sugar substitutes.

1. **Sugarcane** *(Saccharam officianarum):* **kingdom: Plantae Division: Angiospermae; Class: Monocotyledonae; order: Poales family: poaceae; genus and species:** *Saccharam officianarum.* **2n = 80.**

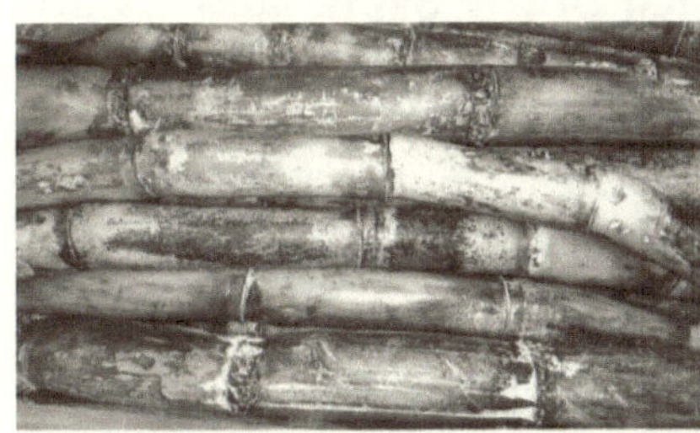

Sugarcane

The sugarcane plant is a tropical perennial of the grass family and grows to a height of 6 to 20 feet. They have segmented thick stems that are fibrous and contain large quantities of sugar juice. Each plant produces lateral shoots that give rise to multiple stems that contain soluble sugars, fiber and water. The leaves are long with parallel veins. Sugar is extracted from the Juice. Sugarcane plants are very efficient C4 plants capable of fixing incident solar energy into biomass. Additionally, sugarcane plants fix atmospheric nitrogen in association with specific bacteria present in the cells of the plant. **Health:** sugar is a high source of energy for all forms of life. However, the consumption of large quantities of sugary foods leads to glucose intolerance and development of diabetes. High sugar consumption also leads to obesity, dental diseases.

2. **Sugarbeet** *(Beta vulgaris):* **kingdom: Plantae; Division: Angiospermae Class: Eudicots; order: Cayophyllales; Family: Amaranthaceae. Chromosome number 2n = 4x = 36.**

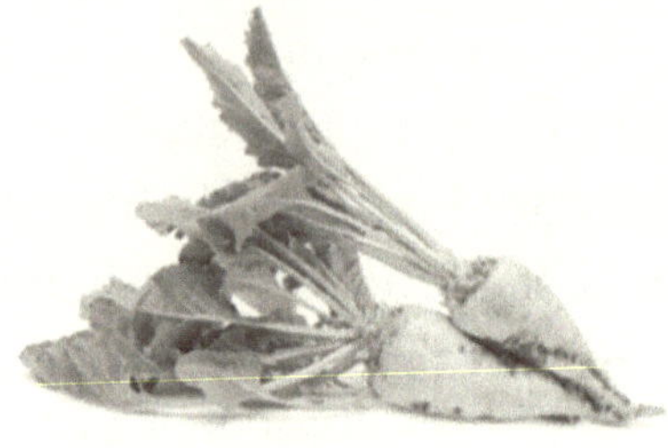

Sugarbeet

Sugarbeet along with garden beet and chard are all different varieties of *Beta vulgaris* and have been described earlier. Unlike the garden beet and chard, sugarbeets have thick conical white fleshy taproots with a flat crown. Sugar formed in the leaves is stored in the taproots that at the time of harvest contain about 20% sugar and rest being water and pulp. Sugar is extracted from the juice of taproots. The pulp is mainly used as animal feed. **Health relevance:** same as that for cane sugar.

3. **Maple sugar** *(Acer saccharam):* **kingdom: Plantae; Division: Angiospermae, Class: Eudicots; order: Sapindales family: Aceraceae. Genus and species:** *Acer saccharam.* **Chromosome number, 2n = 26.**

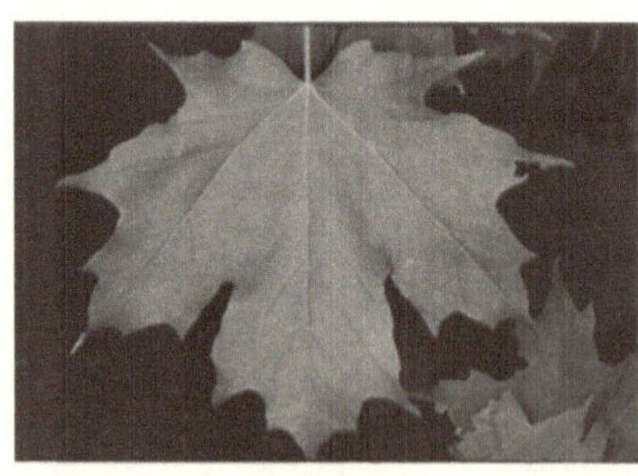

Maple

Sugar maple trees are deciduous trees reaching a height of almost hundred feet or more. The leaves are palmate with five lobes. In the autumn, the leaves turn yellow to red and fall to the ground. The flowers are formed in clusters of 5 to 10 without petals. The fruit is a samara with two winged globose seeds. The sugar formed in the leaves is transported down into the stem towards the root and the sap containing the sugar is tapped by ringing around the bark. The sugar is then processed from the sap and is known as maple sugar. Unlike cane and beet sugar, maple sugar is mainly used in the preparation of candy, maple syrup and other flavored sugar products.

4. **Stevia *(Stevia rebaudiana)*: kingdom: Plantae; Division: Angiospermae Class: Eudicots; order: Asterales family: Asteraceae; Other Names: sweet leaf, sugarleaf, ka'a he'ē "sweet herb." Chromosome number, 2n = 2x = 22**

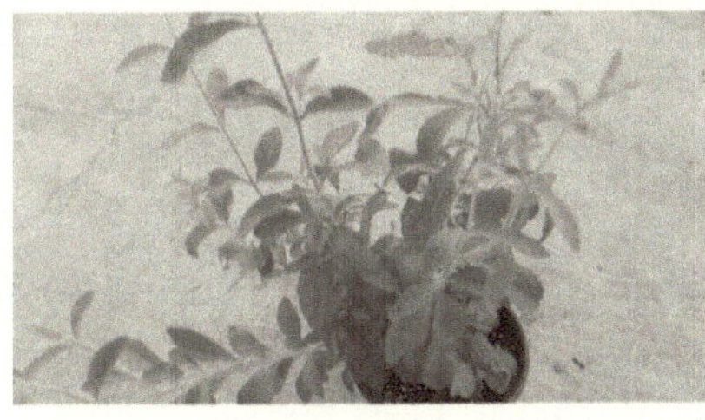

Stevia

Stevia rebaudiana is cultivated and used to sweeten food in China, India, Korea, Taiwan, Thailand and Malaysia. It can also be found in Saint Kitts islands, Brazil, Colombia, Peru, Paraguay, Uruguay and Israel. It is an herbaceous annual plant, with small white flowers. The plants can be grown indoors as houseplants on windowsills or in glass houses. The plants are generally grown from leafy shoots and not from seeds. Stevia is widely grown for its sweet leaves that are the source of sweetener products known generically as stevia and sold under various trade names. The active compounds are various steviol glycosides – mainly stevioside and rebaudioside that have 250–300 times the sweetness of sugar. The leaves can be eaten fresh or put in teas and foods. Currently, after some initial concerns about its safety, the FDA has allowed the use of Stevia as a sugar substitute and stevia sugar is now sold in supermarkets everywhere. **Health:** Apart from being a no calorie sugar substitute, the leaves of Stevia are reported to contain compounds that kill the tick-borne spirochete *Borrelia burgdorferi*. Experiments showed that the leaf extracts killed all the different stages of the spirochetes.

Other sugar substitutes

Brazzein and Pentadin/Oubli *(Pentadiplandra brazzeana)*: Kingdom: Plantae; Group: Angiospermae, Dicotyledonae, Class: Eudicots, Order: Brassicales; Family: Pentadiplandraceae. Chromosome number, 2n = 44.

Brazzein and Pentadin are two naturally occurring sweetener proteins found in the West African plant *Pentadiplandra brazzeana*. Both proteins have a low molecular weight. Brazzein has a molecular weight of 6.5 Kilo Daltons whereas; pentadin has a molecular weight of 12 Kilo Dalton. The sweet taste of Brazzein is closer to that of Sucrose and is comparatively heat stable. The structure of Brazzein is known and recombinant E. coli, Corn and wheat plants expressing the gene have been generated. The plant *P.brazzeana* is a native of Cameroon and Gabon in Africa and both Apes and humans have been consuming this long before the discoveries of Pentadin and Brazzein.

1. **Mabinlins/Mabinlang** *(Capparis masaikai):* **Kingdom: Plantae; Group: Angiospermae, Dicotyledonae, Class: Eudicots, Order: Brassicales; Family: Capparaceae. Chromosome number, 2n = 40.**

Mabinlins are four homologs of proteins with sweetener characters. All have similar amino acid sequences but Mabilinin 2 is the most thermo stable of the four. Mabilinin 2 has an A chain of 33 amino acids and the B chain has 72 amino acids with 2 intramolecular and two intermolecular disulfide bridges which confer greater stability to the protein. The sweetness of mabinlin-2 is unchanged after 48 hours incubation at 80°C. The protein has been experimentally synthesized by solid phase chemistry and has also been expressed in potato plants by recombinant DNA techniques. The protein is not yet marketed as a sweetener.

2. **Marasi/Lumbah/Lemba** *(Curculigo latifolia):* **Kingdom: Plantae; Group: Angiospermae, Class: Monocotyledonae, Order: Asperagales; Family: Hypoxidaceae. Chromosome number, 2n = 18.**

The plants are found in the rain-fed regions of India, Malay Archipelago, Indonesia, New Guinea, and Australia, other parts of Asia, Africa and South America.

There are at least 15 different species of *Curculigo* of which *C. latifolia* is the one most known for the sweetener. Plants of *Curculigo* look very similar to Ginger and Canna with long elongate leaves. The fruits of *Curculigo latifolia* taste like sweetened cucumber and increase the appetite. Though the fruits are not extremely sweet themselves, they produce a very sweet after-taste when a drink is taken after eating the fruit. This also occurs when a sour substance is taken after the fruits, so native people eat the fruits to give a sweet taste to sour foods. The taste-modifying properties of the fruits of *Curculigo latifolia* (Marasi) are due to the presence of the protein curculin. Curculin is a dimer of two identical polypeptides of 114 amino acid residues. It has a sweet taste, which disappears rapidly. When taken after curculin, water tastes sweet, and sour substances likewise seem to taste sweet. For instance, a lemon eaten after taking curculin elicits a sweet taste lasting for about 10 minutes. Curculin is denatured upon heating and hence the sweetener is mainly usable for table sugar applications that do not involve cooking (eg; lemonades, juices). **Health:** In Peninsular Malaysia, infusions of the leaves, stem-tips and roots of Marasi are all used internally against fever. Decoctions of the flowers and roots are taken as a stomachic and diuretic, the rhizomes are also used against eye diseases in North-Eastern India. In Borneo, the leaves of Marasi play a role in magical healing ceremonies. Curculin is considered to be a high-intensity sweetener, with a reported relative sweetness of 430–2070 times sweeter than sucrose on a weight basis. In view of this, it is a good sugar substitute for diabetics.

3. **Miraculin: From, Miracle berry/agbayun, /taami, asaa, / ledidi** *(Synsepalum dulcificum)*: **Kingdom: Plantae, Division: Angiospermae, Class: Eudicots Order: Ericales Family: Sapotaceae. Botanical synonyms:** *Bakeriella dulcifica;* **Bumelia dulcifica;** *Pouteria dulcifica; Richardella dulcifica;* **Sideroxylon** *dulcificum.* **Chromosome number, 2n = 26 Or 28.**

Syncepalum dulciferum is a shrub that grows between 6 to 15 feet in height and has dense foliage. This evergreen plant produces small, red berries, while white flowers are produced for many months of the year.

The glycoprotein sweetener Miraculin is a component of the fruits of the miracle berry tree that is a native of West Africa.

Miraculin is a glycoprotein (MW. 24.5 Kda) which is not sweet by itself. However, the protein generates sweetness by binding to sweet receptors in the tongue under acidic conditions. The glycoprotein is not heat stable. The sweetener has not been marketed except as a food additive in Japan. The sweetener has been experimentally expressed in tomato plants by recombinant DNA technology.

Health: The sweetener may be useful as a food additive for diabetic patients. There is also a possibility of it being used to help cancer patients undergoing chemotherapy since Miraculin counteracts the metallic taste generated by chemotherapy agents.

4. **Mogorosides: From Monk fruit/Buddha fruit/Longevity fruit/Arhat fruit/luohan guo *(Siraitia grosvenorii/Momordica grosvenorii)*: Kingdom: Plantae; Division: Angiospermae, Class: Eudicots, Order: Cucurbitales; Family: Cucurbitaceae. Chromosome number, 2n = 28.**

The sweetener character in the fruits of this plant comes from the presence of Mogorosides that are tri-terpene glycosides. The plants are perennial vines that are mainly grown in Southern China, Thailand, Cambodia and Viet Nam. It is now grown commercially in mountainous regions elsewhere. The melon-like fruit has been a part of Chinese traditional medicine as a treatment for diabetics since the fruit juice that is 300 times sweeter than sugar has a low glycemic index. The fruit extract is now marketed as a sugar sweetener under the name Norbu. Although, the fruit contains fructose and glucose, only the sweet mogroside is extracted from the fruit while manufacturing the sweetener. Norbu is a 100% natural sweetener, sugar substitute derived from Monk Fruit. Norbu can be used as a sweetener for teas and coffees but also in baking and cooking as a sugar substitute. It is currently marketed in Australia. **Health:** The sweetener is considered as generally recognized as safe (GRAS).

5. **Monellin: From serendipity berry (*Dioscoreophyllum cumminsii*): Kingdom: Plantae, Division: Angiospermae, Class: Eudicots Order: Ranunculales Family: Menispermaceae. Botanical synonyms: *D. fernandense, D. podandrium, D. tenerum*. Chromosome number, 2n = 16.**

Monellin is a sweetener protein of 10.7 Kda found in *D. cumminsii*. It is 800–2000 times sweeter than sucrose but is unstable at high temperatures. However, it is soluble in water and can be used as a tabletop sweetener and as a low calorie sweetener in preparation of cold beverages. Monellin protein has been expressed in yeasts by recombinant methods.

6. **Thaumatin/Miracle berry/African serendipity berry (*Thaumatococcus daniellii*): Kingdom: Plantae; Division: Angiospermae, Class: Monocotyledonae, Order: Zingiberales; Family: Marantaceae. Botanical synonyms: *Donax danielii; Monostiche daniellii; Phrynium daniellii*. Chromosome number, 2n = 20.**

Thaumatococcus daniellii is a rhizomatous perennial herb that is closely related to ginger and turmeric plants… It is a native of Western Africa rainforests that is now grown in Australia, Malaysia, Indonesia and other rain forest regions as a source plant for the sweetener Thaumatin. Plants have elliptic leaves that are about 1.5–2 ft long with parallel veins. Flowers are located in spikate inflorescences. Fleshy dark brown fruits contain 3 black seeds enveloped by sticky arils in each fruit. The arils contain two proteins Thaumatin I and II that are about 3000 times sweeter than sugar w/w. Both Thaumatins belong to the class of proteins known as Pathogenesis related proteins (PR proteins) and are made of 207 amino acids with a molecular weight of 22,000 Daltons. Many plants produce small quantities of Thaumatin in response to stress.

Health: Used as a substitute for sugar and hence of value for control of diabetic conditions.

References

Ali, R., Ghizan, S., Nur, A., Psyquay, A., and Pedram K., (2014): Genetic diversity of lemba (Curculigo latifolia) populations in Peninsular Malaysia using ISSR molecular markers AJCS 8(1): 9-17 (2014). Australian Journal of Crop Science

Bezbaruah, H.P. (1971): Cytological Investigations in the Family Theaceae—I. Chromosome Numbers in Some Camellia Species and Allied Genera, Caryologia, 24: 4, 421-426, DOI: 10.1080/00087114.1971.10796449. http://dx.doi.org/10.1080/000 87114.1971.10796449.

Cecilia A.F. Pinto-Miglio,(2006): Cytogenetics of coffee, Citogenética de café (Coffea L.), Brazilian Journal of Plant Physiology, On-line version ISSN 1677-9452, Braz. J. Plant Physiol. vol.18 no.1 Londrina Jan./Mar. 2006, http://dx.doi.org/10.1590/S1677-04202006000100004.

Desai, B.B. and Sanunke, D.K. (1991): Sugar crops, In Foods of Plant origin; Production, Technology and Human Nutrition, Eds. Salunkhe, D.K.M and Deshpande, S.S. Pp 413-489. Van Nostrand, Reinhold, New York, Pp 499.DOI: 10.1590/S0100-84551996000400013.

Duke, J.A. (1983): Camellia sinensis (L.) Kuntze, Handbook of Energy crops, https://www.hort.purdue.edu/newcrop/duke_energy/Camellia_sinensis.html

Duke, J.A. (1983): Coffea arabica L. Hand book of Energy crops. https://www.hort.purdue.edu/newcrop/duke_energy/Coffea_arabica.html

Duke, J.A. (1983): Theobroma cacao L. Hand book of Energy crops. https://www.hort.purdue.edu/newcrop/duke_energy/Theobroma_cacao.html

Figueiredo, G.S., Melo, C.A., Souza, M.M., Araújo, I.S., Zaidan, H.A., Pires, J.L. and Ahnert, D., (2013): Karyotype variation in cultivars and spontaneous cocoa mutants (Theobroma cacao L.). Genet Mol Res. 2013 Oct 18, 12(4): 4667-77. Doi: 10.4238/2013.October.18.5

Frederico, A.P., Ruas, P.M., Marin-Morales, M.A., Nakajima, J.N. (1996): Chromosome studies in some Stevia. Cav. (Compositae) species from Southern Brazil, Brazilian Journal of Genetics 19(4) November 1996

Gelardi, Robert C.; Nabors, Lyn O'Brien (1991): Alternative sweeteners. New York: M. Dekker. ISBN 0-8247-8475-8

Goyal, S.K., Samsher and Goyal, R.K. (2010): Stevia (Stevia rebaudiana) a bio-sweetener: A review. International Journal of Food Sciences and Nutrition, 61, 1, 1-10.

http://indiabiodiversity.org/species/show/32077

http://ntbg.org/plants/plant_details.php?plantid = 3120

http://www.coffeereview.com/coffee-reference/coffee-basics/ introduction/the-good-the-bad-and-the-bland/

http://www.flowersofindia.net/catalog/slides/Wild%20Caper%20 Bush.html

http://www.kew.org/science-conservation/plants-fungi/coffea-arabica-arabica-coffee

http://www.uniprot.org/uniprot/P30233

Inglett, G.E., May, J.F. (1968): "Tropical plants with unusual taste properties." Economic Botany 22 (4): 326. Doi: 10.1007/ BF02908127

Kim, N.C, Kinghorn, A.D. (December 2002):"Highly sweet compounds of plant origin." Arch. Pharm. Res. 25 (6): 725–46. Doi: 10.1007/ BF02976987. PMID 12510821

Kinghorn, A.D and C.M Compadre, (1991): Less common high-potency sweeteners. In Alternative Sweeteners: Second Edition,

Revised and Expanded, L O'Brien Nabors, Ed., New York, 1991. ISBN 0-8247-8475-8

Kocyan, A., (2007): the Discovery of Polyandry in Curculigo (Hypoxidaceae): Implications for Androecium Evolution of Asparagoid Monocotyledons. Ann Bot. 2007 Aug; 100(2): 241–248.Published online 2007 Jun 12. Doi: 10.1093/aob/mcm091. PMCID: PMC2735314

Lim, T.K. (2012): Edible Medicinal and Non-Medicinal Plants, Volume 3, Fruits, Thaumatococcus danielli, Springer, p259

Nabors, L.OB. (2001): Alternative sweeteners/edited by Lyn O'Brien Nabors. New York, N.Y: Marcel Dekker. ISBN 0-8247-0437-1

Perties, J.E. Brandle, A.N. Starratt, and M. Gijzen, (1998): *Stevia rebaudiana*: Its agricultural, biological, and chemical properties. Can. J. Plant Sci. 78: 527–536.

Ravi Kant (2005): Sweet proteins – Potential replacement for artificial low calorie sweeteners. Nutr Jv.4, 2005 PMC549512, and online 2005 Feb 9, Doi: 10.1186/1475-2891-4-5

Chapter 13
Culinary Spices and Condiments

Spices are used mainly to add specific flavors to foods and in many cases as preservative agents. They are also components of various condiments used to flavor food. As such, they are used in small quantities. In general, although some of these spices do contain certain toxic chemicals, they are not harmful because the quantities used are small. Yet, even the small quantities contain beneficial chemicals that help as phytomedicines. As in all cases, caution should be exercised while using these spices in quantities that are larger than usage as spice-agents.

Ajwain/Carum/Bishops weed/Omum *(Trachyspermum ammi/ Carum copticum/Ammi copticum):* **Kingdom: Plantae; Division: Angiospermae, Class: Eudicots Asterids Order: Apiales Family: Apiaceae. Chromosome number, 2n = 18.**

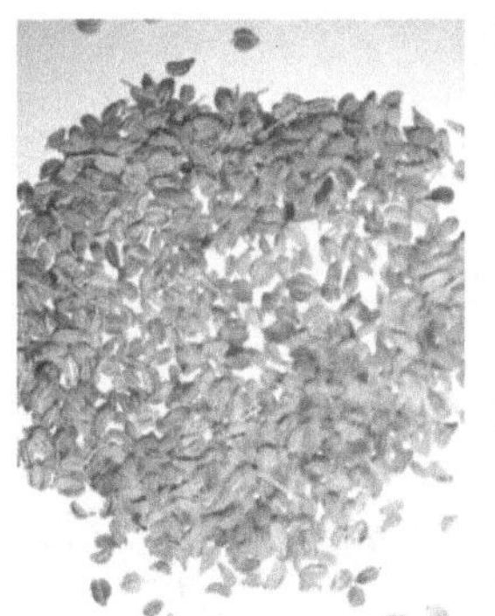

Ajwain

Ajwan plants are annual herbs belonging to the Apiaceae family. Plants are natives of the Mediterranean region but grown extensively in the Indian sub-continent. The plants produce fruits that are botanically called schizocarps. The fruits that are popularly called seeds are dried and used as a spice. The Fruits are dry roasted or fried in butter or sprinkled while making breads and bakery products. It is an anti-flatulent and antispasmodic. The dry fruits are also chewed after food to help digestion. Seeds are also soaked in water and the water extract known as gripe water is drunk to reduce colicky conditions especially for babies. The oil has anti-bacterial properties. It is used as an anti-inflammatory agent for control of arthritic pain.

Anise: *(Pimpinella anisum):* **Kingdom: Plantae; Division: Angiospermae, Class: Eudicots Asterids Order: Apiales, Family: Apiaceae. Chromosome number, 2n = 18 or 20.**

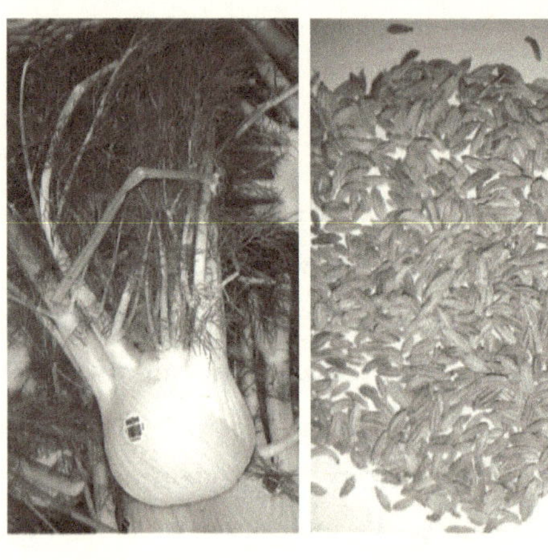

Anise plant   **Anise seeds**

It is an herbaceous annual plant native to Middle Eastern countries growing to a height of 3 ft or more. The plants have simple leaves at the base and at the top the leaves are feathery pinnate, divided into numerous leaves. The flowers are yellow or white approximately 1/8 inch produced in dense umbels similar to those of carrots. The fruit called aniseed is an oblong dry schizocarp 1/8–1/4 in long. The seeds contain the phytoestrogen known as anethole. Anise is used to flavor various liqueurs like the Greek ouzo and the French anisette.

Health: Eating a few seeds help digestion, reduces intestinal spasms and bloating and reduces menstrual cramps. It is given to colicky babies to control intestinal distress. Anise is also used to treat unproductive cough to loosen phlegm and is a constituent of many cough lozenge formulations. The anise seed oil is also used to treat hair lice and to control bad breath. Large dosages have a narcotic effect and can also cause bleeding.

Asafoetida *(Ferula asafoetida):* **Kingdom: Plantae; Division: Angiospermae, Class: Eudicots Asterids Order: Apiales Family: Apiaceae; Genus: Ferula Species:** *F. asafoetida.* **Chromosome number, 2n = 22.**

The asafoetida plant is a perennial herb growing in Afghanistan, Iran, Pakistan and India. It is a monoecious plant with separate male and female flowers. Plants grow to a height of about 5 ft with hollow stems about 5 inches in diameter. Flowers are produced in clusters of umbels and individual flowers are greenish yellow. Stem cortex contain resinous ducts. Fruits are oval and reddish in color. The rhizome and taproot produce a white gummy resin that dries to a dark brown color. It has a fetid smell but when added as a spice with turmeric can give a more pleasant smell like leek. The gum was known as devils dung or food of the Gods or Hing in Hindi. Asafoetida is a common spice used in the Indian sub-continent. **Health:** Asafoetida contains Ferulic acid that is being considered as an anti-ageing chemical and is used in certain skin cosmetics. It also contains numerous other phytochemicals such as di-allyl-sulfide, umbelliferone, isopimpinellin and other chemicals that have anti-cancer, anti-inflammatory, anti-neoplastic, anti-bacterial and other properties. In alternative medicine, it is used as an anti-flatulent digestive aid that eases colic and aids in treating irritable bowel syndrome. In the nineteenth century, it was a common prescription for treating hysteria and mood swings. It was also used for treating abdominal injuries and also for treating influenza. There is evidence that asafoetida repels certain insects. Excessive and prolonged usage can trigger lip swelling and throat irritation. Further, external use of asafoetida for controlling abdominal pain as is used in certain south East Asian countries can cause genital swelling.

Basil/Holy Basil *(Ocimum tenuiflorum/O.sanctum):* **Kingdom: Plantae; Division: Angiospermae, Class: Eudicots, Family: Lamiaceae/Labiatae; Chromosome number. 2n = 32.**

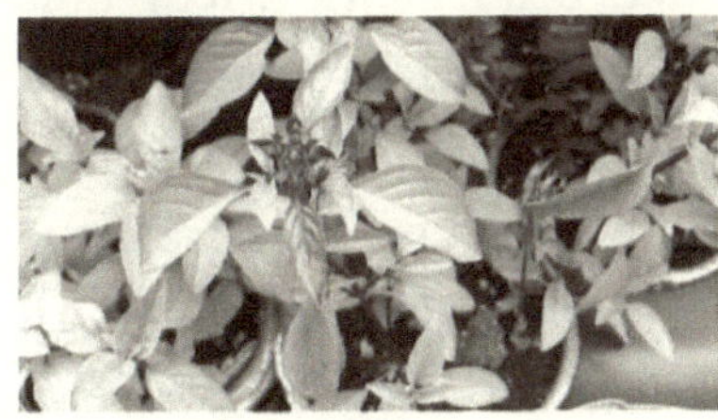

Basil

The Thai basil (*O.basilicum*), the hybrid Thai lemon basil and the hoary basil (*O.americanum*) are close relatives. Holy Basil also known as Thulasi in India is an aromatic shrub with green (Lakshmi Thulasi) or purplish green leaves (Krishna Thulasi) and small racemate pink/white flowers. The entire plant is aromatic due to the presence of an essential oil. **Health:** The holy basil Thulasi has been used for thousands of years in Ayurveda for its diverse healing properties. It is considered to be an adaptogenic and elixir of life. It is said to increase longevity and is used to treat multiple diseases including coughs and colds, respiratory illnesses, skin and digestive diseases. Basil is used for stomach spasms, loss of appetite, intestinal gas, kidney conditions, fluid retention, head colds, warts, and worm infections. It is also used to treat snake and insect bites. Women sometimes use basil before and after childbirth to promote blood circulation, and also to start the flow of breast milk. Basil is a good source of vitamin C, calcium, magnesium, potassium, and iron. The basil plants contain teratogenicity and cancer causing chemicals in low amounts.

Black Pepper: *(Piper nigrum)*, **Kingdom: Plantae, Class: Magnoliids, Order: Piperales, Family: Piperaceae. Chromosome number, 2n = 46, 52, 104 and 128.**

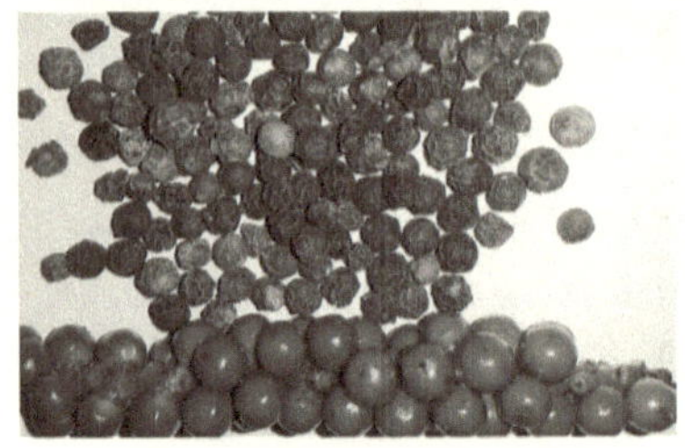

Black Pepper

Black pepper (*Piper nigrum*) is a flowering vine in the family Piperaceae, cultivated for its fruit, which is usually dried and used as a spice and seasoning. When dried, the fruit is known as a peppercorn. When fresh and fully mature, it is approximately 5 millimeters (0.20 in) in diameter, dark red, and, like all drupes, contains a single seed. Several pearl-like fruits are borne on the flower stalk called as a catkin. The fruit along with seed is boiled briefly and dried. This results in black pepper. If the fruit skin is removed and then dried without the skin, it results in white pepper. If the fruit along with seed, is used fresh or in brine then, you have green pepper and likewise if the ripe red fruit is used as such without drying, it results in red pepper. All the different types are used in preparing various foods and as pickle or as a garnish.

The pepper plant is a perennial woody vine growing up to 13 ft in height on supporting trees, poles, or trellises. It is a spreading vine, rooting readily where trailing stems touch the ground. The leaves are alternate, entire, 5 to 10 centimetres (2.0 to 3.9 in) long and 3 to 6 centimetres (1.2 to 2.4 in) across. The flowers are small, produced on pendulous spikes 4 to 8 centimetres (1.6 to 3.1 in) long at the leaf nodes, the spikes lengthening up to 7 to 15 centimetres (2.8 to 5.9 in) as the fruit matures. The fruit of the black pepper is called a drupe and when dried is known as a peppercorn. **Health:** *Piper nigrum* fruits/seeds are used to treat constipation, diarrhoea, earache, gangrene, heart disease, hernia, hoarseness, indigestion, insect bites, insomnia, joint pain, liver problems, lung disease, oral abscesses, sunburn, tooth decay, and toothaches. Pepper contains many phytochemicals, including amides, piperidines, and pyrrolidines and trace amounts of Safrole that may be carcinogenic in laboratory rodents. The Long Pepper (*Piper longum*) is morphologically very similar to *Piper nigrum* and is used as a flavoring agent. Now, it is used mainly in traditional Ayurvedic, Siddha and Unani medicines

Cardomom *(Eletteria cardomom)*: Kingdom: Plantae, Group: Angiospermae, Class: Monocotyledonae Order: Zingiberales Zingiberaceae. Chromosome number Mysore varieties: 2n = 48, 52, Malabar varieties 2n = 48, 50.

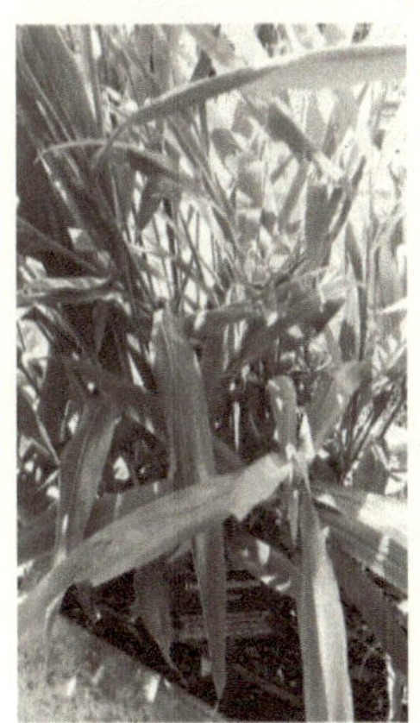
Cardomom

The brown – black seeds, found in seedpods or the green pods with seeds inside are used to spice-up foods and used in medicinal preparations. *Elettaria cardamomum* is a perennial bushy plant native to tropic regions, and can grow to heights of 10' or more, with the tall stems showing long, alternate leaves.

The plants have an underground rhizome from which many shoots arise. The shoots are similar to Ginger. Cardamom requires a steady supply of moisture and will not tolerate drought. If growing in a greenhouse, it should be kept humid and maintained carefully. Cardamom is not cold

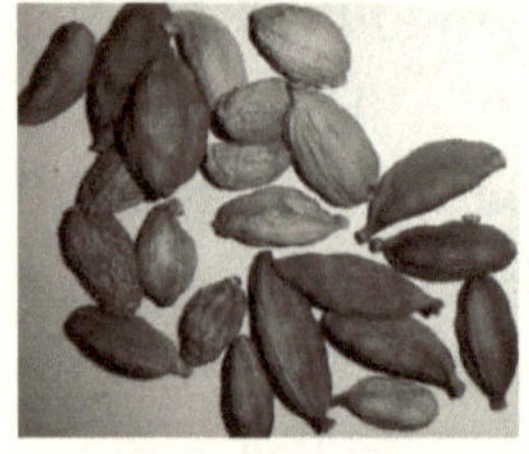
Pods

tolerant and it should be kept in a location with many hours of partially occluded sunlight. The cardamom plants can grow to be large bushes consisting of long, straight, slender stems with numerous symmetrical, dark green, pointed leaves. **Health:** The seeds contain terpineol, limonene, menthone, cineol, myrcene and other phytochemicals. The seeds are chewed as breath fresheners. They are also used in formulations to control pulmonary congestion and to break-up kidney stones.

Caraway/Kala Jeera/Perum Jeerakam *(Carum carvi):* **Kingdom: Plantae; Division: Angiospermae; Class: Eudicots Order: Umbelliferae, Family: Apiaceae. Chromosome number, 2n = 20.**

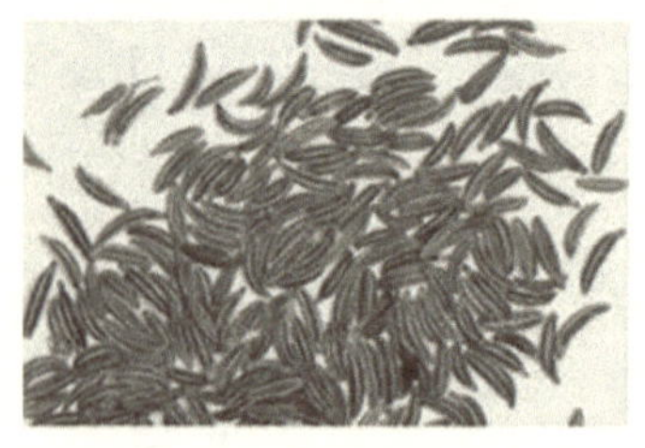
Caraway

Caraway seeds are used to flavor baked foods, liquors, rice dishes and in cosmetic preparations. Caraway plants are biennial with feathery leaves and small pink or white flowers in umbels. The plants look very similar to Carrot, Dill, and Cumin. **Health:** Caraway oil might improve digestion and relieve spasms in the stomach and intestines. Traditionally, Caraway is used for digestive problems including heartburn, bloating, gas, loss of appetite, and mild spasms of the stomach and intestines. Caraway oil is also used to help people cough up phlegm, improve control of urination, kill bacteria in the body, and relieve constipation.

Chives: *(Allium schoenaprasum):* **Kingdom: Plantae; Division: Angiospermae, Class: Monocotyledonae; Order: Asperagales; Family: Amaryllidaceae. Chromosome number, 2n = 16, 2n = 4x = 32.**

Allium schoenoprasum is a small bulbous perennial that is commonly used as a culinary herb to impart mild onion flavor to many foods, including salads, soups, vegetables and sauces. They feature thin, tubular, grass-like, dark green leaves that typically grow in dense clumps to 12." Flower heads can be used as a garnish for soups and salads. **Health:** Bulbs contain organosulfur compounds such as allyl sulfides and alkyl sulfoxides. Chives are reported to have a beneficial effect on the circulatory system.

Cinnamon *(Cinnamomum sp.):* **Kingdom: Plantae; Division: Angiosperms, Class: Magnoliids Order: Laurales Family: Lauraceae Genus: *Cinnamomum* Binomial name *Cinnamomum cassia* (Chinese Cinnamon), *C. vera/C. Zeylanicum* (Sri lankan *Cinnamon*), *C. burmannii* (Indonesian cinnamon), *C. loureiroi* (Vietnamese cinnamon), *C. tamala* (Malabar cinnamon/tamalapatram/Malabathrum/Indian bay leaf/ tejpat). Chromosome number, 2n = 24.**

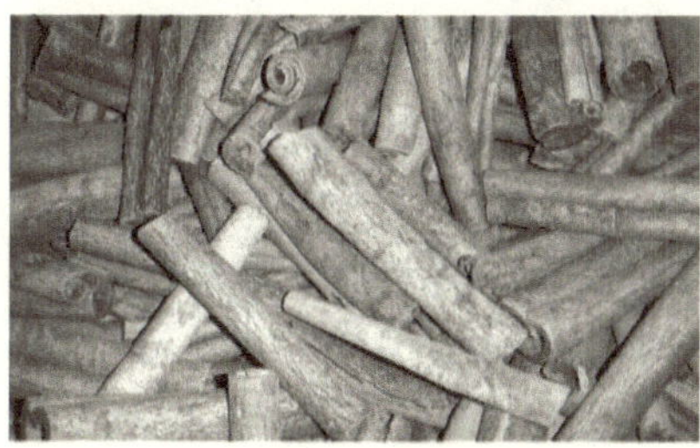

Cinnamon sticks

Cinnamomum cassia called Chinese cassia or Chinese cinnamon is the most common species of Cinnamon that is marketed as Cinnamon. However, most connoisseurs consider SriLanka or Ceylon Cinnamon as the most authentic type of Cinnamon. All species of Cinnamon are evergreen trees and widely cultivated in China, in southern and eastern Asia, India, Sri Lanka, Indonesia, Laos, Malaysia, Taiwan, Thailand, and Vietnam and in the Seychelles and Madagascar in Eastern Africa. The tree grows to 10–15 m tall with greyish bark and hard elongated leaves that are 10–15 cm long and have a decidedly reddish colour when young. The dried bark is carefully stripped from the stems and used as the spice after drying and processing. The different species can be distinguished by the nature of the bark (thickness, stiffness, ability to powder) and aroma. The bark and oil contain cinnamic aldehydes. Pieces of bark powder and oil are used as flavoring spices in foods and in flavored alcohol. **Health:** The bark powder is used to control insulin resistance and as a supplement for treating Type 2 Diabetes. However, it should be noted that Cinnamon bark contains substantial amounts of the blood-thinning agent Coumarin and hence people with liver problems and those on blood thinning agents should use caution if using Cinnamon health supplements.

Cloves *(Syzygium aromaticum)*: Kingdom: Plantae: Angiosperms, Class: Eudicots, Rosids Order: Myrtales, Family: Myrtaceae Genus: Syzygium Species: S. *aromaticum*, **Binomial name:** *Syzygium aromaticum*

Synonyms: *Caryophyllus aromaticus, Eugenia aromatic, Eugenia caryophyllata, Eugenia Caryophyllus.* **Chromosome number, 2n = 22.**

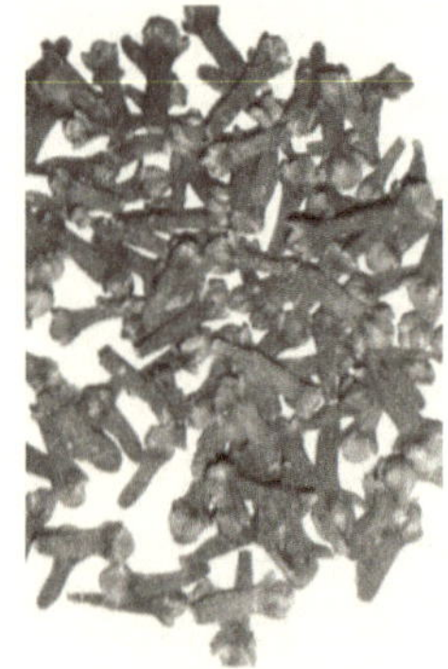

Cloves

The flower buds of the clove tree that are mainly grown in India, Indonesia, Zanzibar/Madagascar and Sri Lanka and in other parts of Africa are used as the clove spice to garnish foods spice up wines and liquors and certain medicinal preparations. The clove trees are evergreen trees that grow to a height of 40 ft. It has large leaves and flowers borne in terminal clusters. The flowers have a long calyx with 4 sepals and 4 petals. The flowers are harvested in the bud stage and generally sun and air-dried. The dried buds are brown in color and are aromatic. They contain the chemical eugenol. **Health:** Cloves and clove oil are used in Ayurvedic and Chinese traditional medicine mainly as an anesthetic to control toothache.

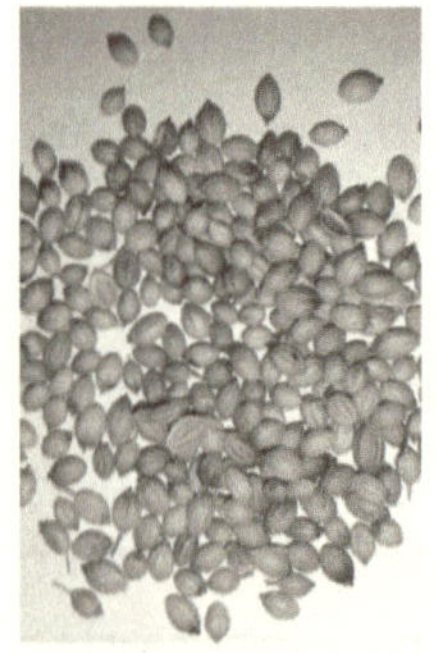

Coriander

Coriander/cilantro *(Coriandrum sativum)*: Kingdom: Plantae; Division: Angiospermae Class: Eudicots Asterids Order: Apiales Family: Apiaceae, Genus and species: Coriandrum sativum. **Chromosome number, 2n = 22.**

Coriandrum known also as Chinese parsley is an annual herb commonly grown in China, India, Sri Lanka and other south East Asian countries as well as Mexico and Central America. It is an annual herb with very tender stems, serrated leaves and small hermaphrodite white or pink flowers in umbels. The fruits are aromatic and are known as schizocarps. In order to germinate, the seeds have to be split in two before sowing. Fresh as well as dried seeds as well as the leaves are used to spice up foods. Seeds and leaves contain the terpenes linalool and pinene that gives the special aroma. **Health:** The seeds as well as leaves contain dietary minerals such as calcium, selenium, iron, magnesium and manganese. Seeds are rich in Oxalic acid and as such, consumption of large quantities may cause kidney stone formation.

Cumin *(Cuminum siminum)*: Kingdom: Plantae; Division: Angiospermae, Class: Eudicots Order: Apiales Family: Apiaceae. Chromosome number, 2n = 14.

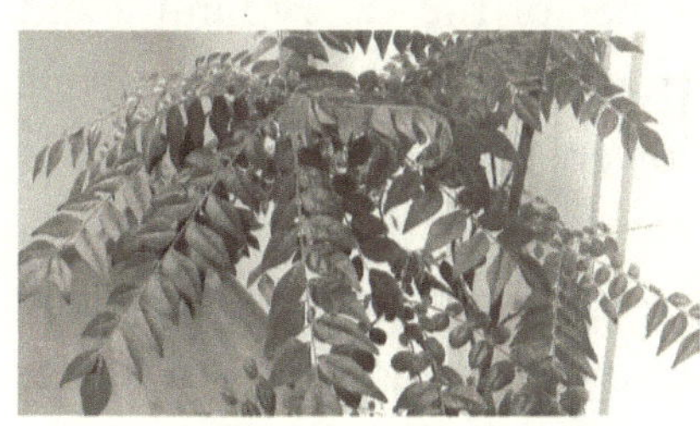

Cumin

Cumin is a culinary and medicinal herb seed that is related to parsley. Plants are annual herbs with branched stems and pinnate or bi-pinnate leaves. Flowers are borne in umbels. Fruits are achenes with a single seed. Seeds are ridged and similar in appearance to caraway seeds. Dried seeds are used as such or after powdering for culinary purposes. Seeds contain cuminaldehyde, cymene and terpinoids. **Health:** Decoctions, infusions, tablets and seeds as such are used as digestive aids and are also components of various Ayurvedic and Siddha formulations. Seed extracts have anti-microbial properties.

Curry leaves *(Murraya Koenigi)*: Kingdom: Plantae, Division: Angiospermae, Class: Eudicots Order: Sapindales Family: Rutaceae. Chromosome number, 2n = 18.

The leaves of the curry tree are used as a garnish in various food preparations of the "curry type" popular in India, Sri Lanka, Cambodia, Myanmar and other countries including the USA where the Indian diaspora have spread. The plants are small trees growing in

Curry Leaves

tropical and sub-tropical countries. The leaves on the tree branches are pinnate with 10–20 glabrous aromatic leaves. Flowers are white in color and are self-pollinated. Fruits are small and globular. Only the leaves are used to garnish foods. Fresh, dry or fried leaves are used.

Health: The leaves and leaf powders are used in Ayurvedic medicine for treating gastrointestinal distress as well as for diabetic control. The leaves contain many alkaloids including girinimbine that shows apoptopic qualities in experimental hepatic cell lines.

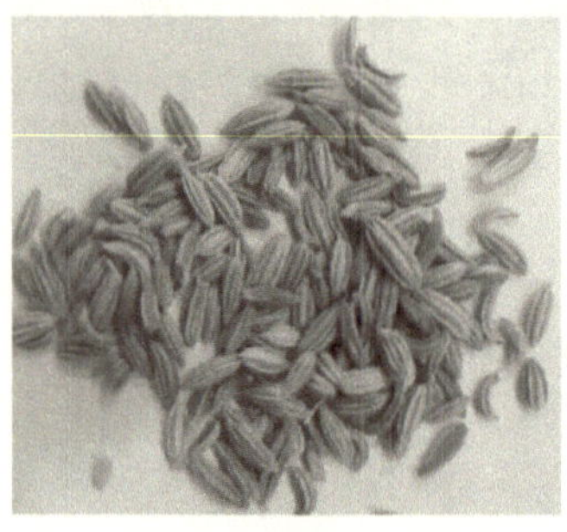

Dill

Dill *(Anethum graveolens):* **Kingdom: Plantae; Division: Angiospermae, Class: Eudicots Order: Apiales; Family: Apiaceae. Chromosome number, 2n = 20.**

Dill seeds are used to spice up foods in many countries. Plants are herbaceous, growing to a height of 2 ft with slender stems and feather-like narrow leaves. Flowers grow on umbels. Seeds contain an aromatic essential oil. **Health:** Chewing Dill seeds help digestion and are anti-flatulent. Seeds and oil have anti-microbial properties.

Fennel *(Foeniculum vulgare):* **Kingdom: Plantae; Division: Angiosperms; Class: Eudicots, Asterids, Order: Apiales Family: Apiaceae, Umbelliferae Genus:** *Foeniculum,* **Species:** *F. vulgare.* **Syn:** *F. officianalis, F.dulce.* **Chromosome number, 2n = 22.**

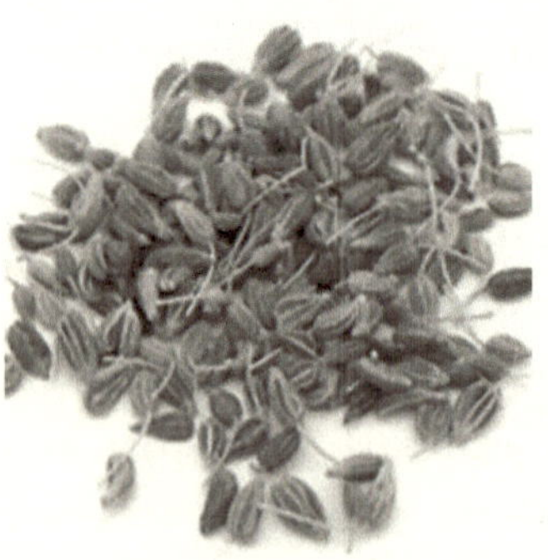

Fennel

It is a member of the celery family and is a hardy perennial herb with a bulbous stem, yellow flowers and feathery leaves. It is indigenous to the shores of the Mediterranean but has become widely naturalized in many parts of the world especially on dry soils near the seacoast and on riverbanks. The plants are highly aromatic and the oil of fennel is a component of the popular liqueur absinthe. Plants grow to a height of about 10 ft. Leaves are divided into threadlike blades. Flowers are tiny, produced in umbels. Seeds are very tiny about 10 mm long. About 5% of the dried seed is made of an essential oil that contains the stilbenoid foeniculoside. The seeds are used as a flavoring agent in foods.

Health: It is known to have carminative properties. It has Anti-gas and digestive stimulant properties. It is a component of many cough syrups, juices, lozenges to control cough and bronchitis. It is also a component of some anti-asthma syrup because of its anti-spasmodic properties.

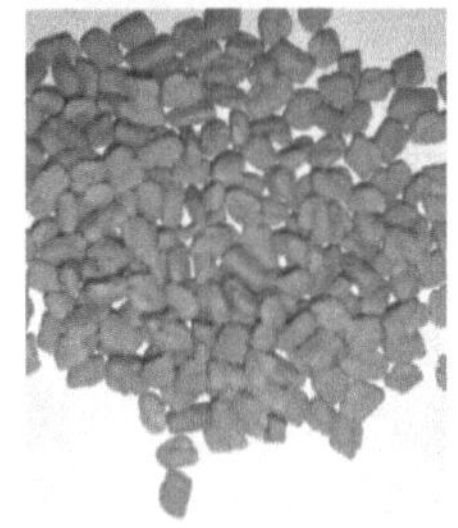

Fenugreek

Fenugreek *(Trigonella foenum-graecum)*: Kingdom: Plantae, Division: Angiospermae, Class: Eudicots, Order: Fagales, Family: Fagaceae/ Leguminosae. Genus and species: *Trigonella foenum-graecum*. Chromosome number, 2n = 16.

Fenugreek is an annual herbaceous plant in the family Fabaceae with leaves consisting of three small obovate to oblong leaflets. It is cultivated worldwide as a semiarid crop and its seeds are a common ingredient in dishes from the Indian Subcontinent. Both fresh and dried leaves are used as vegetables and the yellow seeds are used as a spice mainly in the Indian subcontinent.

Seeds are often roasted to reduce bitterness and enhance flavor. When sold as a vegetable in India, the young plants are harvested with their roots still attached and sold in small bundles in the markets and bazaars. The distinct flavor is due to the presence of the alkaloid trigonelline and the Saponin yamogenin.

Health: Whole seeds, powdered seeds and leaves appear to slow absorption of sugars in the stomach and stimulate insulin. Both of these effects lower blood sugar in people with diabetes. It is commonly used in Ayurvedic medicine to control blood sugar. Fenugreek is also used for digestive problems such as loss of appetite, upset stomach, constipation and inflammation of the stomach (gastritis). It is also used for conditions that affect heart health such as "hardening of the arteries," atherosclerosis and for high blood levels of certain fats including cholesterol and triglycerides. Other popular uses include correcting erectile dysfunction and as a poultice to control inflammation.

Ginger *(Zingiber officinale)*: Kingdom: Plantae Division: Angiospermae; Class: Monocots Commelinids Order: Zingiberales Family: Zingiberaceae. Chromosome number, 2n = 22. Many polyploid varieties exist.

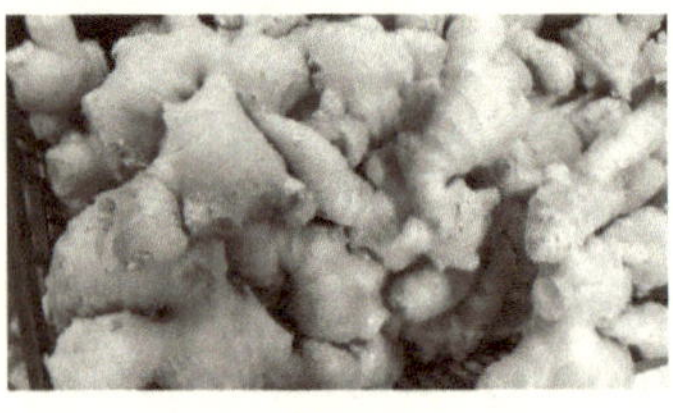

Ginger

Ginger is a perennial herb that grows well in tropical and semi tropical countries. Plants have branched swollen underground stems that are the rhizomes. These rhizomes look like a swollen hand and are the main source of the aromatic spice used in cooking and in medicinal preparations. The underground stems are topped above ground by the leafy pseudo stems that grow from the buds of the rhizome. Flowers grow in cone shaped spikes with yellow flowers. Both the pseudo stems and the true stem (rhizome) are used as spice. The pungent principles in ginger are the non-volatile phenolic compounds gingerol, gingeridione and shogaol. **Health:** Ginger rhizome is used in traditional medicine to control nausea and vomiting due to vertigo, motion sickness and pregnancy. However, some reports indicate potential for miscarriage if used by pregnant women. It is a sialagogue (stimulating saliva). The rhizome contains an essential oil namely, gingerol, which is used as a flavoring agent. There are unconfirmed reports of its use as an anti-cancer agent.

Lavender *(Lavendula angustifolia)*: Kingdom: Plantae Division: Angiosperms, Class Eudicots Division: Asterids Order: Lamiales Family: Lamiaceae Subfamily: Nepetoideae Tribe: Lavanduleae Genus: Lavandula, Type species *Lavandula spica*. Chromosome

number, 2n = 10, 12, 14, 16, 18, 20, 22, 26 depending on variety, possibly due to ploidy levels.

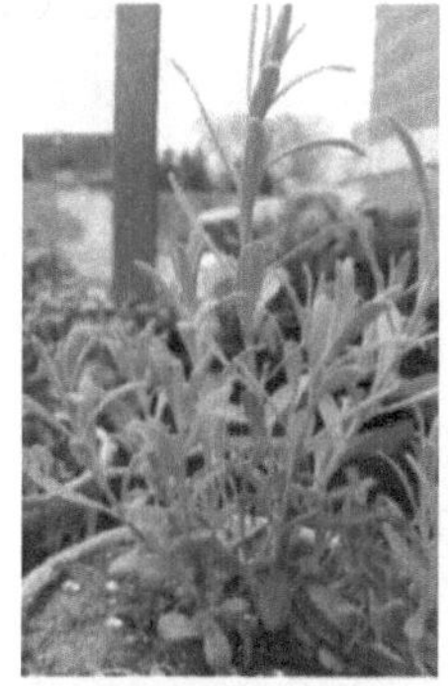

Lavender

The genus includes plants that are annuals, perennials or shrubs. The plant is mainly used for extracting Lavender oil used in aromatherapy and as an anti – anxiolytic agent. Flowers are used in formulations for preparing herbal tea and used as a condiment to flavor baked goods. **Health:** Oil is used in aromatherapy and in sleep formulations.

Lemon balm *(Mellissa officianalis)*: **Kingdom: Plantae, Division: Angiosperms, Class: Eudicots, Asterids, Order: Lamiales Family: Lamiaceae Genus: Melissa Species: M. officinalis Binomial name** *Melissa Officianalis.* **Chromosome number, 2n = 28.**

Lemon balm plants are related to mint. Plants are herbs growing to a height of about 2 ft. In the spring and summer, clusters of small, light yellow flowers full of nectar grow where the leaves meet the stem. The leaves are very deeply wrinkled and range from dark green to yellowish green in color, depending on the soil and climate. When the leaves, are rubbed, aromatic vapors that smell like lemons are released. **Health:** Lemon balm leaves and oil are used as mild sedatives and as anti-anxiolytic agents. Lemon balm contains chemicals that seem to have a sedative, calming effect. It might also reduce the growth of some viruses like Herpes. The leaf juice has mosquito repellant properties.

Marjoram *(Origanum marjorana, Origanum majorana, syn. Majorana hortensis Moench, Majorana majorana):* **Kingdom: Plantae; Division: Angiospermae Class: Eudicots; Order: Lamiales Family: Lamiaceae. Chromosome number, 2n = 54. Ploidy Variations of 6 x, 12 xs, 24 x and 48 xs have been noted.**

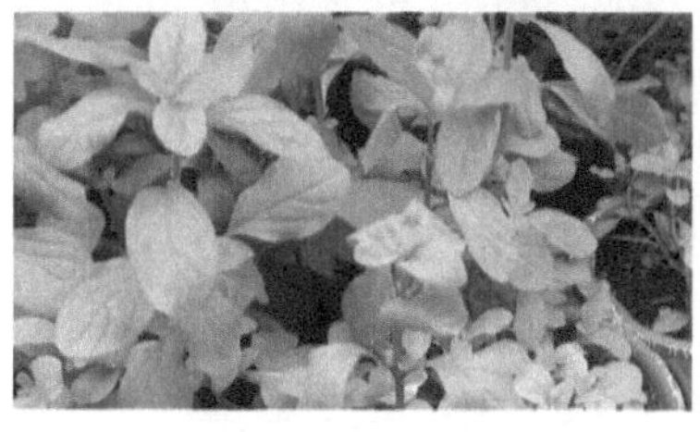

Marjoram

It is a perennial plant growing in temperate climates. Plants grow to about 2 ft and have dark green leaves similar to those of basil. Leaves contain many phytochemicals. **Health;** Flowers, leaves, and oil are used for medicinal purposes. Tea made from the leaves or flowers is used as a treatment for runny nose and colds in infants and toddlers, Marjoram tea is also used for various digestive problems including poor appetite, liver disease, gallstones, intestinal gas, and stomach cramps. Some women use marjoram tea for relieving symptoms of menopause, treating mood swings related to menstrual periods, starting menstruation, and promoting the flow of breast milk. Other uses include treating diabetes, sleep problems, muscle spasms, headaches, sprains, bruises and back pain. It is also used as a "nerve tonic" and a "heart tonic," and to promote better blood circulation.

Mustard (Brassica Nigra)

Mustard seeds and seed paste are used as a spice-condiment to flavor foods. Details of the Mustard plant are given elsewhere under oil seeds.

Nutmeg *(Myristica fragrans)*: Kingdom: Plantae Division: Angiosperms, Class, Magnoliids, Order: Magnoliales, Family: Myristicaceae. Chromosome number, 2n = 38.

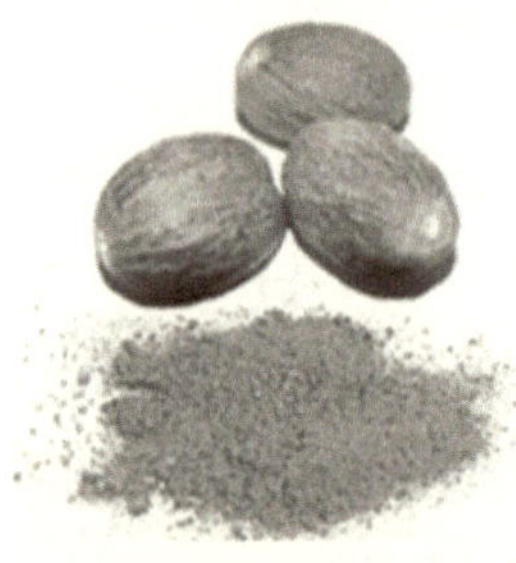

Nutmeg

This is an evergreen tree growing in tropical weather that is the source of the spices nutmeg as well as mace. The tree grows to an average of 20 ft tall to an upper limit of 60 ft. Leaves are dark green, glabrous and alternately arranged. Plants are dioecious with staminate male flowers and pistillate female flowers on different plants. Flowers are borne in groups of 10–15. The pistillate female flowers develop into fruits after pollination. Fruits are globular about the size of a small egg, Fruits split open into two halves revealing a seed covered by an aril. The seed proper is the source of nutmeg whereas, the aril is the source of mace. Both nutmeg and mace are used to flavor foods. An essential oil that is used for culinary purposes is obtained from the nutmeg seeds. **Health:** Nutmeg and mace have no known medicinal properties. However, in large doses, nutmeg has psychoactive properties and can cause serious mental disturbances and behavioral changes including delirium. It can cause nausea, convulsions and palpitations.

Oregano *(Origanum vulgare):* **Kingdom: Plantae Division: Angiosperms, Class, Eudicots Division: Asterids Order: Lamiales Family: Lamiaceae Genus:** *Origanum* **Species:** *O. vulgare.* **Chromosome number, x = 5–11, 13, 17, 20, Polymorphic.**

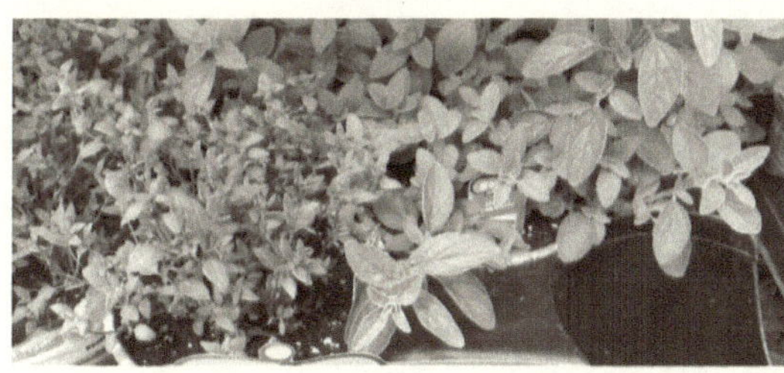
Oregano

Oregano is a perennial herb growing from 20–80 cm tall with opposite leaves 1–4 cm long. The flowers are purple 3–4 mm long produced in erect spikes. Oregano is related to the herb Marjoram sometimes being referred to as wild marjoram. Oregano is an important culinary herb used for the flavor of its leaves that can be more flavorful when dried than fresh.

Health: Among the chemical compounds contributing to the flavor are carvacrol, thymol, limonene, pinene, ocimene and caryophyllene. Oregano contains polyphenols including numerous flavones. Oregano contains chemicals that might help reduce cough and spasms. Oregano also might help digestion by increasing bile flow and fighting against some bacteria, viruses, fungi, intestinal worms, and other parasites.

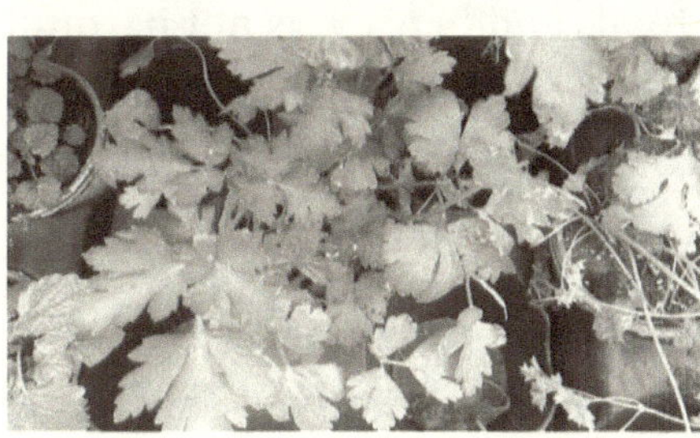
Parsley

Parsley *(Petroselenium crispum):* **Kingdom; Plantae; Group: Angiosperms, Class Eudicots Asterids Order: Apiales, Family: Apiaceae. Chromosome number, 2n = 12.**

Parsley is an annual or biennial plant that is a native of Mediterranean countries but now grown in most temperate climatic conditions as well as in subtropical areas. It produces small tri pinnate leaves. When flowers are produced, they are in umbellate crowns with multiple flowers. The leaves are rich in anti-oxidants, beta-carotene, lutein and lycopene.

Health: Parsley is a good source of anti-oxidants and hence considered good for cardiovascular health. Because of its uterotonic effects, it is not safe for women to consume large amounts of parsley in salads and other foods.

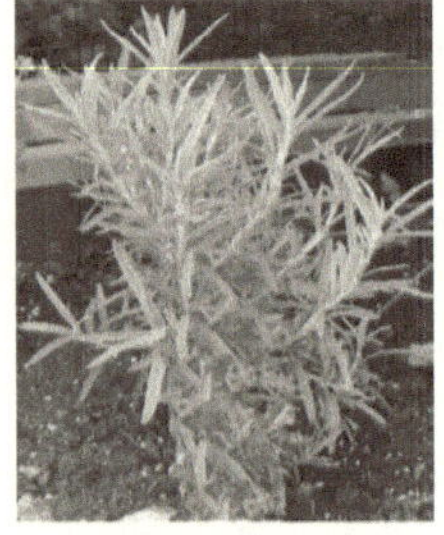

Rosemary

Rosemary *(Rosemarinus officinalis)*: Kingdom: Plantae, Division: Angiospermae, Class: Eudicots, Order: Lamiales, Lamiaceae, *Rosmarinus, officinalis*. Chromosome number, 2n = 24.

The leaves are used as a spice in foods and flavor in herbal tea formulations. Plants are aromatic evergreen 5 ft-6 ft trailing or upright shrubs related to mint. They have a mustard-like slightly bitter taste. **Health:** Leaves contain rosmarinic acid, camphor, caffeic acid, ursolic acid, betulinic acid and the antioxidants carnosic acid and carnosoosem. The oil is used in aromatherapy. Rosemary is used topically (applied to the skin) for preventing and treating baldness; treating circulation problems, toothache, eczema, and joint or muscle pain such as myalgia, sciatica, and intercostal neuralgia. It is also used for wound healing, in bath therapy (balneotherapy), and as an insect repellent. Generally, only a teaspoon of the leaf-powder or oil is used to flavor foods and hence it is not harmful at that amount. Reportedly, it is sometimes used as an abortifacient in large quantities. It can lead to deep coma, spasm, vomiting and even death.

Saffron *(Crocus sativus)*: Kingdom: Plantae; Division: Angiospermae, Class: Monocotyledonae; Family: Iridaceae; Binomial name: *Crocus sativus*. Chromosome number, 2n = 3X = 24.

The style and stigmas (female receptive part of flower) of Saffron flower are used as a spice for various culinary purposes and the golden red dye from it can be used to color foods. The plants are triploid which means that they have 3 sets of chromosomes derived by natural hybridization of different wild species. As with all triploids, the plants are sterile and can be propagated only by vegetative means through the small underground corms that they produce. Corms are modified swollen underground stems. Plants grow to a height of one foot and membrane-

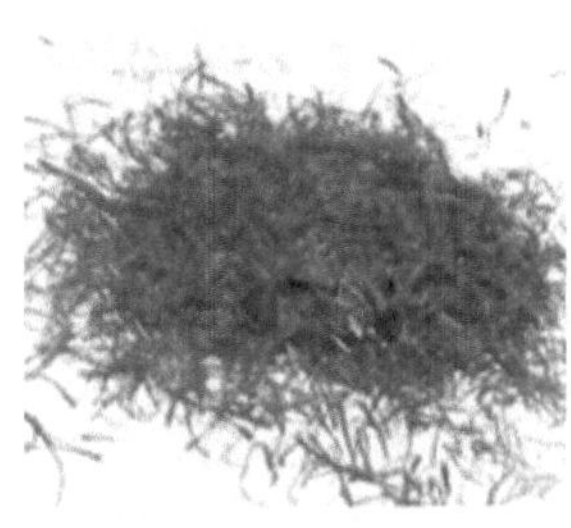

Saffron

like non-photosynthetic leaves known as cataphylls arise protecting the true monocot leaves. During the first year, they produce lilac colored flowers with a long stigma. It is the style and stigma that are used for flavoring and coloring foods. It takes hundreds of flowers to produce a commercially useful amount, which explains why saffron is so expensive. With each successive year, the corms (which look like bulbs) will multiply, the size of the planting will increase, and you will be able to harvest more of the spicy stigmas. **Health:** Saffron contains pre-carotene crocin and chemicals picrocrocin and safranal. The saffron seems to have antidepressive effects and possibly has anti-cancer properties.

Sage *(Salvia officianalis):* **Kingdom: Plantae, Division: Angiospermae, Class: Eudicots, Order: Lamiales, Family: Lamiaceae, Salvia officinalis. Chromosome number, 2n = 14**

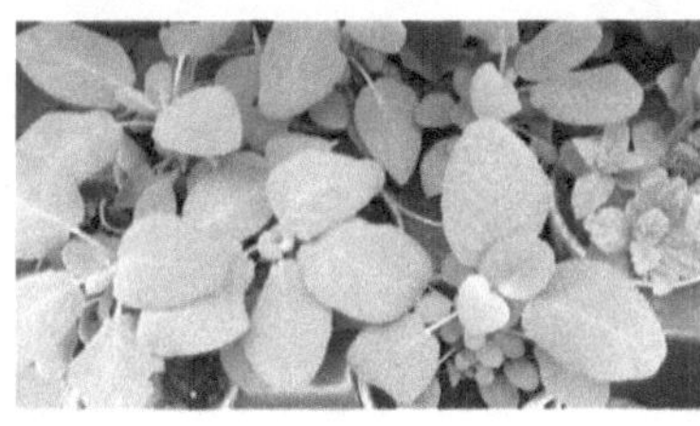

Sage

The dried leaves/leaf powder is used to flavor certain British and European foods but is not generally used in Asian cooking. It is a perennial evergreen shrub with green-grey leaves and bluish-purple flowers. However, many other cultivars grown in gardens have variegated leaves and flowers. Sage is mainly grown in temperate climatic conditions. **Health:** Salvia leaves and oil contains cineol, borneol, thujone, fumaric acid, caffeic acid, various flavones and estrogens. It is highly valued as a healing plant. In India, it is an important component of certain cough syrups and formulations for respiratory conditions. Sage is used for digestive problems, including loss of appetite, gas (flatulence), stomach pain (gastritis), diarrhea, bloating, and heartburn. It is also used for reducing overproduction of perspiration and saliva; and for depression, memory loss, and Alzheimer's disease. Sage leaf extracts seem to enhance memory and attention.

Spearmint *(Mentha spicata):* **Kingdom: Plantae, Division: Angiospermae, Class: Eudicots, Order: Lamiales Family: Lamiaceae, Genus/species Mentha spicata. Chromosome number, 2n = 48.**

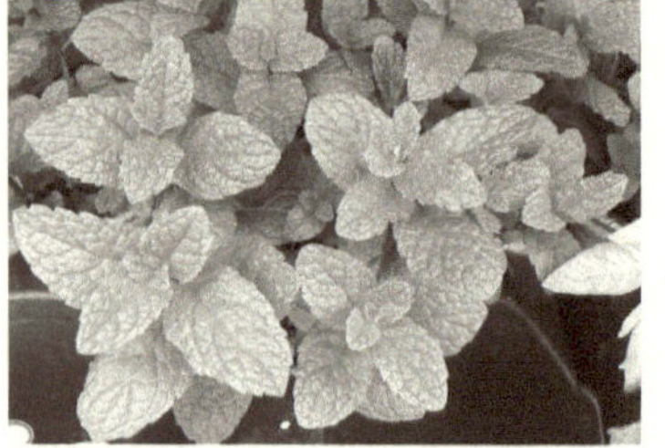

Mentha mint

Mentha leaves are used as flavoring agents, chutney-pickles and as breath-fresheners. They have considerable usage in herbal medicine. Plants are perennials that grow in both temperate and tropical climates. Leaves are serrated and range in colors from deep green to light blue and purple depending on the variety. The plants can spread fast and may be invasive. **Health:** Mint oils are used in cosmetics and insect repellants. Leaves are chewed to help in digestive process and is said to ameliorate stomach illnesses. Mint may cause allergic reactions in some people.

Tarragon/Drago's Mugwort/Estragon *(Artemesis dracunculus):* **Kingdom: Plantae, Division: Angiospermae, Class: Eudicots, Order: Asterales, Family: Asteraceae. Chromosome number, 2n = 18, 2n = 4x = 36, 2n = 6x = 54.**

Tarragon is a green perennial shrub. The shrub is native to the sunny and dry regions north of the tropic of cancer, especially the United States, Asia and Siberia. People in Europe grow this shrub commercially for its perfumed leaves that pass on a licorice-anise essence to salads, sauces and foods prepared with vinegar. Tarragon plants have slender stalks and grow up to a height of two feet and bears glossy green, elongated and slender leaves that are undivided. This shrub is intimately related to wormwood. Tarragon has fibrous roots that are long and extend to all areas where they are grown by means of runners. The shrub bears small flowers that are circular and have a yellow hue with black heads. Flowers of this herb rarely open completely. **Health:** Tarragon contains tannins, coumarins, and flavonoids and also estragole that may be toxic. The plant is closely related to the wormwood plant (*Artemesia*) which contains the anti-malarial artimisin. It remains to be seen if Tarragon also has anti-malarial properties. In herbal medicine, it is recommended for helping digestive processes.

Thyme *(Thymus vulgaris):* Kingdom: Plantae, Division: Angiospermae, Class: Eudicots, Order: Lamiales Family: Lamiaceae. Chromosome number, 2n = 24.

It is a bushy, woody-based evergreen subshrub with small, highly aromatic, grey-green leaves and clusters of purple or pink flowers in early summer. In gardens, it is planted as a ground cover. Leaves contain Thymol that is a disinfectant. **Health;** Thymol is a powerful anti-microbial agent and is a component of many mouthwashes and disinfectants. It is also effective against athlete's foot fungus. It is also used to treat acne and is a component of some cough and cold syrups.

Turmeric *(Curcuma longa):* Kingdom: Plantae, Division: Angiospermae, Class: Monocotyledonae, Order: Zingiberales Family: Zingiberaceae (Ginger family). Common name: Turmeric. Chromosome number, 2n = 62.

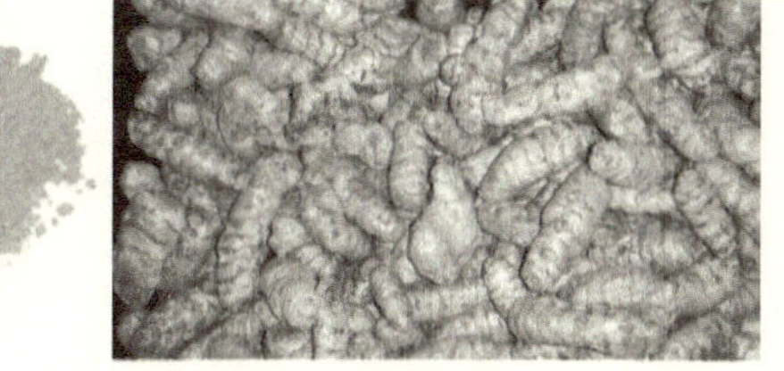

Turmeric powder   **Turmeric**

Curcuma longa is a perennial plant related to ginger growing in tropics and subtropics. They have finger-like rhizomes that are orange-red inside from which long lanceolate leaves that are about 2 feet arise. Flowers are dull yellow, three or five together surrounded by bracteole. It is propagated by cuttings from the rhizome. Fresh roots have an aromatic and spicy fragrance. The rhizomes are dried and powdered for use both as a spice and to extract medicinal Curcuminoids. **Heath:** Turmeric rhizomes contain curcumin and other phytochemicals. It is considered to be very effective in treating gastro-intestinal diseases and is considered to have anti-microbial properties. It is used in many cosmetic preparations. It has powerful anti-oxidant and anti-inflammatory properties that may help protect the circulatory system. Evidence from test tube and animal studies suggests that curcumin may help prevent or treat several types of cancers, including prostate, breast, skin, and colon cancer. Turmeric's preventive effects may relate to its antioxidant properties, which protect cells from damage. More research is needed to verify these claims. There are also reports of its efficacy in adjuvant treatment of type 2 Diabetes and also in treating Alzheimers disease. However, dietary curcumin is poorly absorbed due to poor solubility in water but it is more soluble in alkaline pH. Solubility is also increased if curcumin (turmeric) is taken along with black pepper that contains piperine. Piperine potentiates curcumin absorption. Another approach to increase absorption is to encapsulate the curcumin in liposomes (phytosomes) which are hydrophilic. Liposomes can attach to cell membranes and form vesicles through which the curcumin can be absorbed into cells.

Table 19 – Nutritional profile of Spices

Metabolite	Anise Seeds	Basil Leaves	Pepper Seeds	Cardamom Seeds	Caraway Seeds	Cinnamon Bark	Cloves Buds	Coriander Seeds	Coriander leaves
Water g	9.54	92.06	12.46	8.28	9.87	10.58	9.87	8.86	92.21
Protein-g	17.6	3.15	10.39	10.76	19.77	3.99	5.97	12.37	2.13
Total lipid (fat), g	15.9	0.64	3.26	6.7	14.59	1.24	13	17.77	0.52
Carbohydrate, g	50	2.65	63.95	68.47	49.9	80.59	65.53	54.99	3.67
Fiber	14.6	1.6	25.3	28	38	53.1	33.9	41.9	2.8
Sugar	NA	0.3	0.64	28	0.64	2.17	2.38	NA	0.87
Calcium, mg	646	177	443	383	689	1002	632	709	67
Iron, mg	37	3.17	9.71	13.97	16.23	8.32	11.83	16.32	1.77
Magnesium, mg	170	64	171	229	258	60	259	330	26
Phosphorus, mg	440	56	158	178	568	64	104	409	48
Potassium, mg	1441	295	1329	1119	1351	431	1020	1267	521
Sodium, mg	16	4	20	18	17	10	277	35	46
Zinc, mg	5.3	0.81	1.19	7.47	5.5	1.83	2.32	4.7	0.5
Vitamin C, mg	21	18	0	21	21	3.8	0.2	21	27
Thiamin, mg	0.34	0.034	0.108	0.198	0.383	0.022	0.158	0.239	0.067
Riboflavin, mg	0.29	0.076	0.18	0.182	0.379	0.041	0.22	0.29	0.162
Niacin, mg	3.06	0.902	1.143	1.102	3.606	1.332	1.56	2.13	1.114
Vitamin B-6, mg	0.65	0.155	0.291	0.23	0.36	0.158	0.391	0	0.149
Folate, DFE,	10	68	17	0	10	6	25	0	62
Vitamin B-12, µg	0	0	0	0	0	0	0	0	0
Vitamin A, µg	16	264	27	0	18	15	8	0	337
Vitamin A, IU	311	5275	547	0	363	295	160	0	6748

Metabolite	Anise Seeds	Basil Leaves	Pepper Seeds	Cardamom Seeds	Caraway Seeds	Cinnamon Bark	Cloves Buds	Coriander Seeds	Coriander leaves
Vitamin E, mg	0	0.8	1.04	0	2.5	2.32	8.82	0	2.5
Vitamin D µ g	0	0	0	0	0	0	0	0	0
Vitamin D, IU	0	0	0	0	0	0	0	0	0
Vitamin K µg	414.8	163.7	0.68	0	31.2	141.8	310		
Fatty acids, g	0.59	0.041	1.392	0.87	0.62	0.345	3.952	0.99	0.014
Mono, g	9.78	0.088	0.739	0.43	7.125	0.246	1.393	13.58	0.275
Polyun sat, G	3.15	0.389	0.998	0	3.272	0.068	3.606	1.75	0.04
Cholesterol, mg	0	0	0	0	0	0	0.254	0	0

Table 20 – Nutritional profile of Spices (2)

Metabolite	Cumin Seeds	Dill Seeds	Fennel Seeds	Fenugreek Seeds	Ginger rhizome	Marjoram dry seeds	Oregano dry leaves	Parsley dry leaf
Water g	8.06	0.16	8.81	8.84	9.94	7.64	9.93	5.89
Protein-g	17.81	305	15.8	23	8.98	12.66	9	26.63
Total lipid (fat), g	22.27	15.98	14.87	6.41	4.24	7.04	4.28	5.48
Carbohydrate, g	44.24	14.54	52.29	58.35	71.62	60.56	68.92	50.64
Fiber, g	10.5	55.17	39.8	24.6	14.1	40.3	42.5	26.7
Sugar, g	2.25	21.1	3.39	4.09	4.09	7.27		
Calcium, mg	931	1516	1196	176	114	1990	1597	1140
Iron, mg	66.36	16.33	18.54	33.53	19.8	82.71	36.8	22.04
Magnesium, mg	366	256	385	191	214	346	270	400
Phosphorus, mg	499	277	487	296	168	306	148	436
Potassium, mg	1788	1186	1694	770	1320	1522	1260	2683
Sodium, mg	168	20	88	67	27	77	25	452
Zinc, mg	4.8	5.2	3.7	2.5	3.64	3.6	2.69	5.44
Vitamin C, mg	7.7	21	21	3	0.7	51.4	2.3	125
Thiamin, mg	0.628	0.418	0.408	0.322	0.046	0.289	0.177	0.196
Riboflavin, mg	0.327	0.284	0.353	0.366	0.17	0.316	0.528	2.383
Niacin, mg	4.579	2.807	6.05	1.64	9.62	4.12	4.64	9.943
Vitamin B-6, mg	0.435	0.25	0.47	0.6	0.626	1.19	1.044	0.9
Folate, DFE,	10	10	57	13	274	237	180	
Vitamin B-12, µg	0	0	0	0	0	0	0	0
Vitamin A, µg	64	3	7	3	2	403	85	97
Vitamin A, IU	1270	53	135	60	30	8068	1701	1939

Metabolite	Cumin Seeds	Dill Seeds	Fennel Seeds	Fenugreek Seeds	Ginger rhizome	Marjoram dry seeds	Oregano dry leaves	Parsley dry leaf
Vitamin E, mg	3.33	0	0	0	1.69	18.26	8.96	
Vitamin D, µg	0	0	0	0	0	0	0	0
Vitamin D, IU	0	0	0	0	0	0	0	0
Vitamin K, µg	5.4	0.8	621.7	621.7	1359.5			
Fatty acids, g	1.535	0.73	0.48	2.599	0.529	1.551	1.378	
Monounsaturated, g	14.04	9.41	9.91	1.46	0.479	0.94	0.716	0.761
Polyunsaturated, g	3.279	1.01	1.69	0	0.929	4.405	1.369	3.124
Cholesterol, mg	0	0	0	0	0	0	0	0

Table 21 – Nutritional profile of Spices (3)

Metabolite	Rosemary Dry, leaf	Saffron style-stigma powder	Sage-Leaf	Sp. Mint leaves	Tarragon Dry Leaves	Thyme Leaves	turmeric Powder
Water g	9.31	11.9	7.96	85.55	7.74	65.11	12.85
Protein-g	4.88	11.43	10.63	3.29	22.77	5.56	9.68
Total lipid (fat), g	15.22	5.85	12.75	0.73	7.24	1.68	3.25
Carbohydrate, g	64.06	65.37	60.73	8.41	50.22	24.45	67.14
Fiber	42.6	3.9	40.3	6.8	7.4	14	22.7
Sugar, g	NA	NA	1.71	NA	NA	NA	3.21
Calcium, mg	1280	111	1652	199	1139	405	168
Iron, mg	29.25	11.1	28.12	11.87	32.3	17.45	55
Magnesium, mg	220	264	428	63	347	160	208
Phosphorus, mg	70	252	91	60	313	106	299
Potassium, mg	955	1724	1070	458	3020	609	2080
Sodium, mg	50	148	11	30	62	9	27
Zinc, mg	3.23	1.09	4.7	1.09	3.9	1.81	4.5
Vitamin C, mg	61.2	80.8	32.4	13.3	50	160.1	0.7
Thiamin, mg	0.514	0.115	0.754	0.078	0.251	0.048	0.058
Riboflavin, mg	0.428	0.267	0.336	0.175	1.339	0.471	0.15
Niacin, mg	1	1.46	5.72	0.948	8.95	1.824	1.35
Vitamin B-6, mg	1.74	1.01	2.69	0.158	2.41	0.348	0.107
Folate, DFE,	307	93	274	105	274	45	20
Vitamin B-12, µg	0	0	0	0	0	0	0

Metabolite	Rosemary Dry, leaf	Saffron style-stigma powder	Sage-Leaf	Sp. Mint leaves	Tarragon Dry Leaves	Thyme Leaves	turmeric Powder
Vitamin A, µg	156	27	295	203	210	238	0
Vitamin A, IU	3128	530	5900	4054	4200	4751	0
Vitamin E, µg	NA	NA	7.48	NA	NA	NA	4.43
Vitamin D µg	0	0	0	0	0	0	0
Vitamin D, IU	0	0	0	0	0	0	0
Vitamin K, µg	NA	NA	1714.5	NA	NA	0	13.4
Fatty acids, g	7.371	1.586	7.03	0.191	1.881	0.467	1.838
Monounsat, g	3.014	0.429	1.87	0.025	0.474	0.081	0.449
Polyun sat, G	2.339	2.067	1.76	0.394	3.698	0.532	0.756
Cholesterol, mg	0	0	0	0	0	0	0

References

Archana Shivnaz, Neeraj Tandon, Anand. (2013): somatic chromosomal studies in Ocimum basilicum & Ocimum sanctum International Journal of Phytomedicine, 5, 330-340

Bailer, J.; Aichinger, T.; Hackl, G.; de Hueber, K.; Dachler, M. (2001): "Essential oil content and composition in commercially available dill cultivars in comparison to caraway," Industrial Crops and Products 14 (3): 229–239. Doi: 10.1016/S0926-6690(01)00088-7.

Beckett, K.A. (1987): The RHS Encyclopedia of House Plants, Century Hutchison.

Cobley, L.S. (1976): An Introduction to the Botany of Tropical Crops, Longman Group United Kingdom (1976), ISBN 10: 0582441536 ISBN 13: 9780582441538.

Delaquis, P.J.; Stanich, K.; Girard, B.; Mazza, G. (2002): "Antimicrobial activity of individual and mixed fractions of dill, cilantro, coriander and eucalyptus essential oils." International Journal of Food Microbiology 74 (1–2): 101–109. Doi: 10.1016/S0168-1605(01)00734-6, PMID 11929164.

Garland, S. (2004): The Complete Book of Herbs & Spices, An Illustrated Guide to Growing and Using Culinary, Aromatic, Cosmetic and Medicinal Plants, Frances Lincoln publishers, London.

Hausenblas H.A., Saha D., Dubyak, P.J, And Anton, S.D (2013): Saffron (*Crocus sativus L.*) and major depressive disorder: a meta-analysis of randomized clinical trials," Journal of Integrative Medicine 11 (6): 377–83. Doi: 10. 3736/jintegrmed2013056, PMID 24299602

http://ecoursesonline.iasri.res.in/mod/page/view.php?id = 14910

http://www.indianfoodsite.com/spices.htm

http://uses.plantnet-project.org/en/Carum_carvi_ (PROSEA)

http://uses, plantnet-project.org/en/Elettaria cardamomum_ (PROSEA)

http://uses.plantnet-project.org/en/Pimpinella_anisum_ (PROSEA)

http://www.rjpbcs.com/pdf/2012_3 (2)/[92].pdf

Kalloo, G, G., Bergh, (1963): In Genetic improvement of vegetable crops, Pergamon Press, Tarry town, NY…

Keesing, J.L.S. (1988): Useful plants, *In*, Kew Gardens Book of Indoor Plants, ed. J.B. Simmonds, pp. 186-213. George Philip.

NIIR Board (2010): Handbook on Spices. Asia Pacific Business Press Inc. Pp 416.

NIIR Board of Consultants & Engineers (2013): The Complete Book on Spices & Condiments (with Cultivation, Processing & Uses) 2nd Revised Edition, Asia Pacific Business Press Inc.Pp888.

Parthasarathy, V.A., Kandiannan, K, K, K, K., and Srinivasan, V. (2008): Organic spices. New India Publishing Agency, New Delhi, India, Pp 695

Preedy, V.R. (2015): The Contemporary Encyclopedia of Herbs and Spices: Seasonings for the Global Kitchen (1st ed.), Wiley, ISBN 978-0-471-21423-6.

Purseglove, J.S., Brown, E.G., Green, C.L., & Robbins, S.R.J. (1981): Spices, Volume 2 Longman Tropical Agriculture Series

Bairwa, R., Sodha, R.S., and Rajat, B.S. (2012): Trachyspermum ammi, Pharmacognosy Rev. 2012 Jan-Jun, 6(11): 56–60. Doi: 10.4103/0973-7847.95871. PMCID: PMC3358968.

Ravindran, P.N., NirmalBabu, K, and Shylaja, M, (2005): In Cinnamomum and Cassia, the genus Cinnamomum, CRC Press, Boca Raton, p59.

Seidemann, J. (2005): In World Spice Plants, Springer, Seidemann eds. ISBN: 978-3-540-22279-

Vaughan, J. and Geissler, C. (2009): The New Oxford Book of Food Plants,, OUP Oxford, Aug 27, 2009 – Science – 288 pages (Print) 978-3-540-27908-2 (Online), Pp592.

Weiss, E.A. (2002): Spice Crops, CANI publishers, Wallingford, Oxon, U.K. Pp 429.

Chapter 14

Phytochemicals, Nutraceuticals and Green Chemoprevention

Plants contain many different chemicals that are commonly referred to as phytochemicals. Many of these phytochemicals are also present in the edible parts of the plant such as seeds (rice, wheat, beans etc), oil seeds/fruits (omega fatty acids), leaves (leaf vegetables like amaranth, kale, Spinach), tubers (like potato), edible roots (eg.carrots, Taro, yucca) fruits (apples, mango, berries etc), vegetables (tomato, eggplant etc.), nuts (cashew, pistachio etc.) spices and condiments (anise, cumin, turmeric etc). These chemicals are byproducts of plant metabolism. They have evolved in plants in order to protect themselves against feeding insects, pathogenic fungi, bacteria, nematodes and other agents. However, many of these chemicals have multiple modes of action whereby they can also have beneficial effects in humans. Thus, for example anthocyanins, flavanoids, beta-carotene and various alkaloids protect humans from oxidative damage and provide precursors to vitamins. Some components like Omega 3, 6, 9 fatty acids have cardio protective benefits. In general, plants and their edible parts may contain antioxidant phytochemicals that protect cells from oxidative damage or some contain estrogen like molecules that help in treating postmenopausal symptoms or inhibitors of toxins and mutagens or have antimicrobial/anti parasitic activities, cell-binding activities that prevent bacteria from binding to cell walls etc. A brief description of some of the phytochemicals that could be useful in maintaining good human health is given below.

Alkaloids

Caffeine: Caffeine is a white, water-soluble crystalline powder found in Coffee, tea, cola nuts, cocoa and guarana. Caffeine stimulates the central nervous respiratory and blood circulation systems. Caffeine also acts as a diuretic and helps control some headaches. Excessive ingestion of coffee and hence caffeine can cause sleeplessness as well as increase heartbeats. When used in moderate amounts Caffeine through coffee can help to keep awake and in general increase alertness.

Theobromine: Theobromine is found in Cocoa, tea and cola nuts. Theobromine acts as a diuretic and lowers blood pressure since it dilates blood vessels. Theobromine relaxes bronchial muscles and hence useful for controlling coughs. Thus eating dark chocolates or drinking cocoa helps to relax bronchial muscles.

Theophylline: This alkaloid is found in tea leaves and in much lesser quantities in coffee plants. It is synthesized for medical use. This phytochemical is mainly used to treat Asthma and chronic obstructive pulmonary disease (COPD) since it relaxes the smooth muscles of lungs. It can lower blood pressure and has anti-inflammatory effects.

Trigonelline: Trigonelline found in *Trigonella foenum grecum* leaves (Fenugreek) and seeds are reported to have hypoglycemic, hypolipidemic, neuroprotective, antimigraine, and sedative, memory improving, antibacterial, antiviral and antitumor activities. The alkaloid is closely related to nicotinic acid that is prescribed for treating hypercholestremia.

Carotenoids

Beta-carotene, Provitamin A: Beta carotene which is a water insoluble precursor of vitamin A is found in colored fruits and vegetables such as carrots, yellow squash and pumpkin, sweet potatoes, broccoli, kale, spinach, turnip green, amaranth leaves, brown, red and black rice, mango, peach, apricot and many other colored fruits and vegetables. Beta-carotene has many beneficial health effects including prevention of blindness, anticancer and anti-ageing properties. Beta-carotene is converted to vitamin A after ingestion.

Lutein: Lutein is a fat soluble antioxidant carotenoid found in avacados, carrots, red pepper, mustard greens, broccoli, zucchini, corn, spinach leek, collard greens, kale, Kiwi nuts, pistachio, spinach, amaranth leaves, Zuchini, etc. Lutein is essential for normal vision. The protective role of lutein against eye damage is well documented. Studies have also indicated that lutein improves heart health, protects our skin against UV damage, reduces diabetes induced oxidative stress and possesses antiinflammatory and anticancer properties. Lutein offers eye protection by lowering the risk of age related vision loss. Age related vision loss or age related macular degeneration is caused by steady damage of the retina. Lutein may also reduce cataract development and possibly also photophobia. Lutein can also reduce the risk of skin cancer and sunburn. Under influence of sunlight, free radicals are formed inside the skin. These free radicals can damage the DNA of cells. Lutein can protect against the damaging effects of UV-B radiation. Lutein can also reduce the risk for arterial diseases. Studies have shown that persons with the highest lutein intake showed the lowest artery wall thickening. Lutein also reduces the oxidation of LDL cholesterol thereby reducing the risk of artery clogging.

Lycopene: Lycopene is found in high concentrations in ripe tomatoes and in lesser amounts in pink guava, pink grape fruit, red oranges and watermelons. Lycopene is a very efficient antioxidant that can neutralize oxygen-derived free radicals. Lycopene is generally known for its protective action against prostate cancer. *In vitro* studies have shown the anticancer properties of lycopene against many cancer cells including cancer cells of prostate, stomach, lung, colon and skin. Lycopene inhibits platelet aggregation and reduces the production of foam cells that play an important role in the development of arteriosclerosis. In rats, lycopene helps to prevent arteriosclerosis by reducing inflammation. Lycopene shows antitoxic properties against many toxins such as aflatoxin, cyclosporine and cadmium.

Flavonoids and Bioflavonoids

Vitamin P: These are classified into flavonoids/bioflavonoids, isoflavanoids and neoflavanoids by the International Union of Pure and Applied chemistry. All are ketone-containing compounds. Flavanoids are found in many colored fruits and vegetables. *In vitro*, they have been shown to have anti allergic, anti-inflammatory, antioxidant, antimicrobial, antiviral and anticancer activities. However, it is not clear as to their role in human health. Major flavonoids are Anthocyanins, Epicatechins, Hesperidin, Isorhamnetin, Kaempferol, Myricetin, Naringin, Nobiletin, Proanthocyanidins Quercetin, Rutin and Tangeretin.

Anthocyanins: These are water-soluble flavonoid vacuolar pigments that may appear red, purple or blue depending on the pH. Anthocyanins occur in all tissues of higher plants including leaves, stems, roots, flowers and fruits. Anthoxanthins are clear white to yellow counterparts of anthocyanins occurring in plants. Anthocyanins are derived from anthocyanidins. Plants rich in anthocyanins are blueberry, cranberry and bilberry; Rubus berries including black raspberry, red raspberry and blackberry; blackcurrant, cherry, eggplant peel, black rice, Concord grape, muscadine grape, red cabbage, Zuchini, squash, red and yellow bell peppers, seed coat of soy beans, colored bean seeds, red lentils and purple corn. Anthocyanins are antioxidants. Their exact role in health is not known but fruits, vegetables and leaves containing anthocyanin are considered good for maintaining good health.

Epicatechins: Found in Cocoa, it is a strong antioxidant and improves heart health.

Hesperidin: Hesperidin is a flavanone glycoside found abundantly in citrus fruits, oranges, lemons, lime and other citrus fruits. It is reported to be effective in reducing blood pressure and is generally regarded as being good for cardiovascular health.

Kaempferol: Kaempferol is a type of flavonoid that has been isolated from apples, tea, broccoli, grapefruit, cabbage, kale, beans, endive, leek, tomato, strawberries, grapes and Brussels sprouts. Consumption of foods containing Kaempferol is believed to have pleiotropic effects including antioxidant, anti-inflammatory, antimicrobial, anticancer, cardio protective, neuroprotective, antidiabetic, antiosteoporotic, estrogenic/ antiestrogenic, anxiolytic, analgesic and antiallergic activities.

Myricitrin: It is a flavonoid found in many grapes, berries, fruits, vegetables, herbs, as well as other plants. Walnuts are a rich dietary source. It is found in red wine. Like other flavonoids, plant products containing this flavonoid are considered beneficial for good heart health.

Naringin: It is a major flavonoid in grapefruit and gives the grapefruit juice its bitter taste. It is metabolized to the flavanone Naringenin in humans. Consumption of foods containing Naringin can reduce absorption of many essential prescription drugs used in treatment schedules (e.g. Beta-blockers, Statins, Cyclosporine) and hence drinking grape juice in particular and other citrus fruits along with medications are contraindicated.

Nobiletin: This is found in tangerine and other citrus fruits. It was shown to have anticancer activities *in vitro*.

Pycnogenol: Pycnogenol is marketed in health food stores for treating circulation problems, allergies, asthma, ringing in the ears, high blood pressure, muscle soreness, pain, osteoarthritis, diabetes, attention deficit hyperactivity disorder (ADHD). It is also regarded as a phytomedicine for preventing endometriosis and retinopathy. Pycnogenol is found in grape skin and peanut skin and bark of certain trees.

Quercetin: Is a flavonoid pigment found in many fruits and vegetables particularly Radish (*Raphanus sativus*), Dill (*Anethum graveolens*) Celantero (*Coriandrum sativum*) Kale (*Brassica oleraceae*) Cranberry (*Vaccinium* sp), Blueberry (*Vaccinium* sp) and Onion (*Allium cepa*). There has been no clearcut supportive data although, it has been reported to be effective in treating various diseases including cancer, prostatitis and high blood pressure.

Rutin: is a flavonoid related to quercetin and is found in citrus fruits, mulberries, buckwheat, and asparagus. Many health benefits have been attributed to plants containing rutin.

Tangeretin: Found in citrus fruits, it is commercially marketed as a treatment supplement for treating cancers. It is reported to have anti-mutative, anti-proliferative and anti-invasive properties. At the same time, it is contraindicated in patients being treated with the FDA approved anti-tumor drug tamoxifen.

Terpenes

Geraniol: Found in rose petals, geranium, lemon and citronella oil. It has antibacterial and anti-insecticidal properties but can cause allergies. Rose petals are components of certain jams in India and Middle East.

Limonene: Limonene is found in orange and lemon peels: It has antibacterial and insecticidal properties. Limonene may cause skin allergies. It is marketed as a treatment to relieve gastro-oesophegeal reflux disease.

Ursolic acid: is a triterpene found in apples, basil, bilberries, cranberries, elderflower, peppermint, rosemary, lavender, oregano, thyme, hawthorn and prunes. It is a component of cosmetic preparations and it or its derivatives are potential cancer treatment drugs based on *invitro* studies.

Organo Sulfate and Isothiocyanate Compounds

Allicin: Allicin is an organo sulfur compound found in Garlic and other members of the garlic family that includes onion, shallot, chives and leek. Allicin is the main cause for the many reported effects of garlic in maintaining good health. Allicin through consumption of garlic lowers cholesterol, increases circulation, reduces aggregation of platelets in the blood and has antibacterial effects. Allicin is also regarded as an agent that prevents damage to the liver. The antibacterial activity of Allicin helps in healing ulcers caused by *Helicobacter pylori* and oral and bronchial infections by *Streptococcus* and *staphylococcus*. Allicin may also be effective in preventing colon cancer.

Glutathione: It is a small protein with just three amino acids (Glu-Cys-Gly). It is a powerful antioxidant. The level of glutathione decreases during ageing process. Foods like asparagus, broccoli, Avacados and garlic stimulate glutathione production. Continuous supplementation of glutathione can reduce availability of zinc which is an essential trace metal.

Sulforaphane and Raphanin: These are two isothiocyanates found in the Mustard family – Brassicales that include mustard, cabbage, radish, Brussels sprouts, broccoli, kohlrabi, turnip and watercress. These compounds have antimicrobial and anticancer activities. Sulforaphane is effective against *Helicobacter pylori* that cause gastrointestinal ulcers and hence drinking cabbage juice is often recommended for treating stomach ulcers. Consumption of broccoli is also often recommended as a cancer prevention or treatment option by nutritionists.

Phenolics, Lignans and Xanthans

Capsaicin: Capsaicinoids are found in the fruit pulp of many chili pepper species (*Capsicum chinense C. annum C.frutescens C. baccatum C. pubescens*). Bell peppers do not produce capsaicin. Capsaicin creams and sprays are used to control pain associated with neuralgia, psoriasis and other neuromuscular pain conditions. It has antifungal properties and is an animal repellant. There are contrary reports concerning its effect on cancer. Some studies indicate that it potentiates development of stomach cancers whereas other studies indicate the reverse. Exposure of eyes to Capsaicin causes eye irritation, conjunctivitis and other conditions. Chilli powder containing capsaicin is marketed as a weight-reducing pill without any substantial data.

Curcumin: This is a natural phenolic compound found in the rhizomes of the turmeric plant *Curcuma longa*. It has anti-inflammatory properties and it is also touted to have anticancer activities. It is also reported to be effective in healing gastric ulcers. Curcumin is not very soluble in water and is not readily bioavailable due to its poor absorption but Curcumin is made more bioavailable in its phytosomal form or if taken along with black pepper *Piper nigrum*. Curcumin chelates heavy metals including iron and hence ingestion of large quantities of Curcumin can reduce the availability of iron for synthesis of hemoglobin.

Curcuminoids: are a group of alkaloid compounds found mainly in *Curcuma longa* and a few related plants.

Ellagic acid: This is a phenolic antioxidant compound found in pomegranates, black berries, blue berries, cranberries raspberries, strawberries, myrobalans and in many vegetables. Ellagic acid tablets and capsules are sold as treatment for cancer and heart conditions but have been labeled as a fake anticancer supplement by the Food and Drugs Administration of the USA.

Gallic acid: This is a phenolic acid compound found in walnuts, Indian gooseberry and other plants. It may have antifungal and anticancer properties but no detailed study is available.

Rosmarinic acid: This caffeic acid ester is found in basil (*Ocimum basilicum*), the holy basil (*O. sanctum)*, rosemary (*Rosmarinus officianalis*), marjoram (*Origanum marjorana*), and sage (*Salvia officianale)* thyme (*Thymus vulgaris*) and peppermint (Mentha *piperata*) plants. It is an anxiolytic agent with antiviral properties.

Tannic acid: This is a polyphenolic acid found in oak bark and leaves, black tea, gallnuts, sumac, chestnut and some other tree species. The acid is used in preparations for treatment of burns, rashes, prickly heat and other skin ailments.

Mangostin: This is a phenolic compound with a xanthanoid backbone. The phytochemical is found in *Garcenia mangostana*. Mangosteen is being marketed as a miracle weight reducing agent. It is considered to have antioxidant, anti-inflammatory and anticancer activities. However, none of these claims has been substantiated in control studies. However, products containing mangostin are highly popular in weight reduction programs due to anecdotal claims.

Mangiferin: This is a xanthanoid found in mangoes. Studies in the laboratory using animal models indicate that it may have a role as an antioxidant and antimicrobial agent.

Phytosterols

Phytosterols are steroid compounds similar to cholesterol found in plant mainly in vegetable oils, nuts, vegetables and fruits. Beta Sitasterol, campesterol and stigmasterol are the three main types of phytosterols. Suppements containing phytosterols reduce LDL cholesterol and triglycerides.

Beta Sitasterol is found in avocado, pecans, pumpkin seeds, cashew fruits, rice bran, wheat germ, corn oil, and soybeans. In addition, it is found in many non-food plants such as saw palmetto (*Serenoa repens*). Consumption of foods or extracts containing beta Sitasterol are recommended as herbal treatment of benign prostatic hyperplasia.

Campesterol is a phytosterol that is similar to cholesterol. It is also believed to reduce uptake of cholesterol but at the same time excessive intake of foods, containing campesterol may increase cardiac risk. Banana, pomegranate, pepper, coffee, grapefruit, potato, onion, corn oil, canola, mustard, all contain this phytochemical.

Stigmasterol is also similar to cholesterol and is found in soybean oil, rapeseeds, bitter melon (*Momordica* sp). Stigmasterol is progesterone like sterol and has been reported to have antioxidant, hypoglycemic and anti-hyperthyroid effects. There are also reports that intake of foods containing this prevents breast, prostate, colon and ovarian cancers. It also reduces absorption of cholesterol.

Hydroxycinnamic Acids

Cichoric acid: Cichoric acid is a hydrocinnamic acid belonging to the phenylpropanoid class. It is found primarily in the cichory plant *Cichorium intybus* and in coffee and many others. Cichoric acid has been shown to stimulate phagocytosis.

Coumarin: is a phenylpropanoid phytochemical found in licorice, apricots, cherries, cinnamon, red clover and Tonka beans. It has blood thinning and antifungal functions. It is a vitamin K antagonist. Consumption of products from plants containing coumarins is not indicated in persons on blood thinning agents. The related dicoumarol is an anticoagulant derived from coumarol found in red/sweet clover that is converted by fungi growing on the clover hay.

Ferulic acid: This is a hydroxycinnamic acid found mainly in *Ferula asafoetida* latex resin (Asafoetida). It is also found in smaller quantities in apple, artichoke, peanut, orange, pineapple and water chestnuts. It is also found in wheat grain, flax seeds and barley seeds as well as navy beans and horse gram. Ferulic acid is an antioxidant. *In vitro* and animal studies indicate that Ferulic acid has direct antitumor activity against breast and liver cancers and may also have protective effects against certain carcinogenic compounds.

Saponins

Saponins are glucosides with foaming characteristics. They are found in Chickpeas, peas, soybeans, yucca, quinoa, and members of the Sapindales. They may have many health benefits including cholesterol reduction, prevention of bone loss and antioxidant activities. Saponins in plant foods may cause gastrointestinal distress but since saponins are very soluble in water, grains such as Quinoa, peas, soybeans should be washed and cooked before consumption.

Stilbenes

Resveratrol: Resveratrol is a flavonol antioxidant. It is produced by the plant as a defense against plant diseases. Resveratrol is present in many plants and fruits including red grapes, eucalyptus spruce, blueberries, mulberries and peanuts. The longer the grape juice is fermented with the grape skins the higher the resveratrol content will be. It has anticancer properties, inhibits lipid peroxidation of low-density lipoprotein, and prevents the cytotoxicity of oxidized LDL. Resveratrol also increases the activity of some anti-retroviral drugs in vitro. The antioxidant action of resveratrol helps to prevent damage to DNA. Resveratrol appears to decrease tumor promotion activity by inhibiting the enzyme cyclooxygenase1, which converts arachidonic acid to substances that promote tumor growth. Other experiments show that it has anti glycemic properties and increase life span. However, most experiments were conducted in vitro or in mouse models.

Pterostilbene: This stilbene is closely related to resveratrol. Animal studies show that it reduces cholesterol, triglycerides, and blood pressure. It is a component of red wine that is regarded as having anti-cholesterol and anti-triglyceride activities. It is found in red/black grapes, strawberries, raspberries, blueberries and spinach. It has been shown to reverse age-related decline in cognition. Animal studies show significant improvement in memory loss when rats were fed phytostilbene-containing foods.

Zingiberene and other phytochemicals of ginger roots: Gingerols, zingibain, bisabolenel, oleoresins, starch, mucilage and the essential oils zingiberene, zingiberole, camphene, cineol, borneol, are all found in ginger (Zingiber *officianalis*). All of these together are responsible for the beneficial effects of ginger. Ginger aids digestion and is very effective in controlling nausea.

Other Phytochemicals

Many other phytochemicals are present in plants with potential benefits for good health. These include Damnacanthal, Digoxin and Phytic acid. Damnacanthal that is found in *Morinda citrifolia* is an inhibitor of p56 Ick tyrosine protein kinase. Tyrosine protein kinases are involved in transfer of phosphate from ATP to the tyrosine in the p56 protein that is involved in cell division. Mutations of this protein, can lead to constitutive expression of this protein, leading to cancer particularly in small cell lung cancer. Extracts of the rhizomes of *M. citrifolia* are reported to have anti-cancer activities by blocking expression of this cancer causing protein. Digoxin is a cardiac glycoside found in Digitalis plants. It is used for treating atrial fibrillation flutter and other heart conditions not treatable by other medications. Phytic acid is found in sesame seed, flour, wheat grains/flour, oatmeal, hazel nut and other nuts. phytic acid chelates zinc, lead, cadmium and iron and hence people who depend mainly on vegetarian diets can be deficient in Iron and Zinc and would need supplements of these minerals. However, there are studies that suggest a protective role for phytic acid in prevention of colon cancer because of its ability to chelate toxic minerals such as cadmium and lead.

Glycosides

These are molecules wherein a sugar moety is attached to another functional group through a glycosidic bond. Hydrolysis by glycosidases split the functional group from the sugar. Many plants have such glycosides that protect them from attacks by predators and microbes. These functional groups may have a medical benefit to humans or may be toxic to humans unless they are inactivated by heat or other agents. The glycosides may be classified into: Alcoholic glycosides, Anthraquinone glycosides, Coumarin glycosides, Chromone glycosides, Cyanogenic glycosides, Flavonoid glycosides, Phenolic glycosides, Saponins, Steroidal glycosides or cardiac glycosides,

Steviol glycosides and Thioglycosides. Depending on whether the glycosidic bond lies "below" or "above" the plane of the cyclic sugar molecule, glycosides are classified as α-glycosides or β-glycosides. Some enzymes such as α-amylase can only hydrolyze α-linkages; others, such as emulsin, can only affect β-linkages.

Examples of Glycosides:

Anthroquinone glycosides: Antron and Anthronol are anthroquinones. They are found in Senna, rhubarb, aloe and a few other dicot plants and have laxative properties.

Coumarin glycosides: these are found in many plants like Tonka bean, sweet clover, Cassia cinnamon, strawberries. Coumarins by themselves are not antagonists of Vitamin K but derivatives of Coumarin such as warfarin (Coumadin) inhibit vitamin K and used as blood thinning agents.

Chromone glycosides: Eg. Euchryphin found in *Eucryphia cordifolia*, Chromolin found in *Ammi visnaga*. They have bronchodilator properties.

Cyanogenic glycosides: The aglycone part contains cyanide. These glycosides are stored in plant vacuoles and are released upon infection by microorganisms or wounding. Amygdalin found in bitter almonds, seeds of cherries, apples, and apricots is an example of a cyanogenic glycoside. Dhurrin, linamarin, prunasin are other examples. Roots of tapioca (*Cassava*) also contain cyanogenic glycosides and are toxic if the root tubers are eaten without cooking. Other plants containing cyanogenic glycosides include bamboo shoots and flax seeds.

Flavonoid glycosides: Here, the sugar is bonded to a flavone and both flavone and sugar are released by hydrolysis. Examples are Hesperidin, Naringin, Quercetin and Rutin. These have been discussed earlier.

Phenolic glycosides: These have a phenolic group attached to the sugar. An example is Arbutin that is a glycosylated hydroquinone.

Arbutin found in bearberry plants inhibits tyrosinases and prevents formation of melanin and hence extracts of bearberry can be used in skin creams to lighten the skin.

Steviol glycosides: These are found in the non-sugar sweetener plant *Stevia rebaudiana* and are responsible for the sweet taste.

Thioglycosides: These contain Thiol (sulfur) groups and have anti-microbial properties. These glycosides are found in Mustard and members of the Brassicaceae family.

Momordicosides: They represent a group of triterpinoids cucurbitane glycosides found in the bitter melon Momordica charantia. These have been experimentally shown to have hypoglycemic effects and may be among factors responsible for the known hypoglycemic nature of the fruits of this plant.

Green Chemo prevention: The term green prevention is used to describe the potential benefits of using plant products (food, herbals) to prevent or reduce the chances of cancers, cardio diseases and other health conditions. This is a food-centered approach whereby dietary changes by including specific foods from plants are considered to be a good option for good health. Researchers have concentrated their attention on chemo protective effects of consuming foods containing specific phytochemicals such as Anthocyanins, alkaloids, isothiocyanates, organosulfur compounds on development of cancers and other health conditions. Thus, for example, recent studies have shown that Sulforahenes in broccoli and other crucifers inhibit the development of mouth cancers and other studies have shown that extracts from crucifers inhibit *Helicobacter pylori* the causal agent of stomach ulcers and cancers. Similarly extensive studies on green tea as well as turmeric, garlic, pomegranate and ginger show considerable promise as green Chemopreventive agents for cardio protection, digestive health and various cancers. Chemoprevention by plant-based whole foods offers simple economic opportunities for health care As a result of many observations, statistical data and anecdotal observations, many broad based recommendations on foods that are good for health and those that may be harmful have been put forward. As noted above, many clinical studies have verified and pointed to the usefulness of food-based chemoprevention.

Nutraceuticals: The general term Nutraceutical, was coined in 1989 by Stephen L. DeFelice, for products that range from isolated nutrients, dietary supplements, herbal products, specific diets and processed foods such as cereals, soups, and beverages. Nutraceuticals are products mainly from plants that provide various health benefits including nutritional value, prevention of chronic diseases, delay the aging process, increase life expectancy, prevent obesity and support the structure or function of the body. Nutraceuticals include dietary supplements, which are not meant to treat diseases but only to supplement the better functioning of the body. Nutraceuticals include functional foods that are fortified or enriched natural foods by adding vitamins and other components that are naturally occurring in the concerned foods.

References

Abdullaev, F.I. (2002): "Cancer Chemopreventive and Tumoricidal Properties of Saffron (Crocus sativus L.)," Experimental Biology and Medicine 227 (1), PMID 11788779, retrieved 11 September 2011.

Bauman J, Johnson DE, Zhang Y, Sen M, Normolle DP, and Kensler TW, et al. (2015): American Association for Cancer Research Annual Meeting. 2015.

Boaz, M., Leibovitz, E., Bar Dayan, Y., Wainstein, J. (2011): "Functional foods in the treatment of type 2 diabetes: olive leaf extract, turmeric and fenugreek, a qualitative review" (PDF). Func Foods Health Dis 1 (11): 472–81.

Carroll, R.E, Benya, R.V, Turgeon, D.K, Vareed S, Neuman M., Rodriguez, L, et al. (2011): Phase IIa clinical trial of curcumin for the prevention of colorectal neoplasia. Cancer Prev Res. 2011, 4(3): 354–64. [PMC free article]

Chen, T., Rose M.E., Hwang H, Nines, R.G, Stoner, G.D. (2006): Black raspberries inhibit N-nitrosomethylbenzylamine (NMBA)-induced angiogenesis in rat esophagus parallel to the suppression of COX-2 and iNOS. Carcinogenesis, 2006; 27: 2301–7.

Chen, T., Yan, F., Qian J.M., Guo, M.Z., Zhang, H.B, Tang, X.F, et al. (2012): Randomized clinical chemoprevention trial of lyophilized strawberries in patients with dysplastic precancerous lesions of the esophagus. Cancer Prev Res. 2012: 5.

Cragg, G.M., Grothaus, P.G., Newman, D.J. (2014): New horizons for old drugs and drug leads. J Nat Prod 77: 703–723

De Luca, V., Salim, V., Atsumi, S.M. and Yu, F. (2012): Mining the biodiversity of plants: a revolution in the making. Science 336: 1658–1661

Egner, P.A, Chen, J.G, Wang J.B, Wu Y, and Sun Y, and Lu J.H, et al. (2011): Bioavailability of sulforaphane from two broccoli sprout beverages: Results of a short term, crossover clinical trial in Qidong, China. Cancer Prev Res. 2011; 4: 384–395

Fahey, J.W. (2005): Moringa oleifera: A review of the medical evidence for its nutritional, therapeutic, and prophylactic properties. Part 1, Trees for Life J. 2005; 1: 5. http://www.tfljournal.org/article.php/200512.01124931586.

Fahey, J.W., Kensler, T.W. (2007): Role of dietary supplements/ nutraceuticals in chemoprevention through induction of cytoprotective enzymes, Chem Res Toxicol. 2007; 20: 572–576

Fahey, J.W, and Stephenson, K.K. (1999): Cancer chemoprotective effects of cruciferous vegetables. HortScience, 1999; 34(7): 1159–1163.

Fahey, J.W, Zhang, Y. and Talalay P. (1997): Broccoli sprouts: an exceptionally rich source of inducers of enzymes that protect against chemical carcinogens. Proc Natl Acad Sci U S A. 1997; 94: 10367–72.

Farnham, M.W., Wilson, P.E., Stephenson, K.K., Fahey, J.W. (2004): Genetic and environmental effects on glucosinolate content and chemoprotective potency of broccoli. Plant Breeding, 2004; 123: 60–65.

Georgiev, M.I. (2014): Natural products utilization. Phytochem Rev 13: 339–341.

Goldman, I.L., (2002): Forgotten and future vegetable Phytoceuticals. p. 484–490. In: J. Janick and A. Whipkey (eds.), Trends in new crops and new uses. ASHS Press, Alexandria, VA

Grainger, E.M., Schwartz, S.J, Wang, S., Unlu, N.Z, Boileau, T.W.M, Ferketich, A.K, et al. (2008): A combination of tomato and soy products for men with recurring prostate cancer and rising prostate specific antigen Nutr Cancer, 2008; 60(2): 145–154.

Hardy, G (2000): "Nutraceuticals and functional foods: introduction and meaning." Nutrition 16 (7–8): 688–9. Doi: 10.1016/S0899-9007(00)00332-4. PMID 10906598

Haristoy X, Fahey JW, Scholtus I, Lozniewski A., (2005): Evaluation of antimicrobial effect of several isothiocyanates on Helicobacter pylori. Planta Medica, 2005; 71: 326–330.

http://umm.edu/health/medical/altmed/herb/turmeric#ixzz3oTl6wfFX

Knobloch, T.J., Casto, B.C., Agrawal A., Clinton, S.K, Weghorst, C.M. (2-011): Cancer prevention in populations high at-risk for the development of oral cancer: Clinical trials with black raspberries. (Chapter 14) In: Stoner GD, Seeram NP, editors. Berries and Cancer Prevention, Springer; New York: 2011. pp. 259–280.

Liu, R.H. (2004): Potential synergy of phytochemicals in cancer prevention: Mechanism of action, J Nutr. 2004, 134: 3479S–3485S.

McLaughlin, J.M, Olivo-Marston S, Vitolins, M.Z, Bittoni, M., Reeves, K.W, and Degraffinreid, C.R. (2011): Effects of tomato – and soy-rich diets on the IGF-I hormonal network: A crossover study of postmenopausal women at high risk for breast cancer. Cancer Prevent Res. 2011, 4(5): 702–710.

Milen I. Georgiev, (2016): Phytochemistry Reviews, pp 1-3, DOI 10.1007/s11101-016-9465-1

Pantuck, A.J, Leppert, J.T, Zomorodian, N, Aronson, W., Hong, J, Barnard, R.J, et al. (2006): Phase II study of pomegranate juice for men with rising prostate-specific antigen following surgery or radiation for prostate cancer. Clin Cancer Res. 2006; 12: 4018–4026

Prasad, S; Aggarwal, B.B.; Benzie, I.F.F.; Wachtel-Galor, S (2011): Benzie IFF, Wachtel-Galor S, eds. Turmeric, the Golden Spice: From Traditional Medicine to Modern Medicine; In: Herbal Medicine: Biomolecular and Clinical Aspects; chap. 13, 2nd edition., CRC Press, Boca Raton (FL). PMID 22593922

Priyadarsini KI (2014): "The chemistry of curcumin: from extraction to therapeutic agent." Molecules 19 (12): 20091–112. Doi: 10.3390/molecules191220091. PMID 25470276

Ruhlen R, Sauter E. (2010): Plant based therapies to prevent/treat cancer. Expert Rev Clin Pharmacol. 2010, 3(1): 1–3.

Shapiro TA, Fahey JW, Wade KL, Stephenson KK, Talalay P. (2001): Disposition of chemoprotective glucosinolates and isothiocyanates of broccoli sprouts Cancer Epidemiol Biomarkers Prev. 2001; 10: 501–508

Stoner, G.D, Seeram NP, (2011): Berries and Cancer Prevention, Springer; New York: 2011. p. 313

Stoner, G.D. (2009): Foodstuffs for preventing cancer: the preclinical and clinical development of berries. Cancer Prev Res. 2009; 2: 187–194

Tanaka, S., Haruma, K., Yoshihara, M., Kajiyama, G., Kira, K., Amagase, H, et al. (2006): Aged garlic extract has potential suppressive effect on colorectal adenomas in humans, J Nutr. 2006, 136: 821S–826S.

Thurber, M., Fahey JW., (2009): Adoption of Moringa oleifera to combat under-nutrition viewed through the lens of the "Diffusion of innovations" theory, Ecol Food Nutr. 2009 May-Jun; 48(3): 212-25. Doi: 10.1080/03670240902794598.

Wang, S.Y. (2011): Correlation of antioxidants and antioxidant enzymes to oxygen radical scavenging activities in berries. (Chapter 4) In: Stoner GD, Seeram NP, editors. Berries and Cancer Prevention Springer, New York: 2011. pp. 79–97.

Wildman, Robert E.C., ed. (2001): Handbook of Nutraceuticals and Functional Foods (1st Ed.). CRC Series in Modern Nutrition ISBN 0-8493-8734-5

Yanaka A., Fahey, J.W., Fukumoto, A., Nakayama, M., Inoue, S., Zhang, S., et al. (2009): Dietary sulforaphane-rich broccoli sprouts reduce colonization and attenuate gastritis in Helicobacter pylori-infected mice and humans. Cancer Prev Res. 2009, 2(4): 353–360.

Yang CS, Ju J, Lu G, Xiao H, Hao X, Sang S, et al. (2008): Cancer prevention by tea and tea polyphenols. Asia Pac J Clin Nutr, 2008, 17(S1): 245–248.

Yang, C.S., Wang, X. (2010): Green tea and cancer prevention Nutr Cancer 2010; 2(7): 931–937.

Zick, S.M., Djuric, Z., Ruffin, M.T., Litzinger, A.J., Normolle, D.P., Alrawi, S., et al. (2008): Pharmacokinetics of 6-gingerol, 8-gingerol, 10-gingerol, and 6-shogaol and conjugate metabolites in healthy human subjects. Cancer Epidemiol Biomarkers Prev. 2008, 17(8): 1930–1936.

Zick, S.M, Turgeon, D.K., Vareek, S.K., Ruffin, M.T., Litzinger, A.J., Wright, B.D., et al. (2011): Phase II study of the effects of ginger root extract on eicosanoids in colon mucosa in people at normal risk for colorectal cancer, Cancer Prev Res. 2011, 4(11): 1929–1937.

Chapter 15

Anti-Nutrients and Toxic Phytochemicals in Certain Plant Foods

Unlike animals, plants do not have an immune system. However, plants defend themselves from attack by insects, microorganisms like fungi, bacteria, viruses and other microorganisms by expressing various defense mechanisms that may be physical or chemical in nature. Physical defense mechanisms include thorns, hair, wax coatings and stinging nettle. Chemical defense is based on the expression of phytochemicals such as alkaloids, flavonoids, glycosides, phytates, proteases, oxalates, steroids, stress proteins, carbohydrates and various other anti-nutrients. Edible cereals, pseudo-cereals, legumes, oilseeds, tubers and edible roots as well as Leaf, root, stem and fruit vegetables, culinary fruits, nuts, beverage additives, spices and condiments all contain different kinds of phytochemicals. When consumed as food by humans and animals, some of these phytochemicals are beneficial to human health but other phytochemicals may turn out to be toxic to humans especially when consumed in large quantities without food processing such as cooking. Collectively, harmful molecules found in edible plants are called anti nutrients and toxins. At the same time, it must be pointed out that plants express many different chemicals some of which are harmful and some not harmful and hence, the collective usage of a plant as Food need not result in harm to health just because the plant or plant part used contains harmful chemicals.

Certain anti-nutrients and toxic chemicals are expressed more in certain families of plants than in others. Thus, phytates are found in cereal grains like wheat, protease inhibitors in legume seeds, cyanogenic glycosides in tapioca, solanine alkaloid in Solanaceae, Cucurbitacin in Cucurbitaceae, oxalates in the various yams and Vinca alkaloids in the non-edible periwinkle family. In this chapter, brief characteristics of both phytochemicals and anti-nutrients will be addressed.

There is a general saying that anything consumed in excess will be harmful to health. The anti-nutrients and toxic principles found in plant foods are not a problem for all but, certain specific individuals may react to these anti-nutrients and food phytochemicals. Moreover, most of these anti-nutrients are incapacitated or removed by baking, cooking, fermentation, frying, adding other ingredients like salt and other common food processes that have evolved in various cultures. People who believe that eating raw foods is better for health since cooking removes nutrients should also be aware of the benefits of cooking in terms of removal of anti-nutrients. Juices and smoothies prepared with Kale, broccoli and celery would contain glucosinolates and oxalates that may be harmful to certain individuals. Likewise, eating large helpings of bean sprouts could affect digestive health because of the high lectin content.

The information provided in this chapter is for reference purposes so as to be aware of potential reactions to food. Except for staple foods like cereals, legumes and oils, other foods such as vegetables, fruits, nuts and spices are used only in limited quantities normally. However, in some individuals, even small amounts of any specific food can cause health issues.

Antinutrients

Antinutrients are certain phytochemicals found in commonly edible nutrient plants that contain principles that interfere with absorption of foods.

Amylase inhibitors: Amylase inhibitors prevent the digestibility of carbohydrates and thus affect digestive processes. Such inhibitors are found in most bean and legume varieties.

Glucosinolates: These compounds found in many cruciferous plants such as broccoli, Brussels sprouts, cabbage and mustard, form chelate complexes and educe the bioavailability of iodine. Lack of iodine causes goiters.

Lectins: Lectins are glycoproteins that are found in many seeds and nuts particularly among the legumes. These lectins have evolved in order to protect the seeds from being digested in the intestinal tract of animals so that they may be dispersed intact for germination. They may also have evolved for protection of the seeds from attack by microorganisms. However, since the seeds of legumes, nuts and cereals that contain lectins are also the main source of protein for animals and humans, it is important to know how the lectins react in the digestive system of humans. Lectins are found also in dairy products. Plant lectins are generally known as hemagglutinins since they clump or clot blood. Since, lectins are not fully inactivated in the intestines by the intestinal micro flora; they can cause serious health problems including irritable bowel syndrome and various other colonic diseases if raw unprocessed seeds containing lectins are consumed. Additionally, since lectins can cause leaky intestinal lining, these molecules could enter the bloodstream and cause allergic reactions as well as hemagglutination. Nevertheless, fortunately, lectins can be inactivated by fermentation processes and heat during food preparation. The true health issues due to lectins arise mainly due to consumption of raw nuts including peanuts various types of beans and other unprocessed lectin-containing seed preparations.

Lipase inhibitors: Lipases are enzymes released by the pancreas in order to digest fats. Inhibitors of lipase prevent the breakdown of fats in the intestine and thus reduce body fat but these can cause the pancreas to over-produce lipase in order to compensate and in turn causes pancreatitis. Avacados, Grape seeds, and green apple particularly Granny smith variety are reported to contain these inhibitors.

Oxalates: Oxalic acid is a tri-carboxylic acid produced during the tri – carboxylic acid cycle during normal respiration. Nevertheless, if excessive amounts of oxalic acid are present in foods then, the oxalic acid can combine with calcium in the food and form calcium oxalates that are insoluble and excreted via the stools. This in the end can result in insufficient calcium for bone development or maintenance of bone structure resulting in osteoporosis. When the oxalic acid is absorbed into the bloodstream then, they can combine with calcium ions in the blood and form stones that are deposited in the kidneys. Kidney stones are very painful and can promote kidney and urinary infections. In view of this, foods containing substantial quantities of oxalic acid or oxalates should be avoided. Foods that contain high amounts of oxalates include beets, cashewnuts, chard, celery, coriander seeds, Kiwi fruits, rhubarb, spinach leaves, star fruits, amaranth leaves, the rhizomes and tubers of taro roots, elephant yam and other Dioscorea yams. Soaking the cut vegetables in warm water or lemon juice or cooking by boiling and frying can remove most of the oxalates. The current trend to eat raw spinach and other vegetables in salads could promote oxalate related health issues. In the case of calcium, absorption of this important mineral could be improved by drinking citrus juices or taking calcium citrate supplements.

Protease inhibitors: consuming sufficient quantities of protein is essential for growth and function of all animals and humans. However, it is not enough that the raw protein is consumed but the protein should be digested by bodily enzymes. These enzymes like trypsin and other proteases are secreted by the pancreas. In the case of vegetarians, the bulk of required protein is derived from legumes primarily and to a lesser extent from other plant-based foods. Many seeds that are used in cooking contain anti-nutrients such as protease inhibitors which can reduce or prevent the digestibility of vegetarian proteins such as those derived from soybeans, lentils, Pea, garbanzo beans and various other been types. Therefore, if these protease inhibitors are not inactivated then, the pancreatic cells will be under pressure to increase the productivity of protease that can overcome the anti-proteases for proper digestion. Most of the studies on protease inhibitors have been carried out on soybean proteinase inhibitors. Animals that have been fed exclusively on soybean meal as protein source were shown to have hyperplasia of pancreatic cells that can lead to pancreatic cancer. Since most protease – inhibitor-containing foods are consumed after heat inactivation, cooking, or fermentation, the problems created by protease inhibitors are reduced. However, in recent times, there has been an active movement towards green and raw foods in the belief that cooking and other processes will remove nutrients from the food without realizing that in many cases such as legume seeds, anti-nutrients (protease inhibitors) can pose severe problems. People who drink soymilk, soymilk protein and other soy products should be aware that they might have some digestibility issues if the brand of soy product that they are consuming has not been properly processed to remove protease inhibitors.

Seeds of legumes and nuts that contain protease inhibitors also have other beneficial phytochemicals such as isoflavones that may confer other health benefits or even overcome the effects of anti-proteases in them. Many studies have actually shown that soybean has many beneficial phytohormones that can protect the development of breast cancer in women.

Phytates/Phytic acid: Phytic acid also known as phytate is a high phosphate storage chemical found in the seeds of many plants particularly wheat and rice bran. Its chemical name is inositol hex phosphate, or IP6. The chemical is also found in smaller quantities in many other seeds such as almonds, beans, other legume seeds, corn, sesame, walnuts and many other edible seeds. Phytates act as important phosphate contributors for the germinating seeds and possibly have other roles in the seeds. However, they are strong chelaters of calcium, iron, zinc, copper and other minerals required for human good health. At the same time, it has the capacity to bind toxic metals like lead and cadmium. In view of this, consumption of foods containing phytates will result in loss of calcium needed for bone development, iron for hemoglobin, copper and zinc for various enzymes and immune system activity making them unavailable for absorption. To overcome this problem, it may be necessary to take additional iron and other mineral supplements to overcome the un-availability of calcium, iron, zinc and copper due to phytate binding. On the plus side, consumption of phytate rich foods might be a way to remove toxic heavy metals like lead in detoxification protocols. For people who are on a vegetarian diet and who may be concerned about iron deficiency anemia, the phytate in various grains that form the staple vegetarian diet may be reduced by soaking the grains, sprouting the seeds and fermenting the dough from grain flour. Consuming leavened bread instead of unleavened bread like chapatis, tortillas, Pita bread may be helpful since the fermentation process while making leavened bread removes the phytate. There are also scientific reports in peer-reviewed journals that suggest a role for phytates in reducing colon cancer.

Toxic Phytochemicals

Phytochemicals found in edible plants that have toxic properties if consumed in large amounts and without processing (cooking). These are:

Abortifacients: Celery, parsley, rosemary, garlic, safflower, bitter gourds and snake gourds contain phytochemicals that act as Abortifacients and pregnant women should avoid these.

Arsenic: Rice grown in fields where arsenic pesticides were used tends to accumulate arsenic in the grain. Rice has higher levels of inorganic arsenic than other foods, in part because as rice plants grow, the plant and grain tend to absorb arsenic more readily than other food crops. In April 2016, the FDA proposed an action level, or limit, of 100 parts per billion (ppb) for inorganic arsenic in infant rice cereal. This level, which is based on the FDA's assessment of a large body of scientific information, seeks to reduce infant exposure to inorganic arsenic

Amygdalin: Amygdalin is a glycoside found in the seeds of bitter almonds (*Prunus dulcis*). Seeds of apricot, quince, peaches, plum and black cherry also contain amygdalin. Very small amounts are also found in raw almonds, crushed fruit stones or pips, celery, bean sprouts, carrots, beans – mung, Lima, butter and other pulses, flax seed and various nuts. A semi-synthetic drug known as Laetrile derived from amygdalin marketed in several countries as an alternative treatment for cancer. However, The NIH after extensive tests concluded that laetrile is actually harmful and have banned sale of laetrile although it is available in neighboring Mexico. Both amygdalin and laetrile release cyanide in the body and the cyanide kills both cancerous and normal cells. However, some users claim that the cyanide affects the cancer cells more than normal cells.

Capsaicin: Capsaicin is the active chemical found in hot chili peppers (*Capsicum sp.*) that generate the "heat" when consumed in foods or applied to skin. Liniments containing Capsaicin are used to control pain. While there are many studies that correlate excessive usage of chilly peepers in food with increased risk of colorectal cancer, other studies mostly *in vitro* show that capsaicin kills cancer cells.

Coumarin: Coumarin is a blood-thinning agent. Cinnamon bark and grapefruits contains Coumarin in variable amounts depending on the variety and ecotype. As such, people who are on blood thinning agents should not ingest cinnamon and grapefruit juice.

Cucurbitacin: Cucurbitacin are a family of steroidal glycosides found in species of Brassica, Cucurbita, members of the Rosales and Rubiales. Specifically, substantial amounts of Cucurbitacin is found in various members of the Cucurbitaceae family such as squashes, pumpkins, bitter lemons and other edible fruits and vegetables of this family. They are generally toxic to herbivorous animals but not been shown to have any serious health impacts other than some anecdotal reports. Since Cucurbitacin are cytotoxic, they may prove to have anti-tumor properties.

Cyanogenic glycosides: cyanogenic glycosides are glycosides found in certain plants that converted into hydrogen cyanide upon exposure to air or after ingestion in the body. Bitter almond seeds, apple seeds, bitter pistachio nuts, macadamia nuts, green potatoes (potato tubers that have greened), rutabaga, turnips, and tapioca/Yucca (Manihot) contain these cyanogenic glycosides. Of these, tapioca is a staple food in many countries in Asia, Africa and South and Central America. Consumption of raw tapioca can induce cyanide toxicity that can even result in death. In Africa, a paralytic disease known as konzo is correlated with consumption of untreated tapioca root tubers and even the leaves of this plant. However, the impact of the cyanogenic glycosides is considerably reduced or even prevented by heat treatment, fermentation, cooking and frying processes. Eating raw tapioca should be discouraged. Slicing and sun drying the slices help to remove cyanide. A method known as wetting is used to detoxify the Manihot flour. Herein, the Manihot flour is steeped in water for a period and the wet flour is sun dried thereby releasing the cyanide generated to evaporate.

Fiber: Foods containing both soluble and insoluble fiber are good for general health. However, consuming too much of both types of fiber can speed up the movement of food through the intestines and thus reducing the bioavailability of important nutrients. Additionally, excess fiber can swell in the gastro intestinal pathway and cause food and acid to back up into the gullet causing acid reflux.

Furano coumarins: These are chemical compounds where a furan ring is fused with a Coumarin. Furano-coumarins are produced by certain plants as a defense against insect and animal predators. Grape fruits and Pomelo in the citrus fruit group contain substantial amounts of furano-coumarins that interfere with the uptake and metabolism of a variety of prescription drugs including certain antibiotics and Statin drugs. Certain other citrus fruit hybrids also contain smaller amounts of this chemical. Thus, it is not advisable to drink grapefruit juice while taking specific prescription drugs especially statins. Foods containing furano-coumarins is contraindicated in patients taking blood thinning drugs like warfarin, Coumadin and even aspirin.

Gluten: Gluten is a general name for the proteins found in wheat, rye, barley and triticale. Gluten helps foods maintain their shape, acting as glue that holds food together. Gluten is the composite of two storage proteins, gliadin and a glutenin found in the endosperm of wheat, rye, barley and triticale but not in glutinous rice or corn. Susceptible people who eat foods containing gluten suffer from celiac disease. Gluten sensitive Celiac disease is an autoimmune disease wherein, the villi of the small intestine are damaged and are unable to absorb nutrients and individuals who consume gluten-containing foods react with diahorrea, nausea and other gastrointestinal distress symptoms. In many instances, people who are gluten sensitive do not exhibit outward symptoms but still have nutrition deficiency and growth problems. If not treated by avoiding the offending foods, the celiac disease can trigger other autoimmune diseases, type-1 diabetes, osteoporosis etc. The only treatment at present is to avoid eating foods containing gluten. Certain other gluten sensitive people suffer from gluten sensitive non celiac disease. Such people show symptoms similar to irritable bowel syndrome, headache, chronic fatigue and or fibromyalgia etc.

Myristicin: This phytochemical in Nutmeg *(Myristica fragrans)* has neurotoxic and psychoactive effects. Therefore, consumption of larger than the usual cooking doses can cause hallucinogenic effects including memory mix-up, visual disturbances and other mental conditions.

Neurotoxic amino acids: The Indian pea (*Lathyrus sativus*) expresses a protein containing a toxic amino acid beta oxalyl diaminopropioic acid or ODAP. This toxic aminoacid containing seed protein was a staple food in many regions in India and East Africa and a specialty food preparation in some parts of Italy and Portugal. Consuming this seed protein or seed flour causes a neuro muscular disease called lathyrism. Lathyrism results in wasting of muscles and paralysis. Although banned in India, the lathyrus crop is still grown in many parts of Africa and is a source of protein-food. Recently, there were reports that new varieties of Lathyrus that do not contain the toxic amino acid have been developed.

Phytoestrogens: Phytoestrogens are plant-derived compounds that bind to estrogen receptors in breast and other sites in the human and animal bodies. Most studies have been conducted on soybean seeds but phytoestrogens are also found in fava beans, red clover, flax seeds and sesame seeds. Many studies indicate that phytoestrogens have a positive protective effect in preventing breast cancer. Other studies show that phytoestrogens increase the risk of colorectal and prostate cancer.

Safrole: Safrole is a phenyl propene compound found in the root bark and fruits of Sasafras that was used as a food additive in root beer and sassafras tea. It is currently labeled as a carcinogenic agent by the FDA. Small amounts are found in nutmeg, black pepper, cinnamon and basil. The amounts in these spices are so little that it is not a cause of concern especially since only small amounts of these spices are added to spice up foods. However, this chemical is also found in betel nuts that are chewed like tobacco in India, Bangladesh, SriLanka and other south East Asian countries. Epidemiological studies show a correlation between chewing betel nuts and oral cancer.

Salicylates: salicylates are a group of chemicals found in many plants including edible fruits and vegetables. These naturally occurring salicylates are close cousins of synthetic non-steroidal anti-inflammatory agents like aspirin, methyl salicylates and other NSAIDS. People sensitive to salicylates react with symptoms of asthma, hives, and tinnitus of the ear, irritable bowel syndrome and other gastrointestinal upsets.

Salicylate levels are high in alfalfa sprouts, chili peppers, eggplant, broccoli, olives, spinach, sweet potato, zucchini and other cucurbits. Salicylates found in food are higher in raw fruits, vegetables and salads than in cooked foods. Peeling of the fruits and eating only fully ripened fruits and vegetables can reduce salicylates in the food. Salicylate related health problems are generally inconsequential for the normal population but may have some impact on people who are sensitive to salicylate.

Saponins: Saponins are found in many seeds and are soap like phytochemicals that foam up in water. Examples are soybeans, garbanzo/chickpeas, different bean types, alfalfa leaves, sprouts as well as pseudo-cereals like quinoa, vegetables like asparagus, berries, many other vegetables and seeds. The characteristic feature is the formation of foam when the edible plant part is soaked or washed in water. Most of saponins can be removed by repeated soaking and washing. If they are found foaming during the cooking process, the watery foam can be skimmed off.

Saponins are important because they can bind to cholesterol in the cell membranes and damage the intestinal mucosa thereby allowing various allergens and molecules like lectins to enter the bloodstream through the damaged cell walls. Saponins are also goitrogenic and cause enlargement of the thyroid with the resultant thyroid related health issues. Saponins can also hemolyse red blood cells. In actual usage, saponins containing foods may not be a health issue unless large quantities of saponins containing foods are the main source of energy for various populations.

Solanine: Solanine is a glyco-alkaloid that is found in the leaves and green parts of all members of the Solanaceae family. This includes the leaves of tomato, tomatillo, potato, Turkey Berry/Manathakkali (*Solanum nigrum*) and even the green areas of sprouting potato tubers. Solanine toxicity is expressed as neurological disturbances, gastrointestinal upsets including vomiting, hallucinations and burning of the throat. It may even prove to be fatal if large amounts are consumed. Solanine is soluble in water and hence small quantities of Solanine that may be present in the edible fruits of Solanaceae plants are removed or inactivated by cooking and frying and to a much lesser extent by baking and hence do not pose health problems unless these fruits are eaten raw or used in the preparation of salads. According to a recent report quoted by the FDA, all potato peels contain solanine and hence it is recommended that the skin of potatoes be peeled off before preparing culinary items as food. Fortunately, ripened tomato fruits do not contain this alkaloid.

Urshiol: Mango leaves, stem, inflorescence and fruit peel contain urshiol, which causes contact dermatitis. Another edible plant that contains urshiol is the Cashew nut plant (*Anacardium occidentalis*).

Poison ivy and poison oak, which are non-edible, cause contact dermatitis through Urshiol. When the oil gets on the skin, an allergic contact dermatitis reaction occurs. Most exposed people develop an itchy, red rash with bumps or blisters. Exposure to as little as 50 μg of urushiol is enough to cause a reaction. Depending upon where it occurs and how broadly it is spread, the rash may significantly impede or prevent a person from working.

Other Toxic Principles in Edible Plant Parts

Certain edible fruits, nuts and vegetables contain small amounts of specific toxic compounds. Consuming large amounts of these edibles can cause some health problems. Lychee fruits contain the phytotoxic methylene-cyclopropyl-glycine that is linked to non-inflammatory encephalopathy in children and identified as hypoglycemic encephalopathy by the Centers for disease control, Atlanta, USA. Mangosteen contains hydroxycitric acid, which causes testicular degeneration. The star fruit contains caramboxin and mono oxygenases, which are respectively neurotoxins and anti-statins. Annonacin in custard apples can lead to neurodegenerative conditions. Brazil nuts contain small amounts of radium that is radioactive. Mustard greens may contain cadmium. Consuming large quantities of persimmon can cause blocking of intestines due to formation of a gum called bezoars. Brussels sprouts contain larger than normal amounts of Vitamin K and as such is contraindicated for people who are taking prescription blood thinning agents. Asafoetida resin is a spice and natural medicine used for controlling various gastro intestinal problems. However, excess asafoetida causes throat irritation and genital swelling.

References

Centers for Disease Control and Prevention, (2014): Poisonous Plants
    http://www.cdc.gov/niosh/topics/plants/

Danış O, Ogan A, Anbar D, Dursun BY, Demir S, et al. (2015): Inhibition of Pancreatic Lipase by Culinary Plant Extracts. Int J Plant Biol Res. 3(2): 1038

Ekholm, P., Virkki, L., Ylinen, M., and L. Johansson (2003): The effect of phytic acid and some natural chelating agents on the solubility of mineral elements in oat bran. Food Chemistry Feb 2003. 80. 2, 165–70, 10.1016/S0308-8146(02)00249-2

FDA Poisonous Plant Database: http://www.accessdata.fda.gov/scripts/plantox/detail.cfm?id = 1364

GEO-PIEProject, "PlantToxins and Antinutrients" Cornell University http://everything.explained.today/Antinutrient/

Goldman, I.L., A.A. Kader, and C. Heintz (1999): *Influence of Production, Handling, and Storage on Phytonutrient Content of Foods, Nutr, Reviews, (II) S46-S52 PDF

Hotz C, Gibson RS. (April 2007):"Traditional food-processing and preparation practices to enhance the bioavailability of micronutrients in plant-based diets" J. Nutr. 137 (4): 1097–100. PMID 17374686

http://www.accessdata.fda.gov/scripts/plantox/detail.cfm?id = 1364

http://www.cancerresearchuk.org/about-cancer/cancers-in-general/treatment/complementary-alternative/therapies/laetrile.

https://celiac.org/celiac-disease/what-is-celiac-disease/

Reddy, N.R., Pierson, M.D., Sathe, S.K., and Salunkhe, D.K., (1989): Phytates in cereals and Legumes, CRC Press, Baton Rouge, Florida, 33431.

Reddy, N.R., Pierson, M.D., Sathe, S.K., and Salunkhe, D.K., (1989): Phytates in cereals and Legumes, CRC Press, Baton Rouge, Florida, 33431: Thompson, J.J., Manore, M., Sheeshka, J., Nutrition, A Functional-Approach-Third-Canadian-Edition-Pearson, Benjamin Cummings, Pp768

Chapter 16

Natural Plant Foods for Certain Specific Health Conditions

Many naturally occurring foods contain specific phytochemicals that help to maintain good health. The paragraphs below are only for educational and informational purposes. They are not a substitute for proper medical evaluations and treatment. However, at the same time, it is important to know the specific effects of some of these foods on the human body.

Brain and Cognitive Functions

The relation between brain functions and food intake has been the subject of many research publications. In a recent review, the National library of Medicine of the NIH gave a detailed review of the relationship between food intake and brain function. Thus, cognitive function is improved by intake of: Omega 3 fatty acids (flax seeds, chia grain, walnuts), curcumin from turmeric, flavonoids from cocoa (dark chocolate), green tea, citrus fruits, fat soluble vitamins D and E, fruits and vegetables containing vitamins B-6 and B-12. Of these, vitamin D is obtained by exposure to sun light or through supplementation since plant-oils do not contain this vitamin. Vitamin B-12 is also not available from plant sources but can be obtained from meat and from fermented foods like tofu, buttermilk and yogurt. Vitamin E is found in Asparagus, avocado, nuts, peanuts, olives, red palm oil, spinach, vegetable oils and wheat germ.

Adequate levels of the micronutrient Selenium and iron also help to maintain cognitive functions. However, foods rich in saturated fats and abnormal levels of serum calcium correlate with decline in cognition. With respect to copper, the reports are not conclusive. Some recent studies indicate a higher than normal concentration of copper in serum plasma but not in cerebro-spinal fluids of Alzheimer's disease (AD) patients. Excess copper encourages the formation of amyloid plaques, clumps of proteins in the brain that are thought to contribute to Alzheimer's disease. Other investigators have questioned these findings and so much more needs to be known before the role of copper in AD can be definitively established. Since copper is an essential mineral for many body functions, it is not clear if the high copper found in AD patients is due to an accumulation of this trace mineral which then triggers AD.

Cancer

Cancer is a general term applied to many different conditions wherein, the underlying cause is the abnormal, uncontrolled growth of cells due to inherited genetic factors, mutations and internal and external environmental factors. Mutations may be triggered by viral and bacterial infections as well as toxins, specific food products, additives to food as well was external environmental factors such as radiation and toxic chemicals. Because of multiple research studies, the American Cancer Society, the National Cancer Institute of the NIH and various other research organizations uniformly recommend that foods rich in fiber, antioxidants, adequate vitamins and minerals with simultaneous reduction in high fat, high sugar foods play important roles in prevention and control of various cancers. Foods rich in fiber and anti-oxidants include whole grains, legumes, vegetables and fruits, nuts and certain spices. Details of these foods of plant origin have been listed in earlier chapters. A plant-based diet consisting of lots of fruit, vegetables and legumes, and little red meat, salt and processed carbohydrates may lower the odds of developing estrogen-receptor breast cancer, which accounts for about a quarter of all breast cancers. A study published in the American Journal of Epidemiology found that the likelihood of the cancer was 20 percent less when women followed such a diet. Further, fruits with high levels of carotenoids such as carrots, sweet potatoes, yellow squash, kale, spinach, broccoli, and pomegranate and soybean tofu are all useful preventatives. Some reports suggest that drinking broccoli juice would prevent mouth cancer occurrence.

Diabetes

Foods that are rich in fiber, protein and low in sugars and simple carbohydrates and fats are recommended by the diabetic associations worldwide. Foods and beverages that contain high levels of sugars and simple carbohydrates like starch should be avoided. Foods to be avoided or used in limited quantities are white rice, processed wheat and other grains, Potato and tubers, sugar cane juice, canned fruit and juices. Foods that help to control/reduce diabetes include whole grain cereals, soybean tofu, legumes, vegetables (bitter melon), fenugreek seeds, limited quantities of fresh fruits and juices, limited amounts of nuts like pistachio and walnuts.

Digestive Health

a. Acid reflux: Acid reflux refers to a condition in which stomach acid makes its way up into the esophagus due to a dysfunction of the lower esophageal sphincter. Typical symptoms associated with acid reflux include hiccups, nausea, burping, bloating, bloody stools or vomit, weight loss, acid reflux cough (dry and hoarse) and sore throat. However, the most abundantly present and most bothersome symptoms are often heartburn and regurgitation. Most acidic foods such as citrus juices, coffee, cocoa/chocolates, onion, garlic, oils increase the potential for acid reflux. Plant products that help control acid reflux include Aloe juice, ginger, oatmeal, fennel, bananas and melons, celery, parsley; salads without onion, garlic and tomatoes are helpful.

b. Bowel movements – Constipation: Good digestive health is highly dependent on preventing constipation so that digested foods are evacuated along with built-up toxins. One of the most important components for good digestive health is the consumption of soluble and insoluble fibers in the food. The soluble fibers draw water into the intestines and the insoluble fibers such as cellulose add bulk. Foods rich in fibers are: Staple foods: brown, red or black rice, All whole grain cereals, most legumes, quinoa. fruits: apples, apricots, stone fruits, raisins, figs, prunes, pineapple, strawberries, oranges, watermelon, vegetables: avacados, artichokes, sweet corn, brussel sprouts, carrots, sweet potato, okra, eggplant, all leaf vegetables, tomatoes.

c. Peptic ulcers: The single most important cause of stomach ulcers and pre-cancerous conditions is the bacterium *Helicobacter pylori*. Recent research vindicates the folk medicine recommendation of drinking cabbage juice for controlling the bacterium. Foods containing organo sulfur compounds particularly in broccoli, cabbage and other crucifers are good botanicals for preventing and treating infections of H. pylori.

d. Irritable Bowel Syndrome (IBS): The exact causes of Irritable bowel syndrome cannot be pin pointed. However, genetics, hormonal changes, and environmental factors including stress, food allergies are involved. Coordinated muscle spasms enable movement of food from the stomach through the intestines into the rectum for final disposal of digested food. Irritable bowel syndrome causes faster uncoordinated muscle movements resulting in diarrhea, bloating and gas or the contractions may be slow causing constipation. Foods that are beneficial for control of irritable bowel syndrome include Cooked Artichoke flower heads, okra, hausa potato known as Koorka and the resin of Ferula asafoetida (Hing). Foods that should be avoided include one or more of broccoli, Cabbage, Cauliflower, Onion, Garlic, and Peanuts, other nuts, foods containing gluten, lectins and salicylates.

e. Food allergies: Many plant foods cause allergies in specific individuals. The allergens cause hives, diarrhea, gas and bloating.

These include foods rich in gluten, wheat, oats, Barley, Rye, peanut and many other nut allergens, sesame seeds and oil, celery, onion, garlic, yams and fruits like strawberries.

f. **Non-Gluten foods:** The following foods do not contain gluten and hence could be good sources of nutrition for those who are allergic to gluten. These are Arrowroot, Amaranth seeds, Buckwheat, Sorghum, Millets, Wild rice, White rice.

Ear Nose and Throat (ENT)

There is no direct link between plant foods and ENT health. However, as with other conditions, good ENT health is likely to be benefited by consumption of anti-oxidant rich foods, vitamins and reductions in sugars and fatty acids from the diet. One of the causes of ENT conditions is food allergy. Many foods such as peanuts, tree nuts, gluten, lectins may trigger the release of histamine in specific individuals and hence cause allergic reactions that include sinusitis, rhinitis, dizziness and hearing loss. An important condition in the ear is Meniere disease that exhibits symptoms of vertigo, loss of balance, ringing in the ear and fullness or pressure in the ear. This condition apparently results from accumulation of excess liquid in the inner ear. Such accumulation of fluid could be caused by infection, allergies, stress and some unknown factors. There appears to be no cure but the symptoms could be ameliorated by reducing stress, reducing sodium intake and also reducing simple sugars like honey, refined sugar, high corn syrup, allergens like peanuts and other nuts. Intake of herbal diuretics like pine apple, celery, parsley, dandelion, Juniper berries, asparagus, artichoke, melon and watercress may be useful for getting symptomatic relief.

Eye Health

Cataracts, Glaucoma, night blindness, inflammatory conditions like retinitis, Iritis, Keratitis, Scleritis, Diabetic retinopathy, retinal arterial and venous occlusion, Cystoid macular edema and last but not least Age related macular degeneration (AMD) are among the most common eye conditions that affect good eye health. While most inflammatory conditions are due to allergies and infections, others are both due to genetic factors as well as nutrient related conditions.

Vitamin A, C, E, lutein, zinc, various antioxidents especially zeaxanthin and carotene and omega 3 fatty acids as well as control of diabetes are all important in the control of eye diseases. The following foods provide one or more of the required nutrients for god eye health.

a. **Green and leafy vegetables**: All leafy vegetables (see chapter on leaf vegetables) especially Amaranth, Spinach, mustard greens, Swiss chard, romaine lettuce and Kale leaves as well as broccoli, collard greens, Brussel sprouts, bright colored vegetables, fruits like grapefruit, strawberries, raspberries, bilberries, black berries, currants contain lutein and zeaxanthin which prevent or reduce macular degeneration and reduce photosensitivity

b. **Carotene:** Carrots, pumpkins, sweet potato, green; yellow, red and orange bell peppers contain carotene that is a precursor for vitamin A. Upon ingestion, carotene is converted into vitamin A by the body.

c. **Lutein:** Lutein, xanthophyll carotenoids are important for control of photophobia and macular degeneration. Lutein is found in green vegetables such as Kale, spinach, yellow carrots

d. **Vitamin E:** Sunflower seeds, wheat germ oil, almonds, pecans, walnuts and vegetable oils contain vitamin E.

e. **Zeaxanthin:** Zeaxanthin is a carotenoid alcohol found in yellow corn, saffron, red bell peppers and many green and colored fruits and vegetables. It along with lutein is believed to confer retinal health and prevent macular degeneration.

f. **Zinc:** The trace metal zinc is important for transport of vitamin A from liver to the eye in order to produce melanin that is the pigment needed to protect the eye just as it protects the skin.

High blood pressure and diabetes are conditions that promote poor eye health and hence, it is important to restrict diet to reduce intake of fatty foods and sugars.

Genito-Urinary Health

The genitourinary system includes the kidneys, ureters, bladder, urethra and prostate in males and the ovary and vaginal systems in females.

Natural Diuretics for Water Retention

Natural diuretics are foods, herbs and spices that can be incorporated into everyday diets in order to decrease the amount of excess water that the body may be holding on. Natural diuretics work to increase the output of urine and thus reduce the amount of excessive fluid in the body. Plant foods with diuretic properties are avocado, banana, barley water, celery, chayote squash, bottle gourd, cranberries, coffee, cocoa, Jobs tears (*Coix lacryma-jobi*), parsley, pineapple, pomegranate, pumpkin, fennel, turmeric, water cress and winter melon.

Kidney stones

Calcium oxalate kidney stones are the most common type of kidney stone. The higher the levels of oxalate, the greater risk there is of developing these kinds of kidney stones. Many foods as noted previously contain oxalates that promote formation of kidney stones. These include Amaranth, Spinach, chard and sugar beet leaves, most yams, taro root, Beetroot, Celery, Soybeans, Sweet potatoes, Rhubarb and Cashew nuts. When foods with oxalate are eaten, the oxalate travels through the digestive tract and passes out in the stool or urine. As it passes through the intestines, oxalates bind with calcium and are excreted in the stool and urine. However, when too much oxalate continues through to the kidneys, this can lead to kidney stones. Kidney stones promote urinary tract infections. People who are prone to kidney disease should avoid foods containing high levels of oxalates. Urologists recommend drinking substantial amounts of water to avoid kidney stones. Practitioners of alternative medicine recommend the drinking of banana stem juice as a remedy for dissolving kidney stones but there is no firm clinical evidence to back up this recommendation.

Prostate Health

Enlarged prostate is a common occurrence in men who are seniors. Plants that are considered good for prostate health are tomatoes, watermelons, pink grapefruits, guava and papaya that contain lycopene, which is a powerful antioxidant and helps to shrink or prevent enlargement of prostates. Cruciferous vegetables such as broccoli, cauliflower, cabbage, Brussels sprouts, bok choy and kale also are good choices. Selenium-rich foods such as wheat germ, sunflower and sesame seeds, cashews, mushrooms, garlic and onions are also recommended since some studies show that Selenium reduces risk of prostate cancer.

Ovary

Ovarian cancer is a silent killer. While genetics and hormone levels are critical pre-disposal factors, food might also play a role in preventing ovarian cancers. Intake of anti-oxidant foods is considered good for green chemoprevention. Including tomatoes, red onions, turmeric, green tea and Belgian endive in diets in particular have been recommended by some health food agencies.

Heart Friendly Plant Foods

Occlusion of heart vessels, other arteries and veins can trigger heart attacks and failure. It is increasingly known that stress, improper diet, smoking and genetic factors all play leading roles in proper functioning of the heart and associated blood distribution systems. As for diet, the following foods are recommended for good heart health: Whole grain cereals, nuts, and vegetables, consumption of fiber rich and anti-oxidant foods including oils containing omega 3 oils (Flax seeds, olive oil, Sunflower seeds and oil). Simultaneously, avoiding saturated fats including hydrogenated fats and sugars is important. Diabetic conditions potentiate heart conditions and so it is important to control sugar intake. There are some recent reports that coconut oil that is a highly saturated fat is not bad for heart health but these reports have not been conducted by authentic scientific methods and are mostly anecdotal in nature. Other life style changes such as regular exercise and yoga/meditation are all recommended.

Pain

Pain is a broad term, which includes headaches, migraine, muscular pain, joint pain etc. In general, complementary alternative medicine (CAM) suggests various plant based prophylactic and or treatment options to control pain. Among the most highly recommended plant, foods/spices are turmeric, ginger, red grapes, soybean products, papaya, and foods with high omega 3 fatty acids such as flax oil/seeds.

Turmeric inhibits a protein called NF-kB; when turned on, this protein activates the body's inflammatory response, leading to achy joints. People in Indian subcontinent have been using this spice as an essential component of curries and as a part of Ayurvedic treatments. Turmeric has multiple effects including inflammation control. The active components in turmeric are known as Curcuminoids. Curcuminoids are not easily absorbed from the intestines and hence liposome preparations of turmeric that are better absorbed are being marketed. Mixing turmeric with black pepper is reported to ensure better absorption.

Ginger is increasingly being used as a component in many cuisines. Although mainly used as digestive aid, ginger seems to have anti-inflammation properties.

The isoflavones of Soybeans seem to have anti-arthritic properties. Tofu and other soybean products are being recommended as long-term treatments to avoid joint pain.

Resveratrol in red grapes, blue berries and cranberries is another anti-oxidant that could be an anti-pain agent. It is mostly recommended for cardiac protection.

Cherries are rich in antioxidants such as hydroxycinnamic acid, perillyl alcohol and anthocyanin. Eating cherries and drinking cherry juice considerably reduced arthritis pain in clinical experiments. Their pain scores dropped significantly compared with the scores of those who did not drink the juice. Cherries have a significant effect in reducing and or preventing attacks of gout. Similar pain killing compounds are also found in blackberries, raspberries and strawberries.

Coffee contains caffeine, chlorogenic acid, Quininc acid, cafestol, Kahweol, N. methyl pyridinium and many other chemicals. Of these, Caffeine in coffee and tea are also good for reducing pain. Caffeine is a component of some migraine headache formulations. However, coffee in particular contains acidic principles that can cause digestive problems like reflux disease as well as sleeplessness and is a cardio stimulant.

Papaya contains a proteolytic enzyme, papain that is so potent at fighting pain that it has been used in injections for those suffering from back pain. Today, this enzyme is one of the most popular supplements being sold over-the-counter. However, the supplements do not contain the antioxidants found in the fresh fruit and hence consuming papaya fruit is a better option than supplement capsules.

Skin Friendly Plant Foods

The following are considered good for skin health: Carrots, apricots, and other yellow and orange fruits and vegetables, spinach and other green leafy vegetables, tomatoes, blueberries, beans, peas and lentils, nuts and legumes. Oils such as coconut are held to be very helpful in maintaining and improving skin health. Foods rich in sugars cause obesity and resultant poor skin health.

Remarks

Nature has provided several natural foods through plants that can prevent and or reduce the incidence of various diseases and promote good health. The World Health Organization (WHO) Fruit & Vegetable Intake Guidelines recommend that Adults and children must eat five servings of fruit and vegetables excluding potatoes and tubers daily. Beans and pulses, nuts, dried fruit without added sugars and chemical preservatives are also recommended. In the various chapters in this book, apart from descriptions of the plants that provide the specific food, brief descriptions of nutritional content and health relatedness of various plant-based foods have been included which could be of benefit to the reader. Innumerable research papers in peer reviewed journals, reviews, books and anecdotal reports as well as ethnic medicinal practices all indicate and reiterate the value of plant based foods for nutritional control and therapy of many health situations. However, in the ultimate analysis, a qualified physician is the best judge to decide on specific treatment options including that of alternative medicine.

References

AREDS, report no. 8 (2001): "A randomized, placebo-controlled, clinical trial of high-dose supplementation with vitamins C and E, beta carotene, and zinc for age-related macular degeneration and vision loss: Arch Ophthalmol 119(10): 1417-36.

Arup, M, Cuendet, M., Kondratyuk, T., Croy, Vicki L., Pezzuto, J.M., and Mark Cushman (2007): Synthesis and Cancer Chemopreventive Activity of Zapotin, a Natural Product from Casimiroa edulis, J. Med. Chem., 2007, 50 (2), pp 350–355

Augustsson K, Michaud DS, Rimm EB, Leitzmann MF, Stampfer MJ, Willett WC, Giovannucci, E, (2003): A prospective study of intake of fish and marine fatty acids and prostate cancer. Cancer Epidemiol Biomarkers Prev. 2003 Jan; 12(1): 64-7.

Bays H.E., 92007): Safety considerations with omega-3 Fatty Acid therapy, Am J Cardiol., 200, 99(6A): S35-43

Berbert AA, Kondo CR, Almendra CL et al. (2005): Supplementation of fish oil and olive oil in patients with rheumatoid arthritis, Nutrition, 2005; 21: 131-6.

Berson EL, Rosner B, Sandberg MA, et al.(2004): Clinical trial of docosahexaenoic acid in patients with retinitis pigmentosa receiving vitamin A treatment. Arch Ophthalmol, 2004; 122(9): 1297-1305.

Blasbalg TL, Hibbeln JR, Ramsden CE, Majchrzak SF, Rawlings RR. (2011): Changes in consumption of omega-3 and omega-6 fatty acids in the United States during the 20th century (2011): Am J Clin Nutr. (2011): 2011, 93(5): 950-62.

Boelsma E, Hendriks HF. Roza L. (2001): Nutritional skin care: health effects of micronutrients and fatty acids. Am J Clin Nutr., 2001, 73(5): 853 – 864

Brostow DP, Odegaard AO, and Koh WP, et al. (2011): Omega-3 fatty acids and incident type2 diabetes: The Singapore Chinese Health Study, Am J Clin Nutr., 2011, 94(2): 520-526

Bucks' S1, Ventricle M, Panetta V, Palustris C, Pasqualetti P, Mariani S, Siotto M, Rossini PM, Squitti R (2011): Copper in Alzheimer's disease: a meta-analysis of serum, plasma, and cerebrospinal fluid studies. J Alzheimers Dis. 2011, 24(1): 175-85. Doi: 10.3233/JAD-2010-101473.

Cole, G.M., (2009): Omega-3 fatty acids and dementia. Prostaglandins Leukot Essent Fatty Acids, 2009, 81(2-3): 213-21.

Daniel CR, McCullough ML, Patel RC, Jacobs EJ, Flanders WD, Thun MJ, Calle EE (2009): Dietary intake of omega-6 and omega-3 fatty acids and risk of colorectal cancer in a prospective cohort of U.S. men and women. Cancer Epidemiol Biomarkers Prev. 2009 Feb; 18(2): 516-25.

Dewailly E, Blanchet C, Lemieux S, ET al.92001): n-3 fatty acids and cardiovascular disease risk factors among the Inuit of Nunavik. Am. J. Clin. Nutr, 2001, 74(4): 464-473.

Fernando Gómez-Pinilla (20080: Brain foods: the effects of nutrients on brain function. (2008): Nat Rev Neurosci, 2008 Jul 9(7): 568–578.

Fotuhi M, Mohassel P, Yaffe K. (2009): Fish consumption, long-chain omega-3 fatty acids and risk of cognitive decline or Alzheimer disease: a complex association, Nat Clin Pract Neurol. 2009 Mar; 5(3): 140-52,

Frangou S, Lewis M, and McCrone P et al. (2006): Efficacy of ethyl-eicosapentaenoic acid in bipolar depression: randomised double-blind placebo-controlled study, Br J Psychiatry. 2006; 188: 46-50

Fursova, A., Hz, Gesarevich, O.G, Gonchar, A.M, Trofimova, N.A., and Kolosova, NG. (2005): Dietary supplementation with bilberry extract prevents macular degeneration and cataracts in senesce-accelerated OXYS rats]. Adv. Gerontology., 2005; 16: 76-9.

Galli C, Risé P. (2009): Fish consumption, omega 3 fatty acids and cardiovascular disease, the science and the clinical trials, Nutr Health. 2009, 20(1): 11-20. Review

Gao S, et al. (2007): Selenium level and cognitive function in rural elderly Chinese, Am J Epidemiol 2007; 165: 955–965,

Geelen A, Brouwer IA, Schouten EG et al. (2005): Effects of n-3 fatty acids from fish on premature ventricular complexes and heart rate in humans, Am J Clin Nutr., 2005; 81: 416-20,

Grosso G, Pajak A, and Marventano S, et al. (2014): Role of omega-3 fatty acids in the treatment of depressive disorders: a comprehensive meta-analysis of randomized clinical trials, PLOS One, 2014; 9(4): e96905,

Hall MN, Campos H, Li H, Sesso HD, Stampfer MJ, Willett WC and Ma J. (2007): Blood levels of long-chain polyunsaturated fatty acids, aspirin, and the risk of colorectal cancer. Cancer Epidemiol Biomarkers Prev. 2007, 16(2): 314-21.

Halliwell B (January 2007): "Dietary polyphenols: good, bad, or indifferent for your health?" Cardiovasc Res. 73 (2): 341–7. doi: 10.1016/j.cardiores.2006.10.004. PMID 17141749

Hartweg J, Farmer AJ, Holman RR and Neil A. (2009): Potential impact of omega-3 treatment on cardiovascular disease in type 2 diabetes, Curr. Opin. Lipidol, 2009 Feb; 20(1): 30-8.

http://www.aicr.org/foods-that-fight-cancer/cherries.html?referrer = https://www.google.com/

http://www.aoa.org/patients-and-public/caring-for-your-vision/diet-and-nutrition/lutein?sso = y

http://www.cancer.gov/about-cancer/treatment/cam/patient/prostate-supplements-pdq

http://www.ncbi.nlm.nih.gov/pmc/articles/PMC2805706/

http://www.standup2cancer.org/article_archive/view/foods_that_fight_cancer

https://www.health.ny.gov/publications/0911/

Iso H, Rexrode K.M, Stampfer M.J, Manson J.E, Colditz G.A, Speizer F.E et al (2001).: Intake of fish and omega-3 fatty acids and risk of stroke in women, JAMA 2001; 285(3): 304-312.

Jacques PF, Chylack LT., Jr (1991): Epidemiologic evidence of a role for the antioxidant vitamins and carotenoids in cataract prevention, Am J Clin Nutr. 1991 Jan 53(1 Suppl): 352S–355S. [PubMed]

Jepson, R.G; Williams, G; Craig, J.C Jepson, Ruth G, ed. (2012): "Cranberries for preventing urinary tract infections," Cochrane database of systematic reviews (Online) 10: CD001321. doi: 10.1002/14651858.CD001321.pub5. PMID 23076891

Jeschke MG, Herndon DN, Ebener C, Barrow RE, Jauch KW. (2001): Nutritional intervention high in vitamins, protein, amino acids, and omega-3 fatty acids improves protein metabolism during the hypermetabolic state after thermal injury. Arch Surg. 2001; 136: 1301-1306

Kavanaugh, C.J., P.R. Trumbo, and K.C. Ellwood, (2007): The U.S. Food and Drug Administration's evidence-based review for qualified health claims: tomatoes, lycopene, and cancer. J Natl Cancer Inst, 2007. 99(14): p. 1074-85.

Liva Harinantenaina, Michi Tanaka, Shigeru Takaoka, Munehiro Oda, Orie Mogami, Masayuki Uchida, Yoshinori Asakawa (2006): Momordica charantia Constituents and Antidiabetic Screening of the Isolated Major Compounds. Chem. Pharm.Buil, S4 (7) 1017-1021 (20e6)

Lopresti A.L, Drummond P.D (2014): "Saffron (Crocus sativus) for depression: a systematic review of clinical studies and examination of underlying antidepressant mechanisms of action." Human Psychopharmacology: Clinical and Experimental 29, 517–2.

Murillo G.I, Hirschelman W.H, Ito, A, Moriarty, R.M, Kinghorn A.D, Pezzuto, J.M, Mehta R.G., (2007): Zapotin, a phytochemical present in a Mexican fruit, prevents colon carcinogenesis.

Murray-Kolb L.E, Beard JL. (2007): Iron treatment normalizes cognitive functioning in young women, Am J Clin Nutr. 2007; 85: 778–787

Ortega RM, et al. (1997): Dietary intake and cognitive function in a group of elderly people, Am J Clin Nutr 1997; 66: 803–809 [PubMed]

Pajonk FG, et al. (2005): Cognitive decline correlates with low plasma concentrations of copper in patients with mild to moderate Alzheimer's disease, J Alzheimers Dis. 2005; 8: 23–27.

Seddon JM, Ajani UA, Sperduto RD, Hiller R, Blair N, Burton TC, Farber MD, Gragoudas ES, Haller J, Miller D.T, et al. (1994): Dietary carotenoids, vitamins A, C, and E, and advanced age-related macular degeneration. Eye Disease Case-Control Study Group. JAMA, 1994 Nov 9, 272(18): 1413–1420. [PubMed]

Singh, S., and Aggarwal, B.B. (1995): Activation of Transcription Factor NF-κB is suppressed by Curcumin (Diferuloylmethane). The Journal of Biological Chemistry, 270, 24995-25000.

Singh, J., Sagare A.P., Coma, M., Perlmuttera, D., Geleind, R., Bella, R.D., Deane, R.J., Zhong, E., Parisia, M., Ciszewskia, J.,, Kasper, R.T., and Deane, R. (2013) Low levels of copper disrupt brain amyloid-β homeostasis by altering its production and clearance. PNAS, 110 no. 36, 14771–14776, doi: 10.1073/pnas.1302212110

Sommerburg, O., Keunen, J., Bird, A., and F. J G M van Kuijk (1998): Fruits and vegetables that are sources for lutein and zeaxanthin: the macular pigment in human eyes, Br J Ophthalmol. 1998 Aug 82(8): 907–910.

United States Department of Agriculture Agricultural Research Service, National Nutrient Database for Standard Reference Release 28: https://ndb.nal.usda.gov//

Vanek C, Connor W.E. (2007): Do n-3 fatty acids prevent osteoporosis? Am J Clin Nutr, 2007 Mar. 85(3): 647-8.

West S, Vitale S, Hallfrisch J, Muñoz B, Muller D, Bressler S, Bressler NM. (1994): Are antioxidants or supplements protective for age-related macular degeneration? Arch Ophthalmol 1994 Feb; 112(2): 222–227. [PubMed]

Zhang Z, Wang CZ, Wen XD, and Shoyama Y, Yuan CS (2013): "Role of saffron and its constituents on cancer chemoprevention" Pharmaceutical Biology 51 (7): 920–4. doi: 10.3109/13880209.2013.771190. PMC 3971062, PMID 23570520

Zhang, Y., Neogi, T., Chen, C., Chaisson, c., Hunter, D.J., and Choi, H.K. (2012): Arthritis and rheumatism,, American college of Rheumatology, 64 (12), 4004-4011.